THE STANDARD BIPHASIC-CONTRAST EXAMINATION OF THE STOMACH AND DUODENUM

SERIES IN RADIOLOGY

Radiological Examination of the Gastrointestinal Tract

Volume 1

The Standard Biphasic-Contrast Examination of the Stomach and Duodenum

by

J. Odo Op den Orth

THE STANDARD BIPHASIC-CONTRAST
EXAMINATION
OF THE STOMACH AND DUODENUM

METHOD, RESULTS, AND RADIOLOGICAL ATLAS

by

J. ODO OP DEN ORTH M. D.

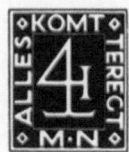

MARTINUS NIJHOFF MEDICAL DIVISION

THE HAGUE / BOSTON / LONDON

1979

ISBN-13: 978-94-009-9314-3   e-ISBN-13: 978-94-009-9312-9
DOI: 10.1007/978-94-009-9312-9

This study was performed at the St. Elisabeth's of Groote Gasthuis, Haarlem, The Netherlands.

Radiology:	Radiological Department
Endoscopy:	Willem Dekker, M.D., Ph.D., Department of Medicine
Histology:	Pathological Laboratory, Municipal Health Service, Haarlem, The Netherlands
Photography:	Meindert G. Popkes
Drawings:	Ronald Bosgraaf
Preparation of the manuscript:	Sonia Dorst

Cases in the atlas presented through the courtesy of others are indicated in the legends of the illustrations.

CONTENTS

PART III. RADIOLOGICAL ATLAS OF COMMON LESIONS OF THE STOMACH AND DUODENUM

ABBREVIATIONS

DC   double-contrast

EGC   Early Gastric Cancer

LPO   left posterior oblique*

PC   positive-contrast

RPO   right posterior oblique*

* Terminology tends to be confusing: sometimes it describes positioning from the tube aspect and at other times from the film aspect. In order to interpret double-contrast studies correctly, it is essential to understand the effect of gravitational forces. The nomenclature then indicates the part of the body closest to the table.

THE STANDARD BIPHASIC-CONTRAST EXAMINATION OF THE STOMACH AND DUODENUM

INTRODUCTION

The rapid growth of fibre-optic endoscopy in recent years has had two consequences for the radiology of the stomach and the duodenum.

1. Radiology has lost its previously rather autonomous position in this field.
2. As a result of the constant feed-back from the endoscopist, which the radiologist can and should have, he is in an excellent position to re-evaluate and improve his own technique of examination.

The author believes that the radiological examination retains its value as a screening technique and a complementary method to gastroscopy and biopsy. Only a sophisticated radiological technique will fulfil these requirements. In 1973 the author developed a standard examination that was called "biphasic", because it combines the advantages of positive-contrast (PC) and double-contrast (DC) techniques. Since that time, an experience of more than 7,500 examinations has been accumulated.

In part I of this study the theoretical background and the technique of examination proper are described. The basic principles of interpretation of DC studies are stated.

Part II deals with the results. Chapter 5 consists of general remarks on the results, and on the complementary rôle of radiological examination and endoscopy. Chapter 6 deals with a quantative study of standard biphasic-contrast examinations in patients over a period of 3 years. This study was restricted to malignant lesions, because it is only in this group that the definite criterion, a histological diagnosis, is obtained. The natural history of malignant lesions also makes follow-up studies possible. Results of the diagnosis of Early Gastric Cancer (EGC) are included.

In part III, an atlas of common lesions of the stomach and duodenum, the results are illustrated.

Part I

METHOD

Chapter 1

A BRIEF REVIEW OF RADIOLOGICAL TECHNIQUES FOR EXAMINATION OF THE STOMACH AND DUODENUM

The main aim of radiological examination of the stomach and duodenum is macroscopic visualization of the anatomy of this part of the gastro-intestinal tract. There are five modes of examination:

1. complete filling studies
2. compression studies
3. mucosal relief studies
4. double-contrast (DC) studies
5. hypotonic studies.

1.1. Complete filling studies

When the stomach is filled with a PC medium, a frontal view provides a picture of its medial and lateral contours. By turning the patient to left and to right, it is possible to see more contours. If the stomach possessed the shape of a cylinder with its axis in the longitudinal axis of the body, it would always be possible to detect a lesion. Because the stomach is not a simple cylinder, this method, while important, possesses only a limited value.

1.2. Compression studies

If the PC filled stomach and duodenum are compressed carefully, it is possible to add "en face" pictures to the contour diagnosis of the complete filling method. This method is also important but it also possesses its limitations. For instance, the upper part of the stomach beneath the thoracic cage cannot be compressed. Even below the costal margin compression is virtually impossible in some patients. In obese subjects the duodenal bulb often points backwards and cannot be compressed.

1.3. Mucosal relief studies

A picture of the mucosal relief is obtained by applying a small volume of PC agent to the mucosa, either acitively (by palpation) or passively (by means of gravity). This method, theoretically sound at first sight, yields very few useful results. The reason is that the stomach is not distended by the small volume of contrast agent swallowed. An everyday practice of pathologists when examining the opened stomach (resected or removed at autopsy) is to stretch it slightly, in order to detect small lesions.

1.4. Double-contrast (DC) studies

A DC picture is obtained by coating the inner surface of a distended hollow viscus with a thin layer of a PC medium. Distension of the viscus can be obtained by using a second contrast agent, usually gas.

Short history of the DC technique
As early as 1911 Von Elisher (61) filled the stomach with a PC agent (zirconium oxide), and then added air through a tube. Fisher (74) in describing the DC technique of examining the colon, advised turning the patient several times on his longitudinal axis in order to achieve a good mucosal coating. Later this manoever proved to be of the utmost importance in DC examination of the stomach as well. In 1923 Baastrup (6) obtained an excellent picture of an air-distended resected stomach with bismuth carbonate coating its inner surface. By means of in vivo studies he attempted to obtain DC pictures by first giving the patients a small quantity of barium suspension followed by 200-250 grams of riceflour porridge.

Many authors adopted techniques of this sort, sometimes slightly modified, using a barium suspension and gas introduced either through a tube or by using an effervescent drug. Such workers were Vallebona (264), Hilpert (114), and Pribram and Kleiber (205).

In 1941 D'Eloia (62) introduced a DC technique

which he called pneumogastroscopy. He passed a Miller-Abbott tube into the stomach and used it to insufflate a large enveloping balloon with 250-400 ml of air and 50-100 ml of water (as ballast). Before and after the balloon had been insufflated, the patient was given a suspension of barium sulphate to swallow. This suspension was then evenly compressed into the gastric musoca by the expanding balloon and used to obtain pictures. This method was complicated and rather impractical, but it demonstrated the essentials of the DC technique excellently.

In 1958 Amplatz (4) described how air could be introduced into the stomach by allowing the patient to aspirate a barium suspension and air together, by using a drinking straw with a midway perforation. Towards the end of the 1960s the use of silicon antifoaming agents became popular to prevent air bubbles in the stomach. They were administered either in tablets or as powders (85, 108, 190, 206) or combined with the barium suspension (243).

In 1973 Pochaczevsky (201) devised the so-called "bubbly barium" technique of introducing carbon dioxide into the stomach. He described the technique of preparing a carbonated cocktail of barium suspension by using a soda syphon.

Thus the concept of the DC method is more than 65 years old. In recent years it has become a popular and perfected method through the work of many authors (39, 84, 86, 87, 94, 100, 101, 105, 107, 110, 116, 123, 143, 148, 150, 151, 192, 207, 220, 225, 245, 254, 257, 258, 260), notably the Japanese, and in particular Shirakabe, Ichikawa and Kawai (237, 238, 118, 124). Although the method can provide a nearly ideal image of the total inner surface of the stomach, it possesses its limitations for routine use.

DC examination of the posterior wall of the stomach is easy to perform. When the patient is supine (fig. 1), the barium excess lies in the fundus.

The walls of the gas-distended corpus and antrum are covered with a thin layer of barium. The layer on the posterior wall is of course thicker than that on the anterior wall. These conditions are ideal for a DC examination of the posterior wall of these segments, using vertical or nearly vertical beam projections. Tilting the table to 30°-40° anti-Trendelenburg and rotating the patient into the Right Posterior Oblique (RPO) position enables the posterior wall of the fun-

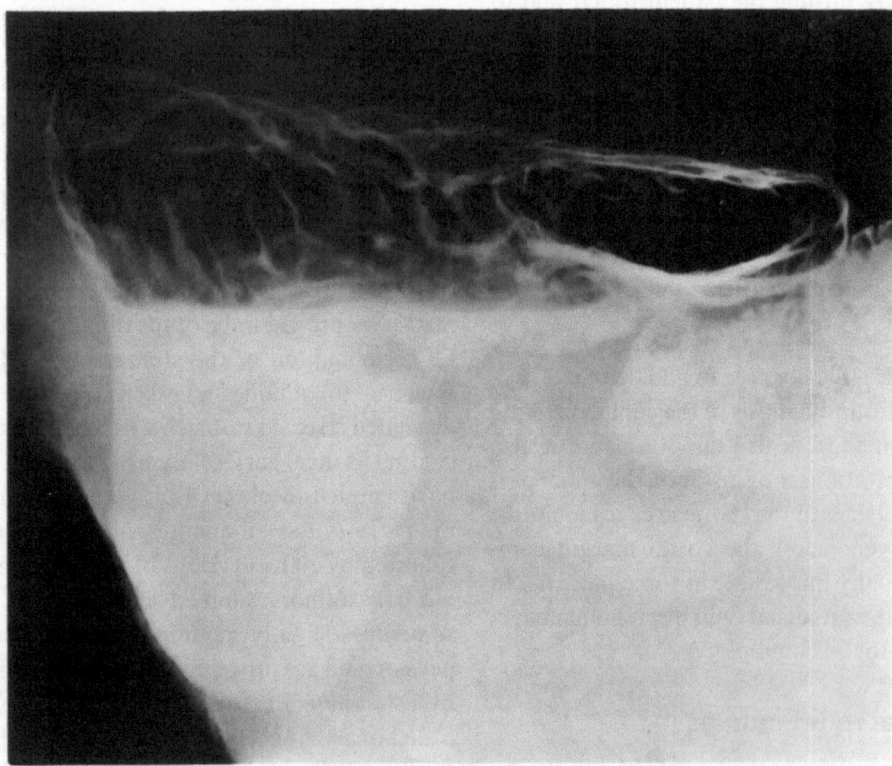

Fig. 1
Patient supine, horizontal beam projection.

dus to be examined in the same way. When the patient is turned prone (fig. 2), the gas moves into the fundus. The corpus and the antrum are now completely filled with barium. DC examination of the anterior wall can be performed only with the patient in a deep Trendelenburg position and by combining a small volume of barium with a large quantity of gas, utilizing a beam direction vertical to the table. These conditions may be obtained simply by passing a nasogastric tube. It is clear that both a deep Trendelenburg position and the use of a nasogastric tube are impractical for routine examinations.

Although only vertical beam projections and the horizontal, Trendelenburg and anti-Trendelenburg table positions have so far been discussed, excellent DC studies of the fundus may be obtained by using horizontal beam projections with the patient erect.

The results of both PC and DC studies can be improved by drug-induced hypotonia.

1.5. Hypotonic studies

Drug-induced hypotonia greatly improves the results of the gastric examination. The technique converts the stomach from a hollow viscus with high muscular tone and vivid peristalsis which is open at least at one end (the pylorus) into a flaccid viscus which is often closed at both ends.

A mucosal surface can be imaged better when it is distended. As stated before, the pathologist stretches the opened specimen of the stomach to inspect the wall.

If the pylorus remains closed for some minutes – as occurs in most patients after the intravenous administration of a drug inducing hypotonia – troublesome duodenal and jejunal superimposition can be prevented. Drugs such as atropine sulphate, propantheline bromide (pro-banthine), hyoscine N butyl bromide (buscopan) and oxyphenonium bromide (antrenyl) possess contraindications. Glaucoma is considered to be an absolute contraindication and prostatism and significant cardiac disease including arrythmias are relative ones. Side-

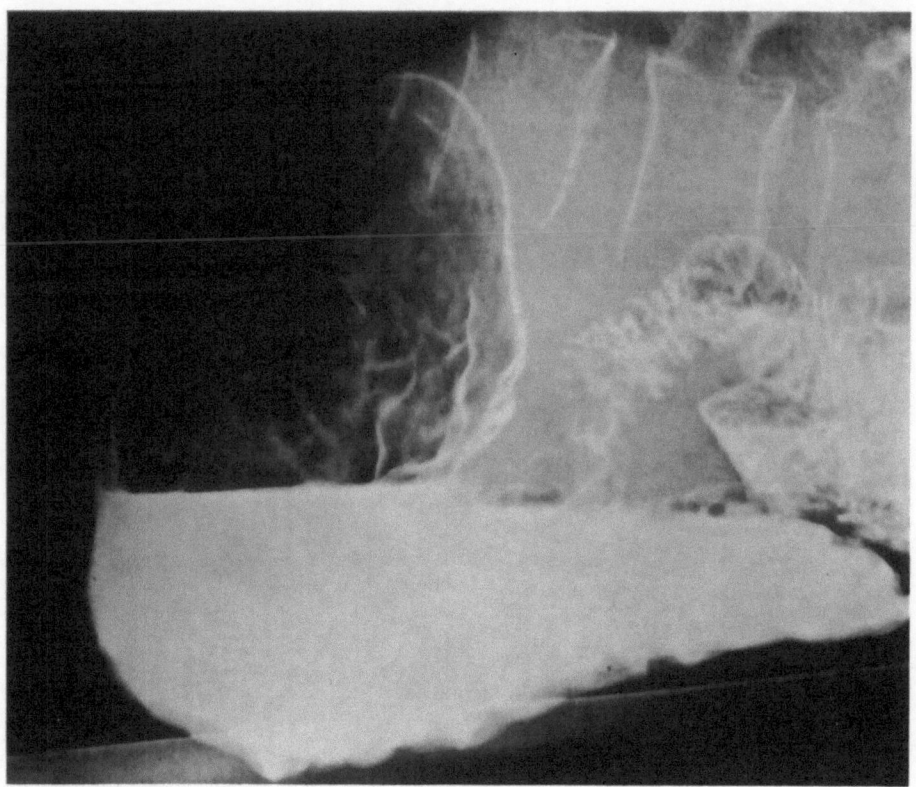

Fig. 2
Patient prone, horizontal beam projection.

effects such as urinary hesitancy and retention, dryness of the mouth, throat and nasopharynx, blurring of near vision and tachycardia have been described (90, 158, 162, 189). Therefore it is not advisable to use these drugs as part of every routine examination.

Glucagon (24, 146, 168, 169, 171) produces very few and only slight side-effects, mainly nausea and vomiting. Contraindications include phaeochromocytoma, insulinoma and warfarin-induced hypo-thrombinemia (90, 189). Another contraindication is brittle diabetes (71), and some consider insulin-requiring diabetes mellitus to be a relative contraindication (200). Currently glucagon is viewed as the drug of choice in hypotonic gastrography (170).

The hypotonic technique also greatly improves the diagnostic yield of the examination of the duodenal loop, as compared with the conventional examination (48).

Chapter 2

WHY IS A STANDARD BIPHASIC-CONTRAST EXAMINATION NECESSARY?

None of the radiological techniques described in chapter 1, viz. complete filling, compression, mucosal relief and DC studies, when used separately can in a simple way provide complete visualization of the lining of the stomach. DC studies made with the patient supine and erect can visualize precisely the posterior wall of the antrum and the corpus, and the total fundus. The supine studies will reveal even tiny lesions, which cause irregularity of the surface of the posterior wall of the stomach, and also lesions with abrupt margins of the anterior wall, as explained in fig. 3. Lesions with gently sloping edges

will be missed. Dedicated DC techniques for the anterior wall are too complicated to use routinely. Therefore PC studies are necessary to visualize lesions with gently sloping edges of the anterior wall of the corpus and the antrum. To avoid blind angles a *biphasic technique* combining the advantages of both DC and PC techniques is required.

Standardization of a technique, although restricting the freedom of the individual examiner, can result in a study of uniformly high quality. Japan with its high rate of gastric cancer leads the world in the standardization of gastric series.

In 1973 the author introduced a standard examination for the stomach and duodenal bulb, which was designed to meet the following requirements:

a. DC techniques must be used to visualize those parts of the stomach that are easy to examine with them.
b. PC studies should continue for the reasons already stated.

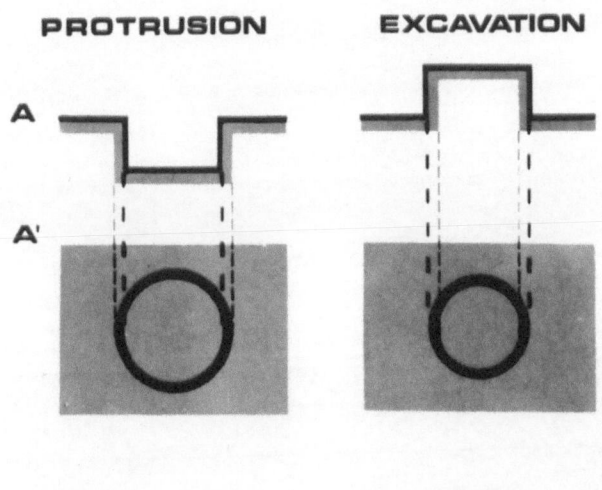

PROTRUSION   EXCAVATION

A

A'

B

B'

Fig. 3
The DC posterior-wall series accurately reveals all posterior-wall lesions, as well as excavations and protrusions of the anterior wall with abrupt margins.

A.   A protruding lesion with abrupt margins on the anterior wall (left) and an excavation with abrupt margins on the anterior wall (right).

A'.   The posterior-wall projections. Both lesions cast a ring shadow.

B.   A protruding lesion with gently sloping edges on the anterior wall (left) and an excavation with gently sloping edges on the anterior wall (right).

B'.   The posterior-wall projections. Both lesions will be missed on a supine DC series.

c. The series must be easily reproducible, even by junior residents and radiologists who have no particular interest in the upper gastro-intestinal tract.

d. Complete examination of the stomach and duodenal bulb should not take too long, say not more than 15 minutes, to complete in a cooperative patient.

e. The study must include examination of the stomach following drug-induced hypotonia (this requirement was added in 1974).

This examination was called "the standard biphasic-contrast gastric series (195)."

Chapter 3

THE STANDARD BIPHASIC-CONTRAST GASTRIC SERIES

3.1. Barium suspension and preparation of bubbly barium

The barium suspension required for a biphasic gastric series must possess several specific properties to be of a sufficient quality to use:

a. a medium-high density
b. a low viscosity (nearly as "thin" as water)
c. good mucosal adherence
d. the suspension must mix well with gastric secretions.

If the bubbly barium method of Pochaczevski (201) is used – as the author strongly advises – another property must be added, viz.:

e. release of the CO_2 gas must be completed within 2 minutes.

Although commercial preparations may comply with one or two of these requirements, they are expensive. The author's barium suspension is prepared by the Hospital Pharmacists according to a recipe given in table 1. The medium-high density (82.5% W/V, SW 1.62) it possesses is required to combine high contrast in DC studies and transparency on PC studies.

Preparation of bubbly barium

A soda syphon* is filled with 2 liters of the barium suspension. Preliminary refrigeration of the syphon

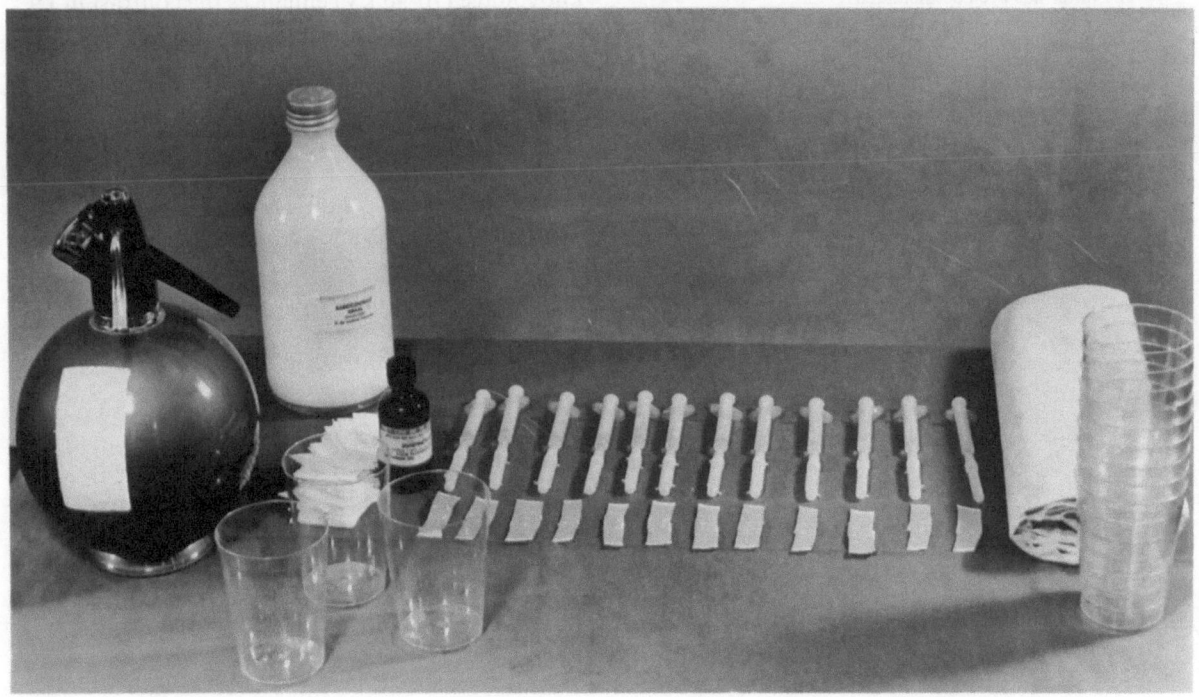

Fig. 4
Preparations required for 12 standard biphasic-contrast gastric series.

* Sparklets Syphon (Globemaster type), Sparklets, Queen Street, London N17 8JA, England (part of British Oxygen Co., Ltd.).

Table 1.

Recipe for barium suspension

Sodium citrate 2 aq	600 g
Natrosol 250 G[1]	275-500 g
mixed with barium sulphate[2]	1,000 g
Corrigentia[3]	300 ml
Antifoam A.F. Emulsion, Rhodorsil	600 ml
Antimousse 70426 or Mylicon[4]	
Water[5] up to	30 l
Barium sulphate[2]	32 kg
Water[5] up to	40 l

[1] Hercules Co. Natrosol 250G is hydroxyethylcellulose. The 2% W/V solution in water has, at 25° C, a viscosity of approx. 200 cP (Brookfield Viscosimeter). The exact quantity needed depends on the batch quality.

[2] Barium sulphate, plain U.S.P. (Mallinckrodt) or Barium Sulphate pro Roentgen (Bayer).

[3] Composition of the corrigentia:

Sodium cyclamate	120 g
Saccharin sodium	12 g
Water	800 ml
Tween 80	320 ml
Sweet orange concentrate	1.2 l
Nipaginesters[6] in alcohol 90%	12.5 ml
Water up to	2.4 l

[4] Antifoam A.F. Emulsion (Dow Corning) or Rhodorsil Antimousse 70426 (Rhône-Poulenc) containing ~3% dimethylpolysiloxane. Mylicon (Stuart Pharmaceuticals) contains 6.6% simethicone so that 2,700 ml is needed if this is used.

[5] The water has been decalcinated.

[6] Composition of nipaginester in alcohol:

Methylparaben	200 mg
Propylparaben	50 mg
Alcohol 90% W/V up to	1 l

For making the suspension, a high-speed mixer is needed.
(Reproduced by permission of Radiology.)

as well as the suspension is an essential feature since the CO_2 gas will not dissolve readily at room temperature. After being tightly screwed down, the contents of 2 cartridges of CO_2 are slowly added, and the syphon is shaken vigorously. Addition of the CO_2 has to be spread evenly over a period of 10 minutes. Experiments have shown that the bubbly barium prepared in this way dissociates in about 90 seconds and produces one part of barium suspension and two parts of CO_2. One syphon is sufficient for 12 standard biphasic-contrast series. If stored in the refrigerator, the bubbly barium will not dissociate. If stored overnight, the suspension should be shaken moderately prior to use.

3.2. Premedication

An intravenous injection of 0.5 mg of glucagon is given immediately prior to the examination. Fig. 4 shows the preparations which are made to perform 12 standard biphasic-contrast gastric series.

3.3. Technical factors

High kilovoltage (120-150 kV) is used for short exposures and transparency of the PC studies. Lower kilovoltage (70-90 kV) enhances the contrast in DC films; by using rare-earth intensifying screens short exposure times can be retained (fig. 5).

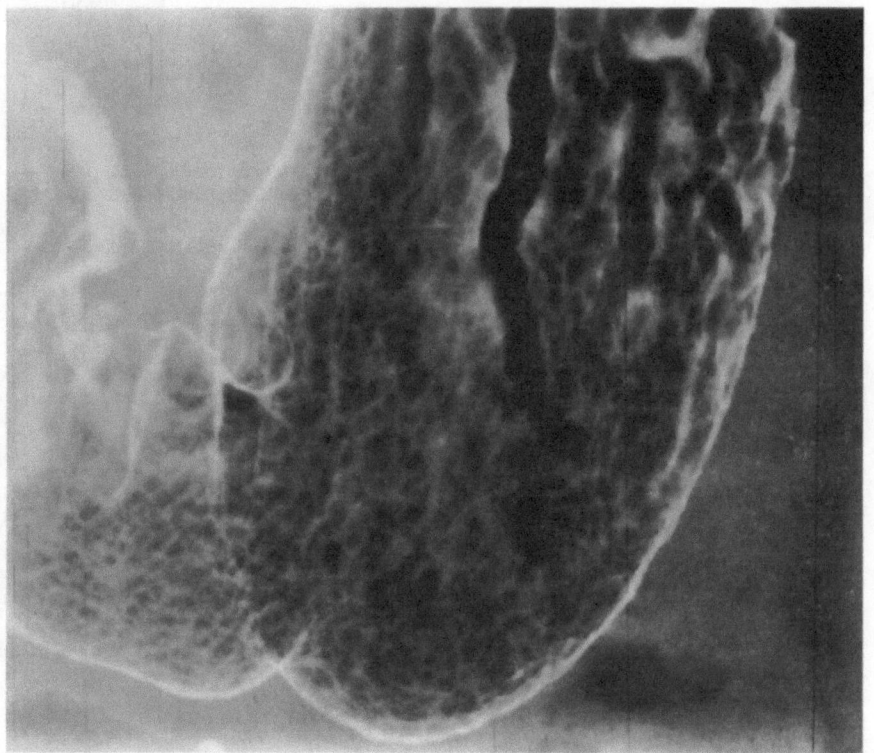

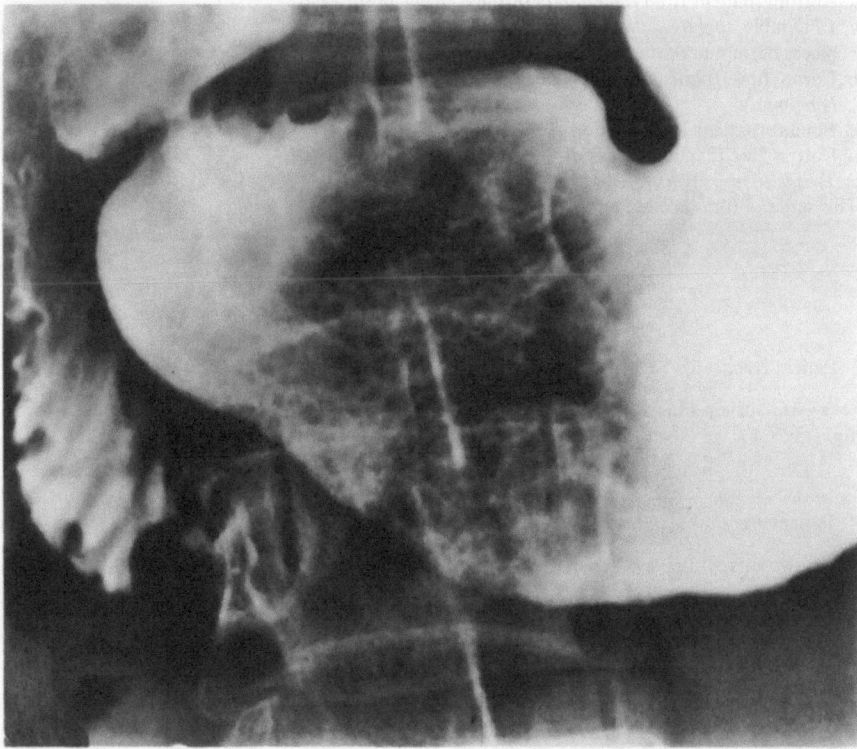

Fig. 5
a & b. Areae gastricae demonstrated in the DC and in the PC (compression) study. The use of a medium-high density barium suspension enables a biphasic examination to be performed. (5a reproduced by permission of Radiology).

3.4. Method proper

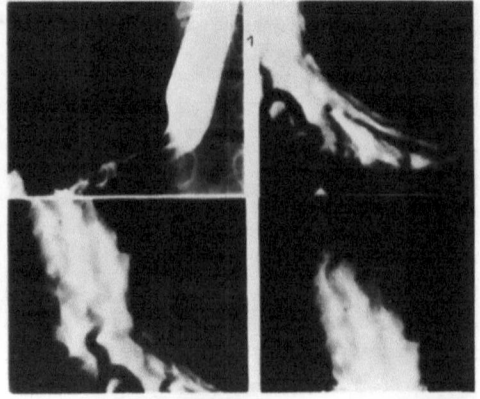

1. Patient *prone*/table *horizontal* or *slightly anti-Trendelenburg*. The patient takes half a mouthful of normal barium suspension (i.e. without CO_2) and swallows it on request.

Spot films:
a. Esophago-cardiac junction. Patient is turned into right lateral position and then prone again.
b. Mucosal relief study.
c. Mucosal relief study.
d. Mucosal relief study (fig. 6a).

Fig. 6a

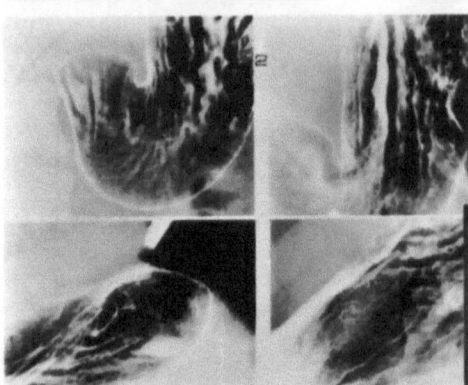

2. Patient *supine*/table *30°-40° anti-Trendelenburg*. Patient instruction: "You will now get something resembling soda water. Try to swallow it all at once. Don't belch...." Then 250 ml of bubbly barium is swallowed under fluoroscopy. The esophagus is inspected. Then the table is placed horizontally and the two-minute period of CO_2 dissociation begins. The patient is asked to turn himself around (if possible 2 or 3 times) in order to obtain a good coating.* He is also instructed about breathing and how to stop on request. The respiratory excursion, i.e. the exact position in ex- or inspiration, greatly influences gastric configuration and thus image quality (fig. 7). DC pictures of the antrum, fundus and corpus. Each picture is made with a fresh coating.

Patient movement between *right lateral* and *LPO*/table movements between *horizontal* and *anti-Trendelenburg*.

Fig. 6b

Spot films:
a. Antrum (patient from *right lateral* through *supine* position to *LPO*/table *slightly anti-Trendelenburg.*) As soon as gas replaces barium in the antrum, the picture is made.
b. Corpus (low) (patient from *right lateral* to *supine* position/table *horizontal*).
c. Fundus (patient *RPO*/table *30°-40° anti-Trendelenburg*).
d. Corpus (high) (patient back to *nearly supine*/table *less anti-Trendelenburg*) (fig. 6b).
This series of films is often repeated.

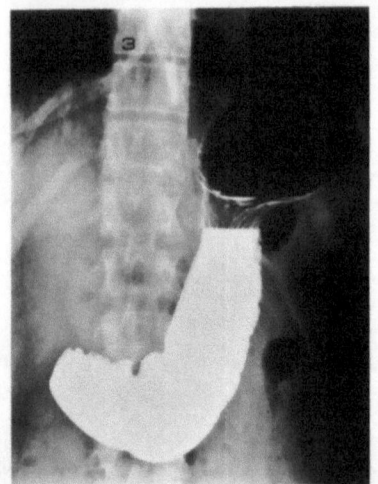

3. Patient *erect*/table *vertical*.

Large-size survey film: Postero-anterior or antero-posterior** (fig. 6c).

Fig. 6c

4. Patient *erect*/table *vertical*.

Large-size survey film: LPO erect film (fig. 6d).

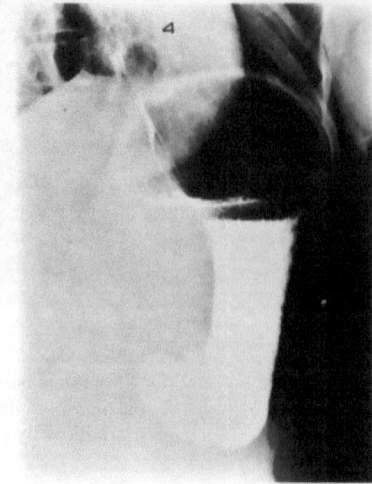

* If, after the bubbly barium has been swallowed, it is seen to pass through the pylorus, the technique has to be adapted to prevent duodenal and jejunal superimposition. DC films with non-optimal coating and some gas bubbles, but without superimposition, can be obtained by turning the patient first into the right lateral and then into the LPO positions.

** depending on whether the X-ray apparatus is of the conventional or remote controlled type.

Fig. 6d

5. Patient *erect*/table *vertical*.

Spot films:
a. Compression study.
b. Compression study.
c. Compression study.
d. Lateral study of the corpus with the patient turned sideways and bending over. Hiatal hernia or gastro-esophageal reflux on fluoroscopy? (fig. 6e).

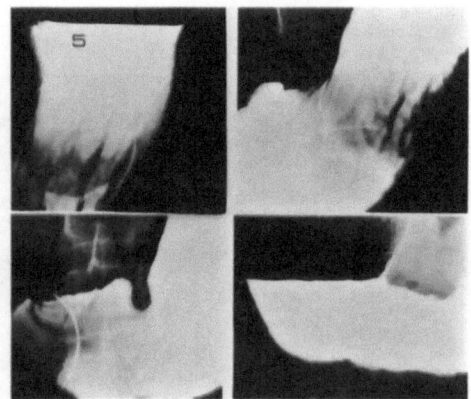

Fig. 6e

6. Patient *prone*, *RPO*/table *horizontal*.

Spot film:
a. Complete filling of the duodenal bulb with a compression paddle between the table and the patient.

Patient *erect*/table *vertical*.

Spot films:
b. *LAO* – compression study of the duodenal bulb (Holzknecht's spoon).
c. *RPO* – compression study of the duodenal bulb (Holzknecht's spoon).

Patient movement from *right lateral* to *LPO*/table *horizontal*.

Spot film:
d. DC film of the duodenal bulb (fig. 6f).

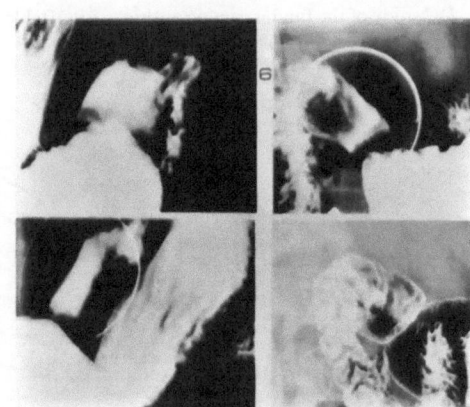

Fig. 6f

7. Patient from *right lateral* to *supine*/table *horizontal*.

Large-size survey film: postero-anterior or antero-posterior** supine film (fig. 6g).

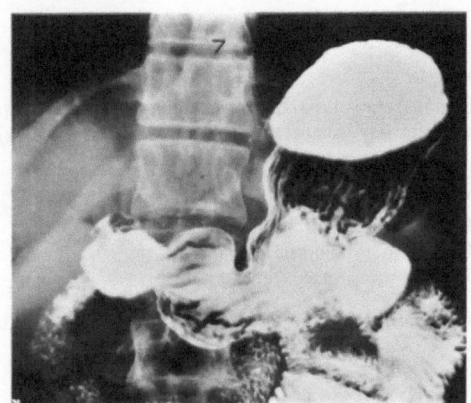

** depending on whether the X-ray apparatus is of the conventional or remote controlled type.

Fig. 6g

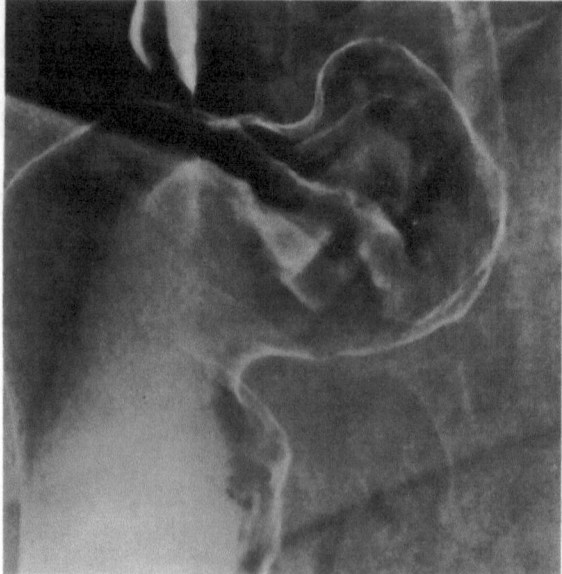 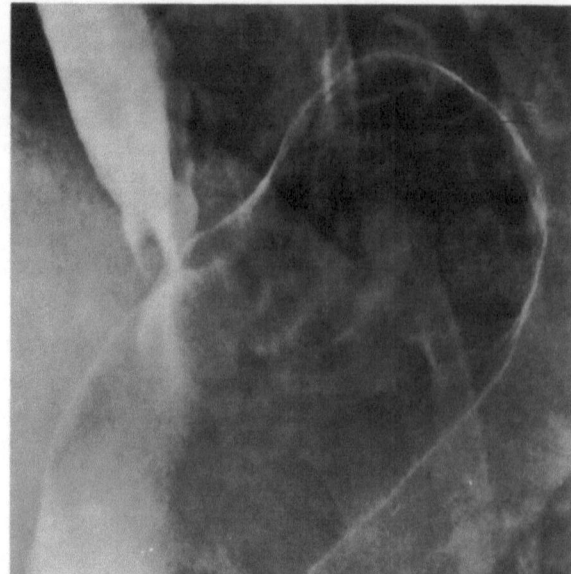

Fig. 7

a. DC study of the fundus, supine position, RPO; table about 35°   b. Patient in the same position: expiration.
anti-Trendelenburg: inspiration.

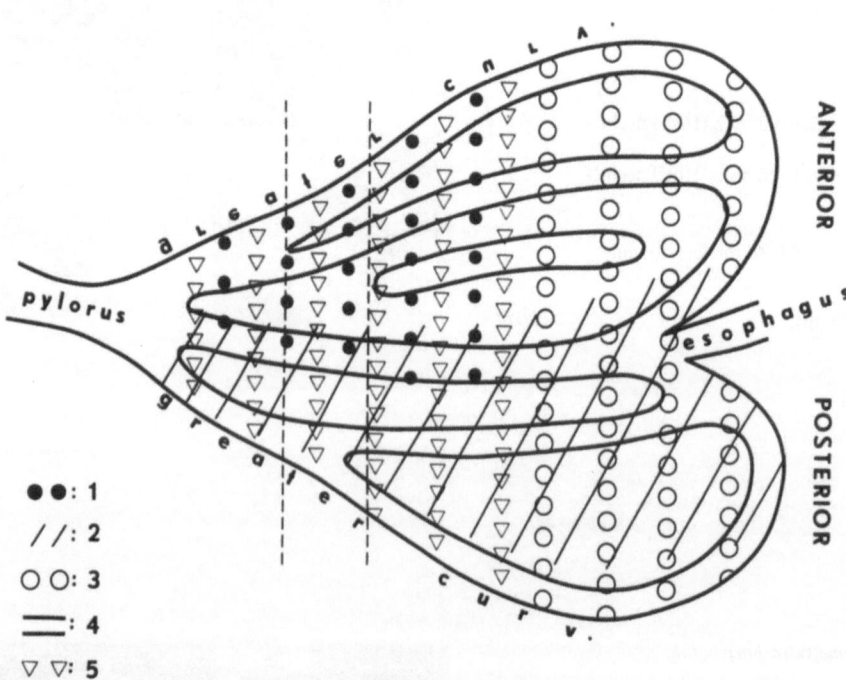

Fig. 8
Regional map of the stomach cut along the greater curvature with the gastric mucosa
exposed. The area between the dotted lines is the gastric angle.

1 = mucosal relief studies (1)
2 = DC vertical beam studies (2)
3 = DC horizontal beam studies (3 & 4)
4 = contour diagnosis (3, 4 and 5)
5 = compression (5).

The numerals in brackets refer to the examination method as described in chapter 3,
section 4. (Reproduced by permission of Radiology.)

Sometimes the examination of the stomach has already been completed, i.e. step 5 above, before the effect of the glucagon has worn off, resulting in inadequate filling of the duodenal bulb. When this occurs, the patient has to wait about 10 minutes – providing enough time for the next patient being examined. After this 10-minute period, films of the duodenal bulb are made and the peristaltic movements of the stomach are carefully studied.

If the patient belches, or if for some other reason additional gas is required, a simple effervescent powder is used, e.g. a mixture of tartaric acid and sodium bicarbonate (11:12). While commercial effervescent granules may be easier to swallow, they are expensive and have not yet been registered by the drug control bodies of several countries.

3.5. Coverage

As fig. 8 shows, coverage of the stomach is excellent, although the posterior wall of the stomach overlaps to a greater degree than the anterior wall. No details are given for coverage of the duodenal bulb since this is complete with compression. If compression is impossible, e.g. in extremely obese subjects, DC studies can still be performed and overpenetrated PC films can exclude gross lesions of the anterior wall with gently sloping edges.

3.6. Complementary hypotonic duodenography

The logical consequence of the method described is that a consecutive hypotonic duodenogram can easily be performed. The indication is provided either by clinical data or by the appearances of the films obtained at the standard biphasic examination.

Technique
Patient right lateral/table slightly anti-Trendelenburg. The patient swallows another cup of bubbly barium and an assistant punctures a vein. When barium is seen in the duodenal loop, 1 mg of glucagon is injected. Immediately after the needle has been withdrawn (the pylorus not yet having closed), the patient turns to LPO to allow the gas to pass into the duodenum. In order to provide a good mucosal coating the patient is turned approximately 135° from the supine LPO position to the prone position and back again (fig. 9). This movement prevents the gas from escaping from the duodenal loop, because of its posterior position. Then films are made in the supine LPO and in the prone positions (fig. 10). Sometimes a compression cone or paddle between the patient and the table is helpful in the prone position in order to eliminate troublesome superimposition of the barium filled antrum and the DC filled duodenal loop (fig. 11).

This technique of tubeless hypotonic duodenography adds only a few minutes to the standard series.

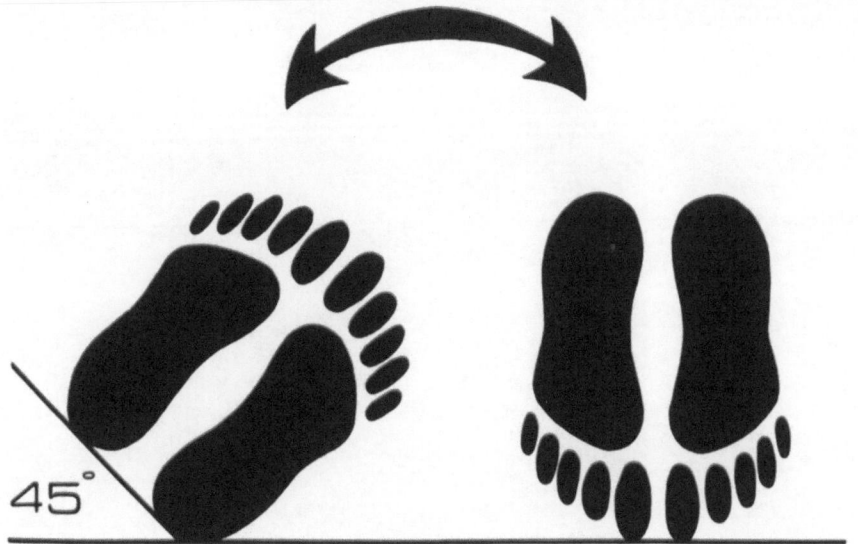

Fig. 9
Diagram to show the movements of the patient necessary for a good mucosal coating.

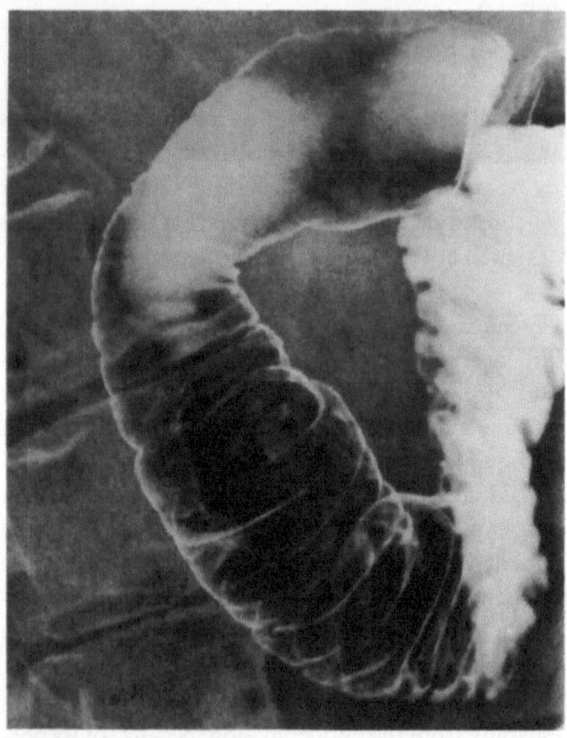

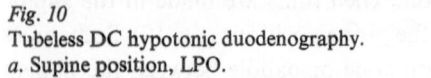

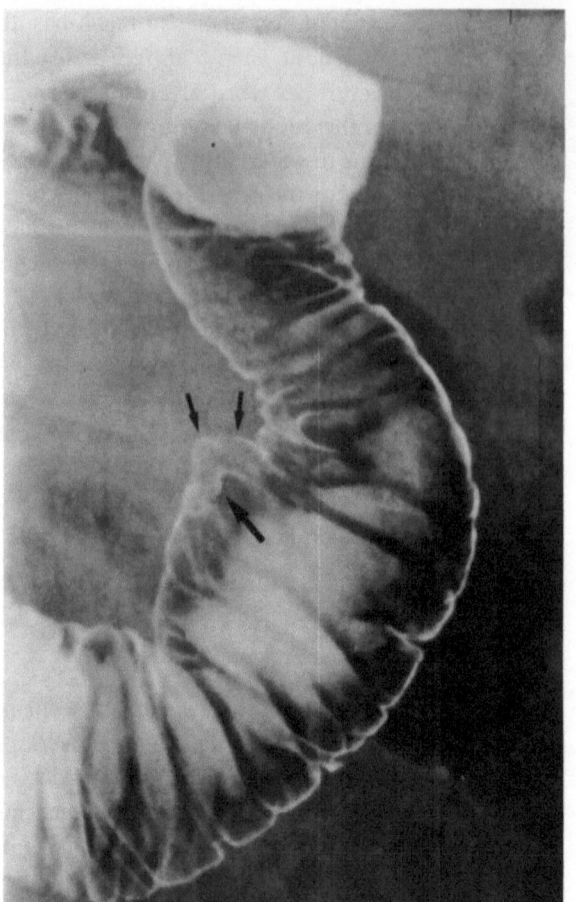

Fig. 10
Tubeless DC hypotonic duodenography.
a. Supine position, LPO.
b. Prone position. The promontory (small arrows) and the major
   papilla (large arrow) are often better visualized in this projection than in the supine LPO position.

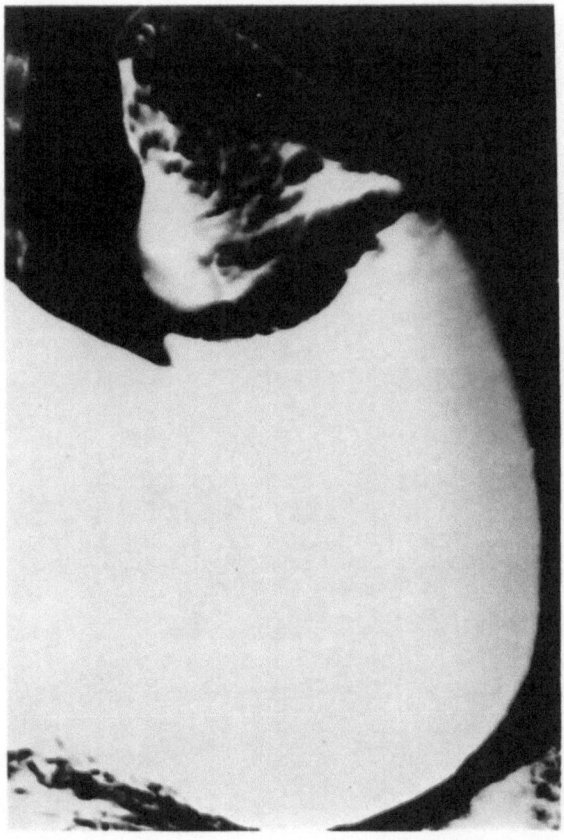

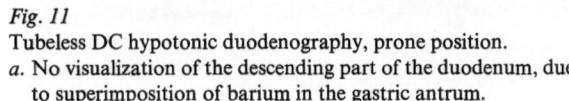

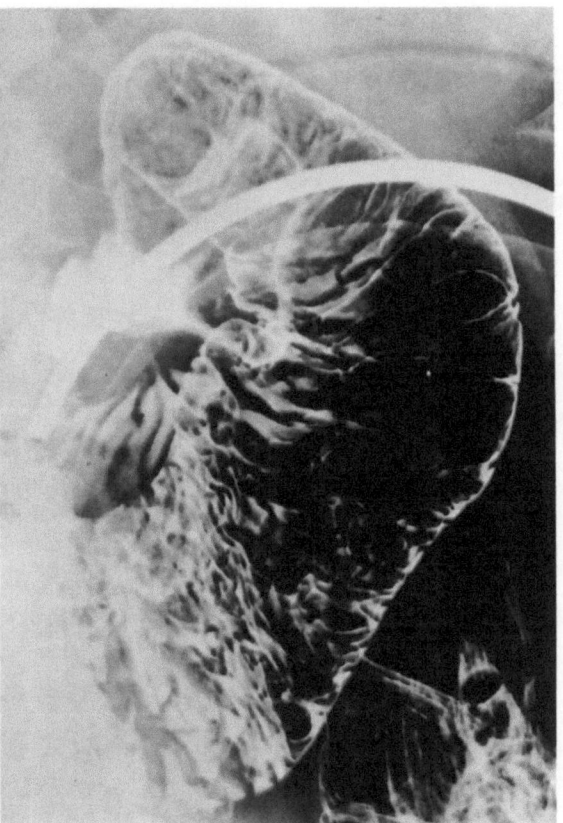

Fig. 11
Tubeless DC hypotonic duodenography, prone position.
a. No visualization of the descending part of the duodenum, due to superimposition of barium in the gastric antrum.

b. Same examination, showing good visualization of the duodenal loop by applying a compression paddle between the patient and the table.

Chapter 4

BASIC PRINCIPLES FOR THE INTERPRETATION OF DOUBLE-CONTRAST STUDIES

Radiography of the stomach and duodenum can be defined as the registration of different levels. Gastric lesions can be classified into protrusions and excavations (127). The changes produced by protrusions and excavations in conventional PC studies are common knowledge to the radiologist. But changes revealed by DC studies are not always properly interpreted and therefore require further elaboration. The impulse for solving many of the problems in the DC diagnosis of gastric lesions – both protruding and excavated – was given by Ichikawa (118). He explained the different appearances of anterior- and posterior-wall mucosal folds in DC studies made in the supine position, using a vertical beam.

Folds in the posterior wall are visualized as radiolucent bands which separate pools of contrast medium. Folds in the anterior wall show two distinct white contrast lines which run parallel to each other. These "railway track" shadows are one-end projections of contrast material coating the two vertical parts of the folds (fig. 12). This appearance can be used to differentiate between protrusions and exca-

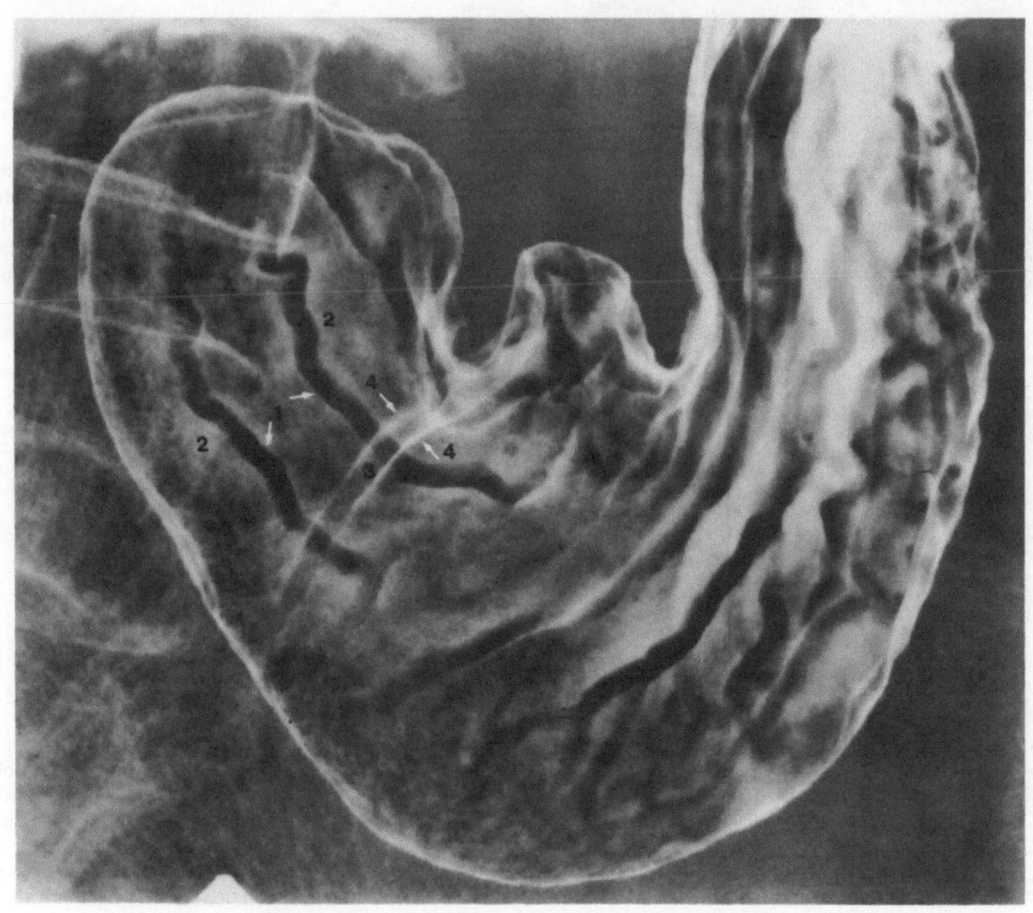

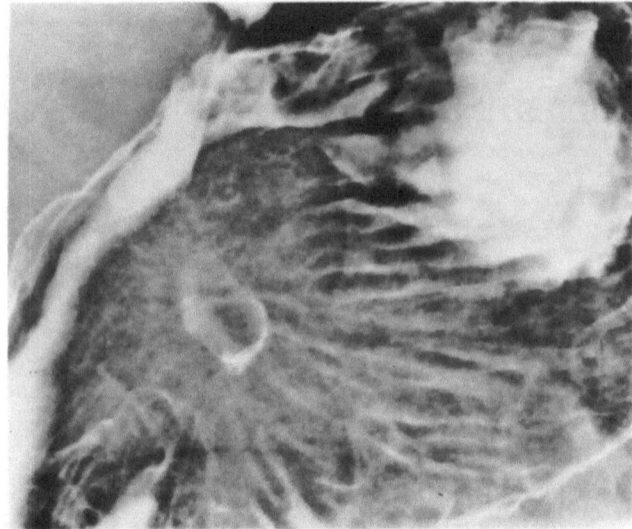

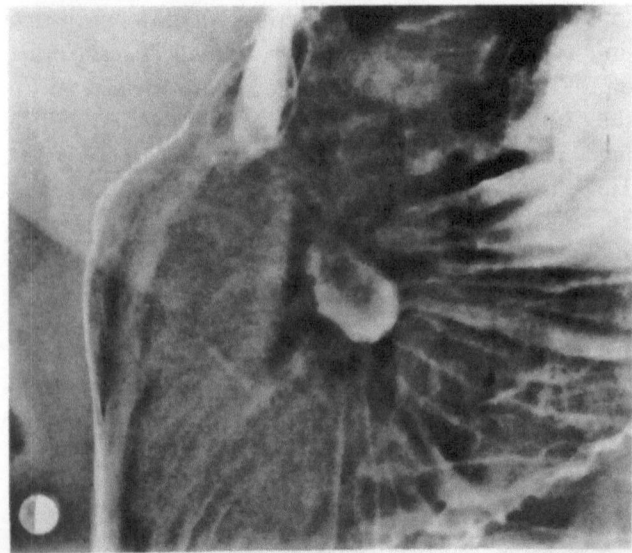

Fig. 13

a. DC study, supine position, RPO; table 35° anti-Trendelenburg. Ring shadow: the barium at the bottom of
   the ring shadow suggests a niche in the posterior wall.
b. Same position. More barium has entered the niche,
   confirming that the lesion is an ulcer of the posterior
   wall.

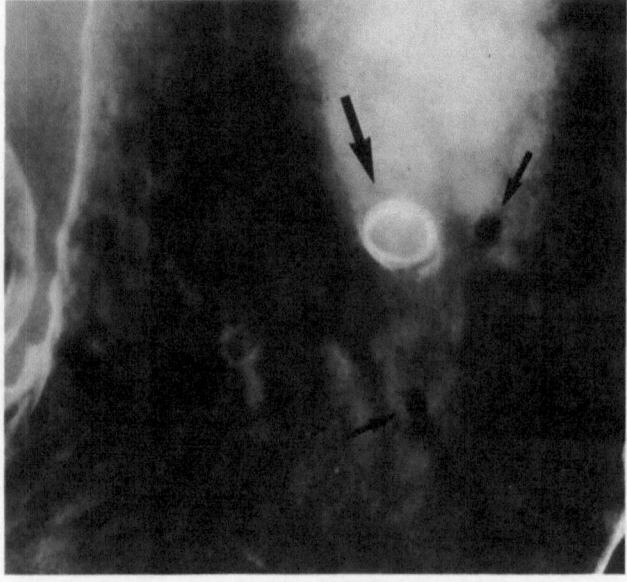

Fig. 14

DC study, supine position. Ring shadow (large arrow)
projected on the corpus of the stomach. The ring sign is
formed by the circular line shadow from an end-on projection of barium coating the cylindrical part of an
abruptly marginated lesion. The lesion must be localized
on the anterior wall, because there is no filling defect in the
pool of barium on the posterior wall or no filling of a
niche. Abruptly marginated polypoid lesion of the
anterior wall. Filling defects (small arrows) in the pool of
barium are polypoid lesions in the posterior wall.

vations on either the anterior or the posterior wall.

Lesions with abruptly-marginated edges can be easily imaged in supine DC studies. For example, round lesions with such edges, either protruding or excavated, will produce a ring shadow if situated on either the anterior or the posterior wall. Differentiating between an excavation or a protrusion of the posterior wall or an abruptly marginated lesion of the anterior wall can be accomplished by manipulating barium suspension along the posterior wall, either through tilting the table or by moving the patient. An excavation of the posterior wall is revealed as a barium-filled niche (fig. 13), and a protrusion as a filling defect. With a lesion of the anterior wall, however, the ring shadow remains unchanged (fig. 14). In the differentiation between abruptly marginated lesions of the anterior wall, it should be remembered that the ring shadow in a deep excavated lesion surrounds a radiolucency (fig. 15). In a highly protruding lesion, the ring shadow surrounds a weak density. Differentiation is easy by means of PC compression studies (fig. 15b). Should this prove impossible, the lesion is projected en profil (fig. 15c).

Posterior-wall protrusions with gently sloping edges can also be visualized on the supine DC pictures by manipulating some barium suspension along the posterior wall. It is sometimes easier to demonstrate such lesions with PC than with DC studies (fig. 16).

As emphasized above, anterior-wall protrusions and excavations with gently sloping edges are usually missed in the supine DC film (fig. 3). On PC compression studies they appear either as a filling defect or as a niche, both without a sharp margin (figs. 17 and 18).

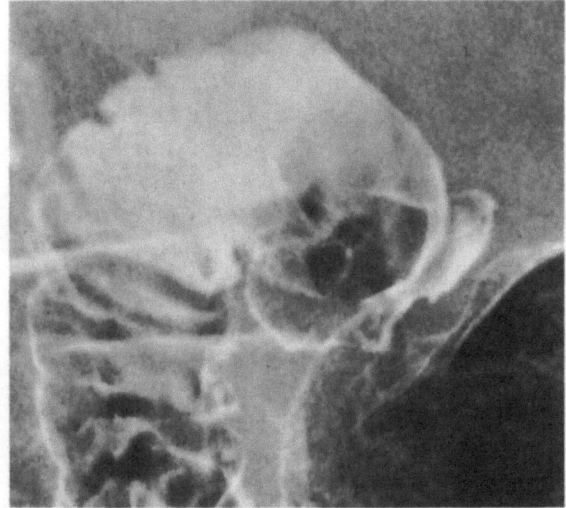
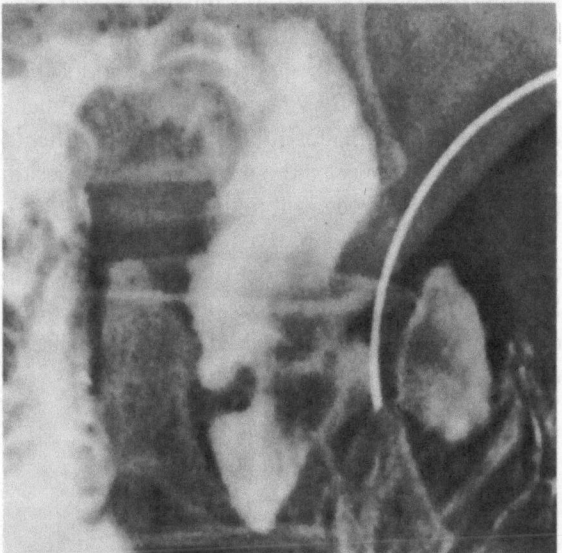
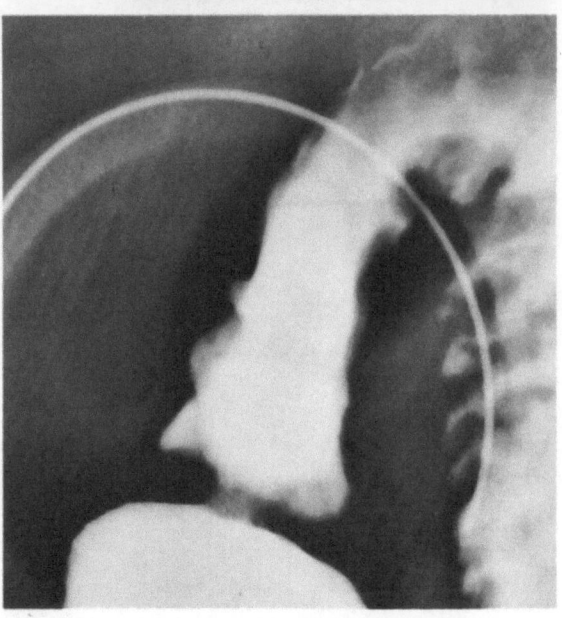

Fig. 15

a. DC study, supine position, LPO. Ring shadow in the duodenal cap. No barium suspension could be caught in the ring shadow by altering the patient's position or by tilting the table. As proved in b and c, the lesion was an abruptly marginated ulcer in the anterior wall.

b. PC compression study, erect position, LPO.

c. PC compression study, erect position, RPO.

DC studies may provide an almost three-dimensional view, as is demonstrated in fig. 19. This film shows a sharp line of contrast medium in the region of the angulus. The image of the stomach above the line is less transparent. At its lateral end this sharp contrast line crosses a barium pool, situated, of course, on the posterior wall of the stomach. Since the line remains sharp, it is not in touch with the barium on the posterior wall – the so-called "silhouette phenomenon (70)." Thus, it may be concluded that the line is formed in the anterior wall of the stomach. In fact, the line represented an external impression caused by the liver.

When performing DC studies of the stomach, the radiologist must beware of barium spots or droplets hanging down like stalactites from polyps and folds of the anterior wall. The author and a colleague have convincingly proved the nature of these spots (193) (figs. 20 and 21). In fig. 22 several of the phenomena described above are illustrated in the same patient.

Thin patients may exhibit a specific pseudo-lesion previously described by Laufer (91, 150) (fig. 23). This phenomenon is observed in DC studies when the anterior and posterior gastric walls touch. Fluoroscopy dispels all doubts and enables this kind of pseudo-lesion to be recognized as such, because its form alters during respiration.

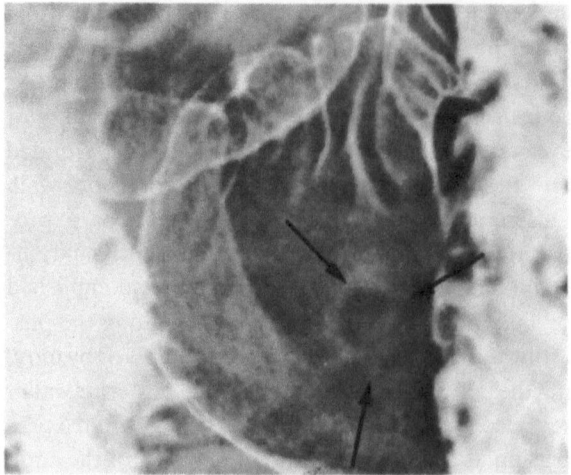

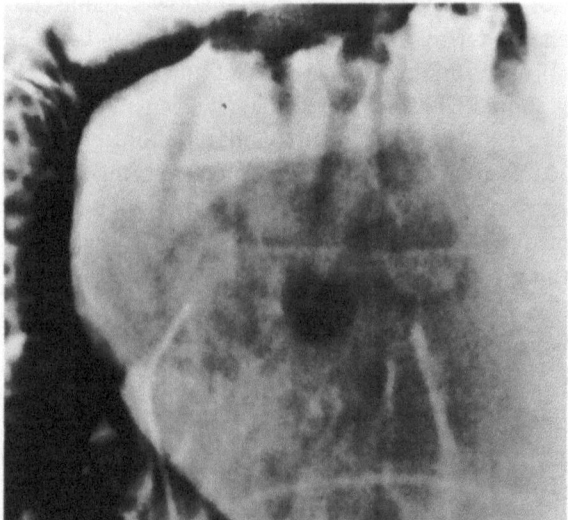

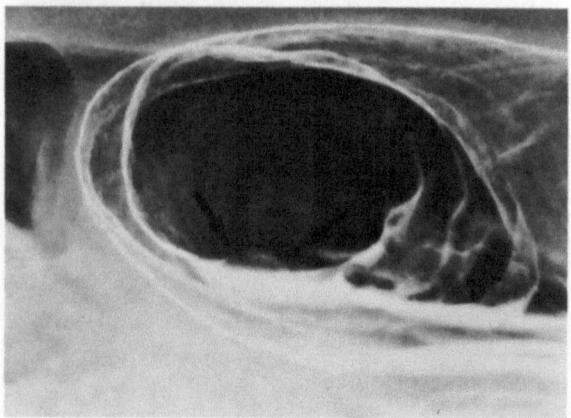

Fig. 16

a. DC study, supine position, LPO. The arrows indicate a protrusion with gently sloping edges on the posterior wall of the gastric antrum. There is no sharp delineation.

b. PC compression study, erect position. The lesion is demonstrated more easily with a PC compression study.

c. Supine position, horizontal beam projection. In this projection the situation on the posterior wall and the form of the lesion which could be predicted from a and b are confirmed (arrows).

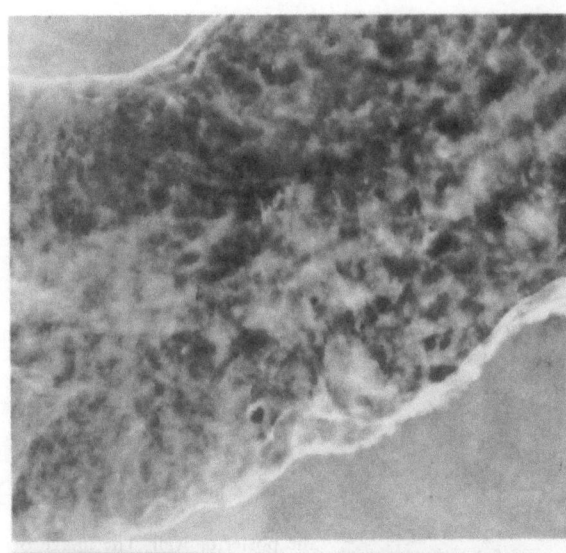

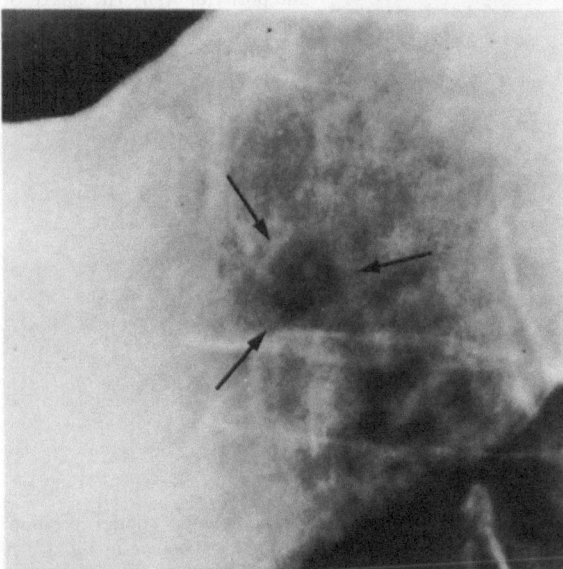

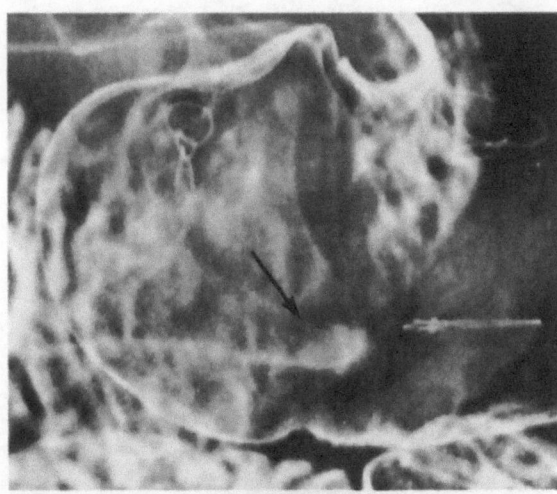

←
Fig. 17

a. DC study, supine position: no abnormalities.

b. PC compression study, erect position, revealing a filling defect (arrows).

c. Supine position, horizontal beam projection confirming that a polypoid lesion with gently sloping edges of the anterior wall is present.

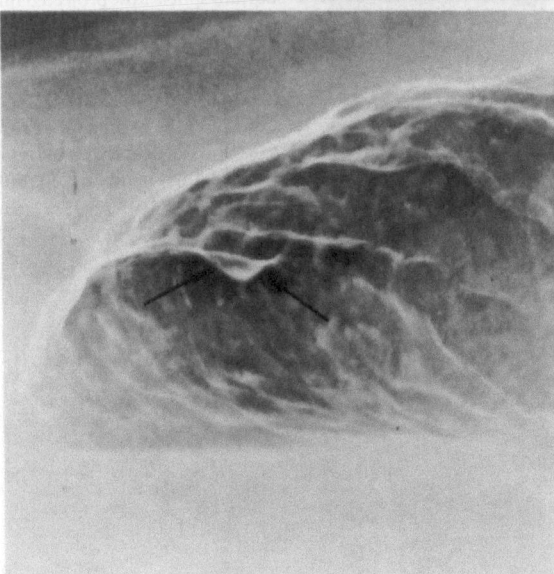

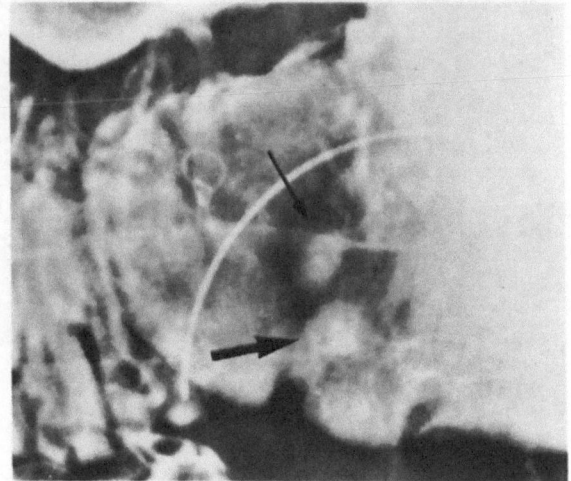

Fig. 18 ↑

a. DC study, supine position, LPO. Contrast fleck (arrow) is caused by a niche in the posterior wall which has gently sloping edges.

b. PC compression study, erect position, revealing a second ill-defined niche (large arrow). This one also has gently sloping edges but it lies in the anterior wall. Lesions confirmed by gastroscopy.

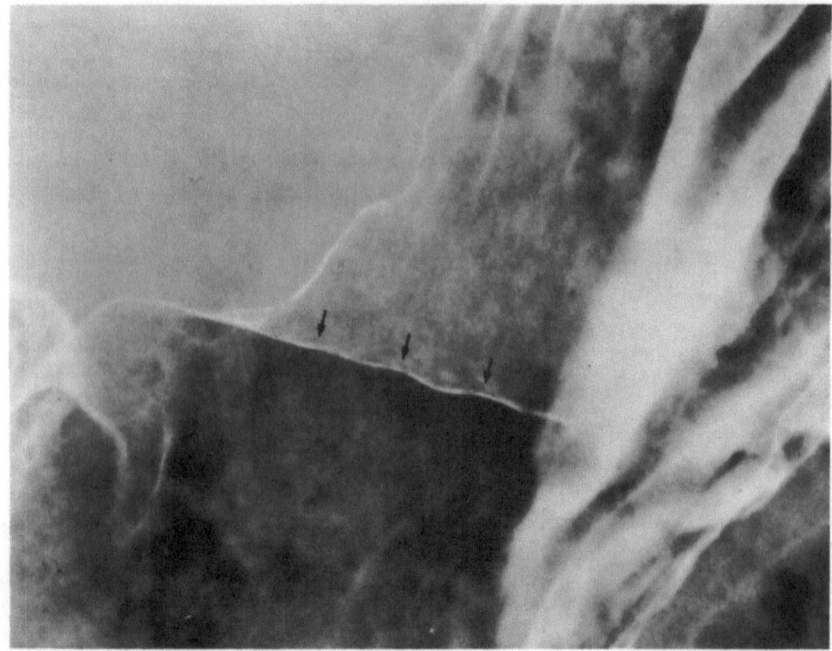

Fig. 19
DC study, supine position. There
is a sharp line in the region of
angulus (arrows). On the lateral
side this line crosses a barium pool
which is of course situated on the
posterior wall of the stomach.
Since the line remains sharp, it is
not in touch with the barium on
the posterior wall. The image of
the stomach above the sharp line is
denser. The line was shown to be
an anterior-wall indentation of the
stomach caused by the liver.

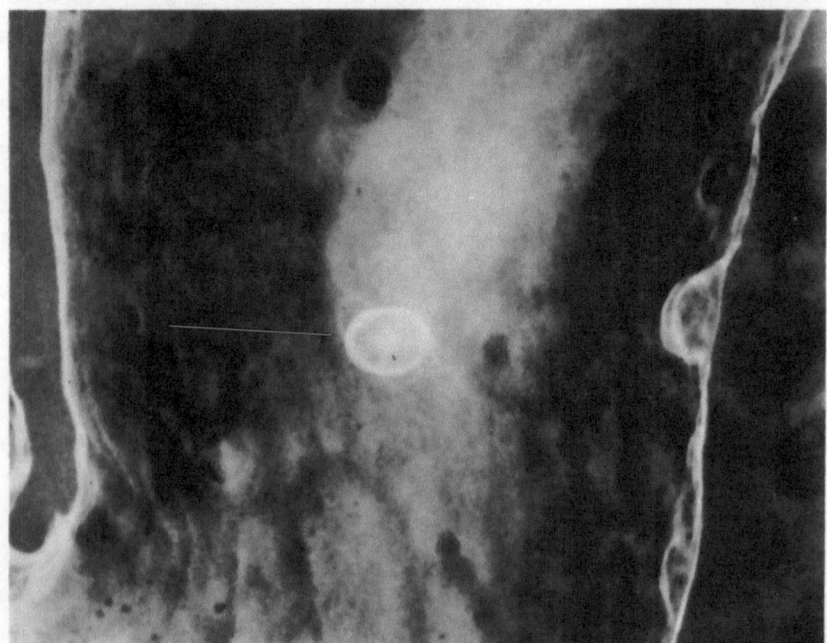

Fig. 20
a. DC study, supine position.
Same patient as in fig. 14. A
barium spot is now projected on
the top of the abruptly marginated cylindrical polypoid
lesion of the anterior wall.
b & c. Horizontal beam projections show the barium spot to be
caused by a droplet of barium
(small arrow) hanging from the
lesion (large arrow).

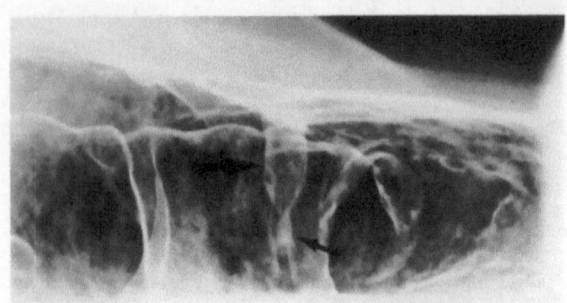

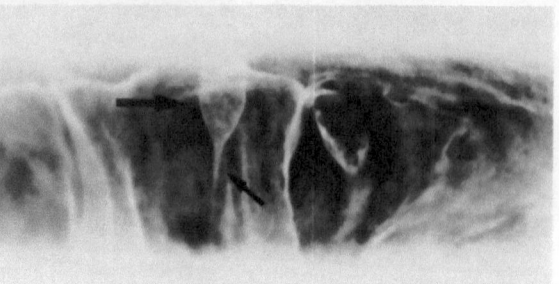

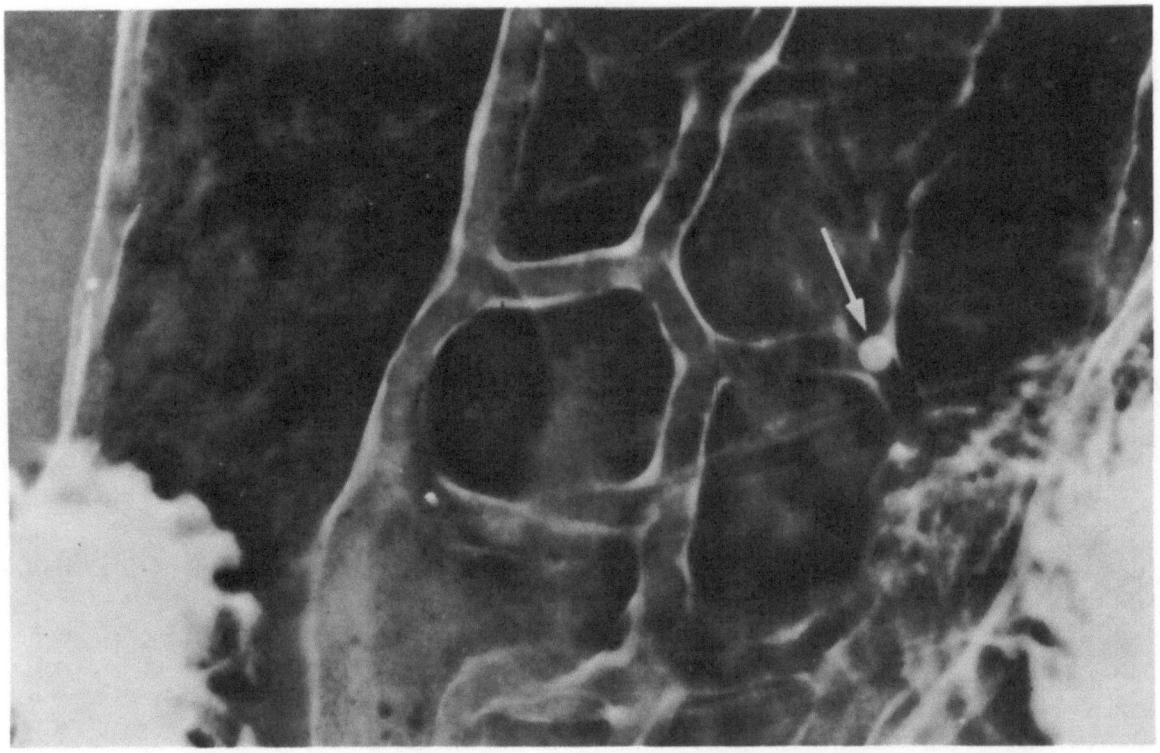

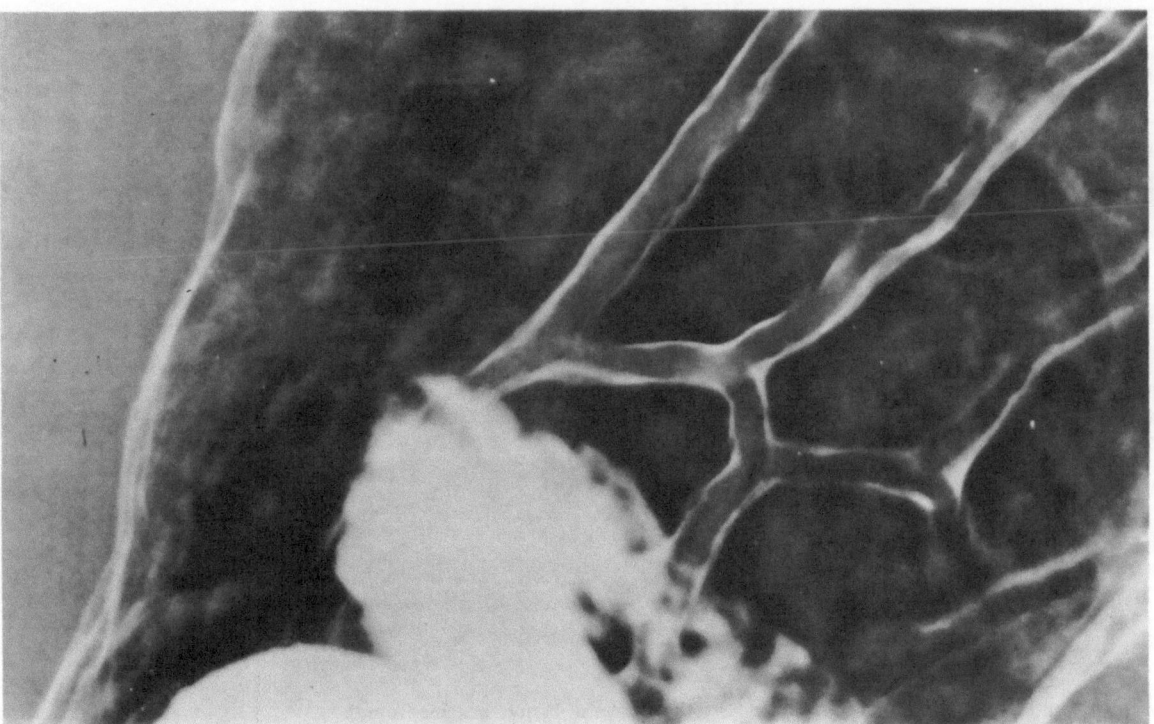

Fig. 21
a. DC study, supine position, partial RPO. There is a droplet of barium hanging from an anterior-wall fold crossing (arrow).
b. Same patient, a few moments later: the barium spot has disappeared, the droplet having fallen by gravity.

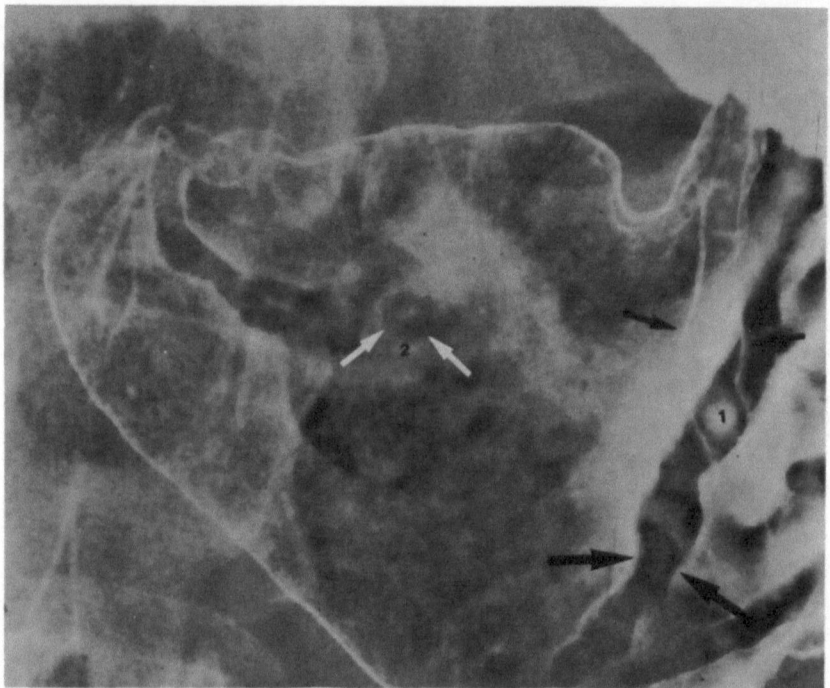

Fig. 22

a. DC study, supine position. Several phenomena are illustrated in this patient. The large arrows point to a typical fold of the posterior wall. The small black arrows indicate an anterior-wall fold. Lesion 1 is a droplet of barium suspended from the anterior-wall fold. Lesion 2 is a slightly elevated protrusion with gently sloping edges and a central excavation on the posterior wall – a typical varioliform erosion.

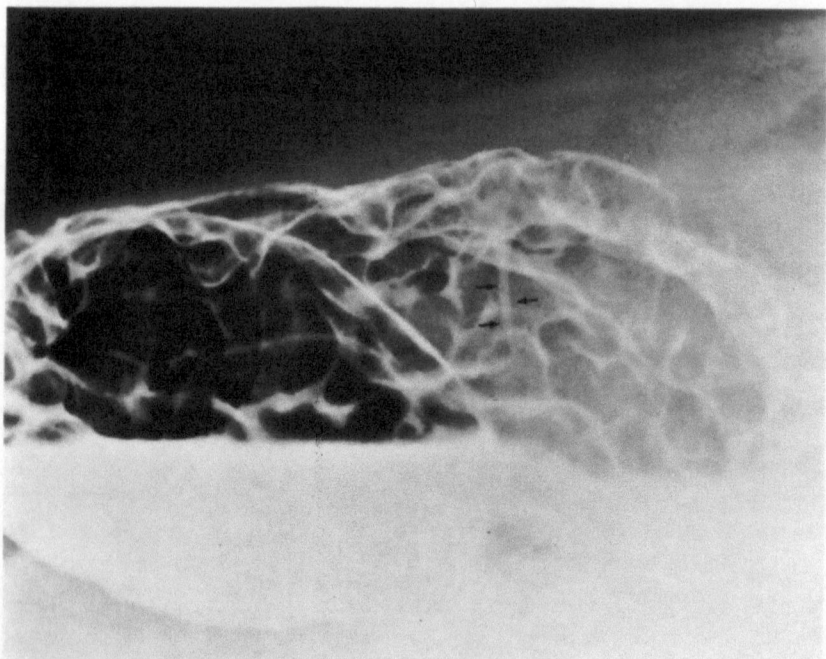

b. Horizontal beam projection. The arrows point to the droplet of barium hanging from the anterior wall fold (lesion 1).

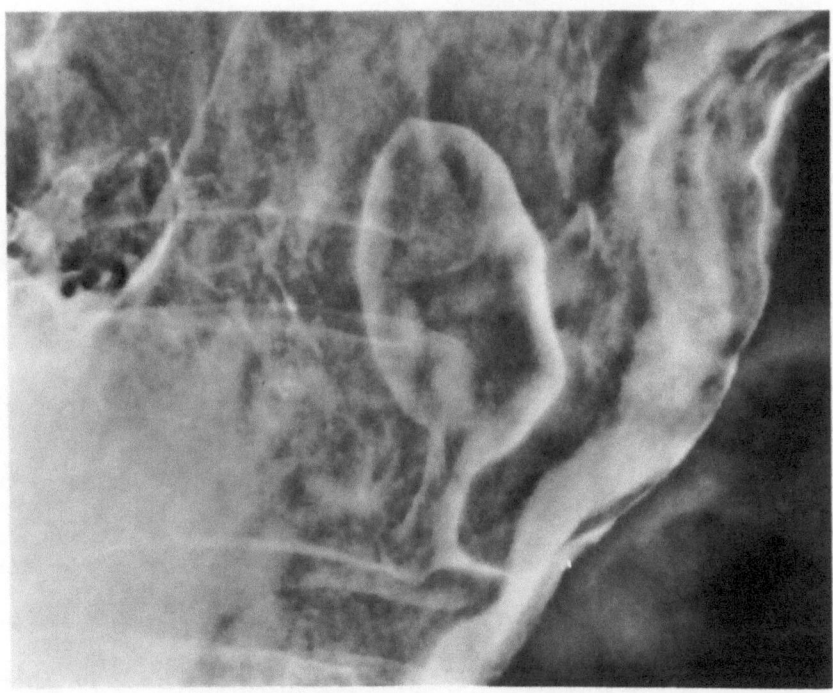

Fig. 23
DC study, supine position. Pseudo-lesion as described by Laufer (91, 150). This "kissing artefact" phenomenon occurs when the anterior wall and posterior wall touch. Under fluoroscopy this kind of pseudo-lesion is easily recognized because its form constantly changes during respiration.

Part II

RESULTS

Chapter 5

GENERAL REMARKS

During the period 1 September 1973 to 1 April 1978 about 7,500 standard biphasic-contrast studies were performed in patients over 18 years of age. The projections described previously (chapter 3) were routinely made – with one exception. Step 5d, viz. study of the corpus of the stomach with the patient turned sideways and touching his toes, proved difficult to execute in elderly patients and impossible to use with remote-controlled machines. In instances in which it was omitted, the presence of a hiatal hernia was determined when the patient initially swallowed the barium in the prone position. Gastro-esophageal reflux was studied while the patient lay in the different horizontal positions.

Series 2 (DC spot films of the stomach) was often repeated.

After the first year, a premedication of glucagon 0.5 mg was given as a routine. Experience showed that this level of premedication significantly improved our results in respect of detailed radiography of the stomach and duodenum. Prior to using glucagon routinely, varioliform erosions were only rarely diagnosed. Following it, they became a frequent diagnosis. Often a varioliform erosion was discovered in the hypotonic phase which could not be demonstrated when the hypotonia had subsided. However, this success is certainly not attributable only to the use of glucagon: personal experience and also the feed-back from the endoscopist contributed greatly.

It became clear that both DC and PC radiography were necessary. In most cases the diagnosis was made on the DC studies or on the PC compression studies, and often by a combination of these two (figs. 18, 53, 59, 68, 70, 89, 126, 149, 151). Only rarely did the mucosal relief studies made in the prone position permit the diagnosis to be made (fig. 24).

Many more lesions which had been seen before only exceptionally, became daily findings once the standard biphasic-contrast examination was introduced. For example, areae gastricae were identified in the antrum in most of the patients. They were also identified in the corpus and gastric fundus in many patients. As stated before, varioliform erosions became a common radiological diagnosis. Since a varioliform erosion is an elevated lesion only a few millimetres in diameter and with a tiny central excavation, the author believes it is a good model for testing the efficacy of the examination. Although varioliform lesions had been radiologically demonstrated as early as 1933 (109), and Frik and Hesse (75) found them in 2 per cent of patients, experienced radiologists have confirmed that they are encountered only exceptionally in personal practice.

Routine DC studies greatly improve the convincing en face demonstration of tiny niches in the upper part of the stomach where compression cannot be applied (fig. 25). Gastric ulcer scars, which appear as a convergence of folds – indicating that the patient had suffered from peptic ulcer disease – were frequently demonstrated. Polyps with a diameter no greater than 2 mm. and cases of polyposis of the stomach appeared to occur more frequently than is generally thought (see chapter 7, section 5.1.). They were most often found in elderly patients with an atrophic gastritis.

Continuous cooperation between the radiologist and the endoscopist soon taught that the radiological and endoscopic examinations are complementary (34). Although radiology can detect even the slightest differences in the level of the mucosa, it does not reveal changes in colour of the mucosa. Gastric xanthelasmata or lipid islands can only be diagnosed by means of endoscopy. The same holds true for small bleeding lesions, e.g. hemorrhagic gastritis. Endoscopy proved to be superior in demonstrating mucosal lesions of the stomach, often small, just below or at the site of the hiatus in cases of hiatal hernia.

Extensive scarring and deformity of the duodenal bulb often makes it impossible radiologically to demonstrate or exclude an active ulcer; this can readily be done by endoscopy (10, 250). On the other hand, radiology gives a better impression of the total degree of deformity of the duodenum (106, 261).

The difficulties of differentiating between an active duodenal ulcer and an ulcer scar are well-known to the radiologist. Improvements in technique resulting in the demonstration of minute gastric niches with converging folds have produced the same problem in gastric radiology. It is not possible by radiological means to distinguish between a very small active ulcer and an ulcer scar that presents itself as a tiny excavation (fig. 25). Only gastroscopy can demonstrate if there is intact mucosa on the floor of a small crater.

Endoscopy also provides the opportunity of biopsy for a histological diagnosis. There are situations in which radiology can suggest the diagnosis more easily, e.g. linitis plastica, in which the failure of segments of the stomach to distend can be more easily documented by the radiologist than the endoscopist. Submucosal neoplastic infiltration and the mucosa, which may be intact, renders gastric biopsy less reliable than in other types of malignancy. Not

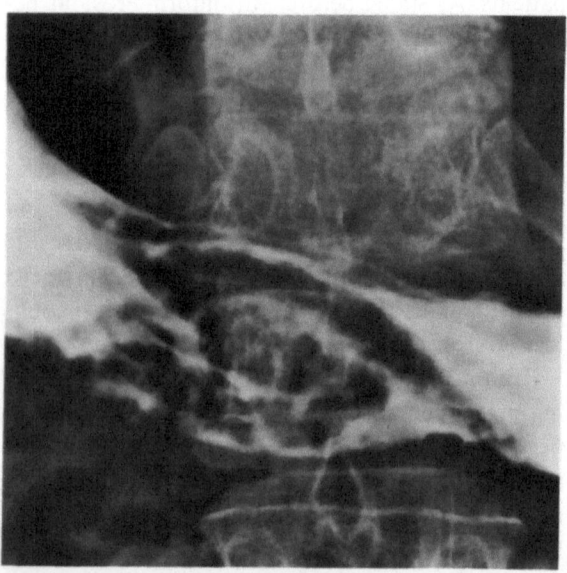

a

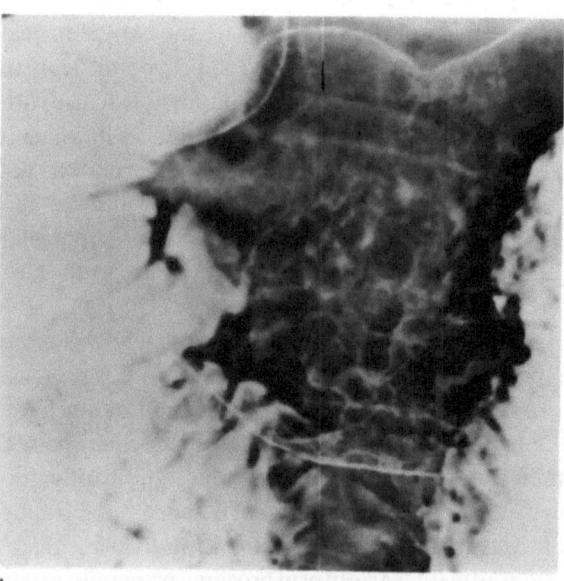

b

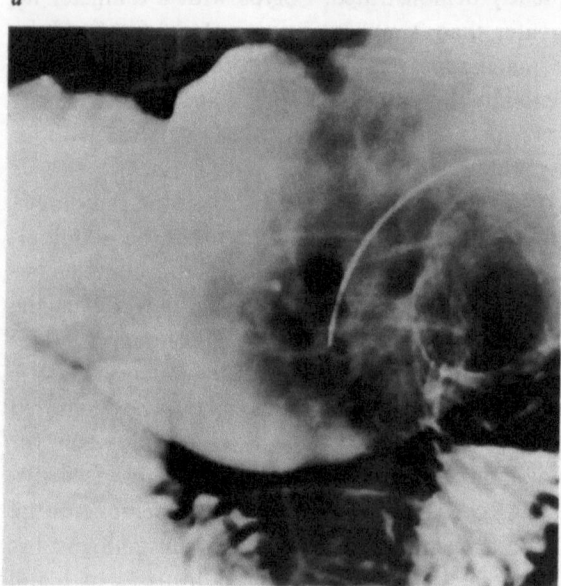

c

Fig. 24

a. PC mucosal relief study, prone position, after the patient swallowed 30 ml of the barium suspension. There is an irregular polypoid lesion of about 4 cm in diameter.

b. DC study, supine position. Owing to troublesome superimposition of the barium suspension in the duodenum this picture was obtained with great difficulty. It indicates that the lesion is situated on the posterior wall. When supplementary CO_2 was given, the lesion effaced nearly completely.

c. PC compression study, erect position. Several polypoid filling defects are visible.

This case illustrates the complementary rôle of the 3 projections. The PC mucosal relief study in this case provided the best impression of the true dimensions of the lesion. Endoscopy demonstrated only one polypoid lesion with a diameter of 5 mm and, in addition, an erosive lesion with a diameter of 8 mm. Biopsy revealed adenocarcinoma. In the resected specimen a polypoid adenocarcinoma restricted to the mucosa (EGC) and measuring $3\frac{1}{2} \times 4\frac{1}{2} \times \frac{3}{4}$ cm was found. This case also indicates the complementary rôle of radiology and endoscopy.

infrequently it results in false-negative bioptic diagnosis.

In stenosing lesions, radiology can reveal the distal boundary of the lesion (fig. 26), e.g. stenosing malignancies of the cardia and antrum, and pyloric stenosis due to peptic ulceration. The areae gastricae in most instances can be visualized radiologically in an easy way – in contrast to routine endoscopy (34, 157). Lesions that are easily effaced by inflation of the stomach, can be visualized better by radiological examination than by endoscopy (see fig. 24).

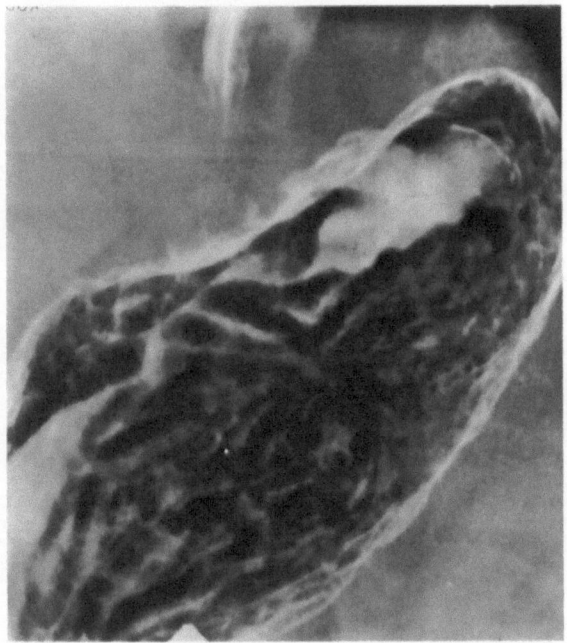

Fig. 25
DC study, supine position, RPO; table 30° anti-Trendelenburg. A small niche with converging folds caused by an ulcer scar is present in the posterior wall, confirmed by endoscopy. (Reproduced by permission of Radiology.)

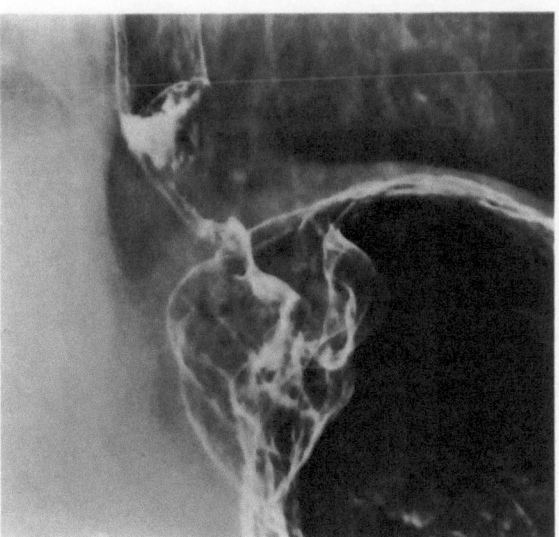

Fig. 26
DC study, erect position. Irregular stenotic lesion of the cardia. Radiology showed the proximal and distal boundaries. The gastroscope did not pass the stricture but biopsy confirmed the radiological diagnosis of adenocarcinoma. The complementary rôle of radiology and endoscopy is illustrated by this case.

Chapter 6

QUANTITATIVE RESULTS IN THE DIAGNOSIS OF MALIGANT LESIONS OF THE STOMACH

6.1. Introduction

The aim of this investigation is to verify the reliability of the standard biphasic-contrast gastric examination as the screening method for the detection of potentially malignant lesions, to determine which patients should be subjected to gastroscopy and biopsy.

This investigation has been restricted to malignant lesions since a more or less objective standard can be applied to this group of lesions, within the meaning of a histological diagnosis. Because of the natural history of malignant lesions, a follow-up study is possible; a long interval between the initial examinations, which may occasionally elapse, does not materially affect the result.

Moreover, it was interesting to investigate if Early Gastric Cancer was present among our group of malignant lesions, particularly because this finding has frequently been reported in the Japanese literature but rarely in the writings of Western authors (33, 63, 65, 72, 89, 98, 111, 156, 166, 167, 183, 217, 229, 237, 240, 241, 248, 258). The designation Early Gastric Cancer refers to a gastric carcinoma that does not extend deeper than the submucosa. The 5-year survival rate is higher than 90 per cent (see chapter 7, section 6.). For a diagnostician to overlook this type of lesion is a tragedy – particularly in view of the 5-year survival rate of only 10 per cent of patients with gastric carcinoma reported in the literature (32).

Since carcinoma of the stomach may present as a wide variety of lesions, ranging from minute alterations in mucosal relief, through ulcers, to large masses, this investigation also tests the sensitivity of the standard biphasic-contrast examination method in demonstrating non-neoplastic lesions of the stomach.

6.2. Methods and materials

Between 1 September 1973 and 1 September 1976, 4,054 standard biphasic-contrast gastric examinations were performed in 3560 patients aged 30 years and over. No gastroenterostomy or partial gastrectomy was performed on any of these patients.

Gastroscopies were carried out in 776 patients of this group one or more times, during the period 1 September 1973 and 1 January 1977. Multiple biopsies were usually taken, followed by histological examination. The indications for the gastroscopies differed: only in the event of acute hemorrhages was a gastroscopy carried out without preliminary radiological examination. In most cases it was dictated by the report of the preceding radiological examination, and it was also regularly carried out in patients with persistent complaints that could not be explained sufficiently by the initial radiological examination.

The 776 patients who had undergone one or more gastroscopies were divided into two groups:
I 733 patients who had been examined radiologically prior to gastroscopy (Table 2), and
II 43 patients in whom gastroscopy preceded radiological examination (Table 3).
Of both groups, the results of the radiological reports, gastroscopies and histological diagnoses were encoded on cards. If more than one radiological and/or endoscopic examination had been performed, the examinations closest together in time were used. If a malignant lesion was finally diagnosed histologically, the data of the initial examinations were also evaluated.

The radiological findings were placed in 11 categories, varying from appearances very suspicious of a malignant lesion (number 1) to normal appearances (number 11). Then these groups were pricked off the card index system, ranking in the

Table 2.
Group I, i.e. radiological examination preceding gastroscopy – 733 patients

radiological diagnosis		histological diagnosis		
categories	patients	malignant non-Hodgkin lymphoma	adeno-carcinoma	of which = EGC
1. definitely malignant lesion, suspicion of malignant lesion, one or more polyps ($\varnothing > 2$ cm), gastric retention suggesting a malignant cause	88	1	42*	6
2. one or more ulcers suggesting malignancy	19	1	6	4
3. one or more ulcers or ulcer scars	129	0	3	1
4. indefinite lesion, gastroscopy desirable	89	0	3	0
5. gastric retention, benign cause	5	0	0	0
6. "réaction antral" without demonstrable ulcer	18	0	0	0
7. one or more polypoid lesions ($\varnothing < 2$ cm), one or more varioliform erosions	68	0	0	0
8. atrophy of the mucosa	24	0	0	0
9. miscellaneous: submucosal lesions, indentations, varices, heterotopic pancreatic tissue, diverticulum	15	0	0	0
10. normal, but slightly coarse gastric folds	32	0	0	0
11. normal	246	2	0	0
total	733	4	54	11

* In one the histological report of the biopsies was most suspicious of adenocarcinoma. Furthermore there was overwhelming radiological, endoscopic and clinical evidence of a malignant lesion. No operation; no autopsy.

order from 1-11, and from every group the number and nature of the eventual malignant lesions determined histologically were recorded.

As a subsequent exercise, data from 3 sources was correlated and examined to determine whether any malignant lesions had appeared up to 1 March 1978 in the original patients. This data (group III) was provided by the Medical Records Department, by the Department of Medicine in which the gastroscopies were carried out, and by the Department of Radiology in which the barium studies were made.

Finally, the records of the Regional Pathological Laboratory were checked. The list of malignant le-

sions of the stomach diagnosed between 1 September 1973 and 1 March 1978 was reviewed (group IV) to find any such lesions that had been missed in patients who had undergone a standard radiological examination during the first 3 years of this period. In this way, an attempt was made to trace patients who had initially been examined in the author's Department but in whom a malignant lesion of the stomach had subsequently been diagnosed in another regional hospital.

All 54 cases of adenocarcinoma of group I were found in categories 1-4, i.e. those in which the definite suspicion of a malignant lesion was present.

Table 3.
Group II, i.e. radiological examination following gastroscopy – 43 patients

radiological diagnosis		histological diagnosis		
categories	patients	malignant non-Hodgkin lymphoma	adeno-carcinoma	of which = EGC
1. definitely malignant lesion, suspicion of malignant lesion, one or more polyps ($\varnothing > 2$ cm), gastric retention suggesting a malignant cause	1	1	0	0
2. one or more ulcers suggesting malignancy	1	0	1	1
3. one or more ulcers or ulcer scars	7	0	2	0
4. indefinite lesion, gastroscopy desirable	1	0	0	0
5. gastric retention, benign cause	0	0	0	0
6. "réaction antral" without demonstrable ulcer	1	0	0	0
7. one or more polypoid lesions ($\varnothing < 2$ cm), one or more varioliform erosions	1	0	0	0
8. atrophy of the mucosa	3	0	0	0
9. miscellaneous: submucosal lesions, indentations, varices, heterotopic pancreatic tissue, diverticulum	2	0	0	0
10. normal, but slightly coarse gastric folds	4	0	0	0
11. normal	22	0	0	0
total	43	1	3	1

Eleven of these 54 belonged to the Early Gastric Cancer category, as ultimately confirmed by the resected specimen. When the file of radiological reports was examined to find instances in which the initial radiological report had not been encoded, it was found that all these lesions had been detected at first examination. In the higher categories, i.e. normal or practically normal, no carcinomas were found but there were 2 cases of malignant non-Hodgkin lymphoma. These two cases require further discussion.

Case 1: The radiological report was normal (see fig. 27a). Gastroscopy 5 weeks later revealed inflammatory changes in the corpus of the stomach and an ill-defined, 3 × 5 cm area on the posterior wall, which had a cobble-stone appearance and a few irregular ulcers. Biopsy showed a malignant non-Hodgkin lymphoma. Repeated radiological examination 12 days after the gastroscopy revealed coarse areae gastricae in the suspected region (fig. 27b).

This is an instance of incorrect radiological diagnosis. It must be pointed out however, that this case dates from the initial few months after the standard biphasic examination was introduced, when sufficient experience had not yet been gained and the pictures obtained were inferior compared with those made later on.

Case 2: The radiologist reported no gross pathology; there was a slightly funnel-shaped antrum (fig. 28a).

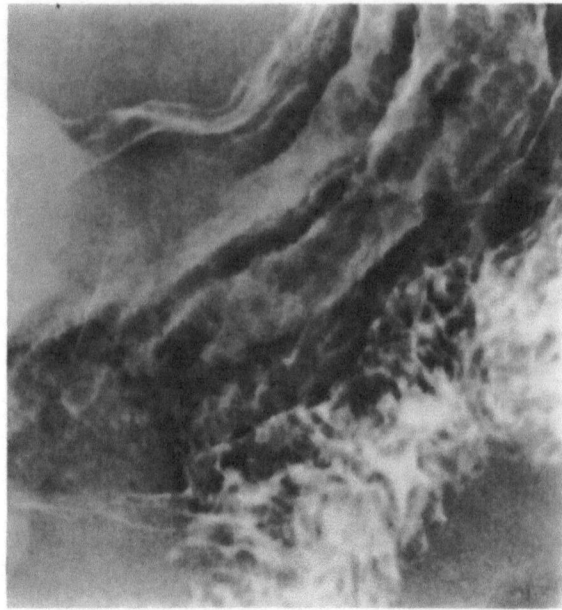

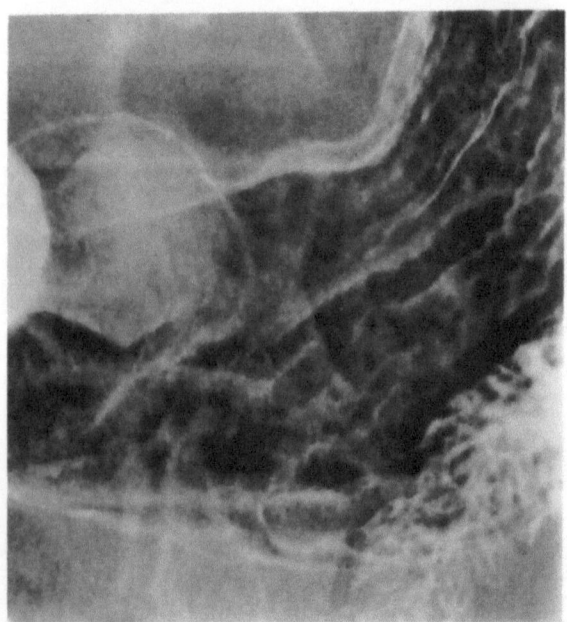

Fig. 27

a. DC study, supine position. This examination was reported as normal.

b. DC study, supine position, about 6 weeks later, following biopsy, which had revealed a malignant non-Hodgkin lymphoma. The radiological report on this examination referred to coarse areae gastricae in the area from which the biopsies were taken.

These studies date from the initial months of the investigation. Retrospectively, an abnormal nodular appearance of the folds can be noticed on both pictures. Also, there are fine nodules between the folds which do not represent areae gastricae.

Gastroscopy, carried out more than three months after the radiological examination, revealed a lesion suggestive of an adenocarcinoma of the antrum. Repeated radiological examination six days after gastroscopy confirmed the presence of a tumor of the antrum (fig. 28b). Biopsy: malignant non-Hodgkin lymphoma.

It is doubtful whether this case – also dating from the initial months of the examination period – was really false-negative. The lesion certainly was rapidly progressive.

In group II the malignant lesions were in categories 1, 2 and 3. Since all the lesions were very obvious, they would not have been missed, even without foreknowledge of the results of gastroscopy. This applied particularly to the only case of Early Gastric Cancer (fig. 85).

Group III covers the investigation made on the basis of data from the Medical Records Department, the Department of Medicine and the Department of Radiology between 1 September 1973 and 1 March 1978.

This investigation produced two cases in which there was overwhelming evidence but not a histological diagnosis of a malignant lesion of the stomach. This evidence was largely radiological. In another patient, autopsy revealed a tiny gastric carcinoma; 12 days previously, a radiological diagnosis of an ulcerating gastric tumor had been made. In yet another case, a carcinoma of the stomach was found at operation. Sixteen days previously, an incomplete radiological examination had shown gastric retention, but a benign rather than a malignant lesion had been considered to be its cause. No gastroscopy was performed.

One true mistake came to light. More than 18 months after a radiological examination of the stomach in a patient, repeated examination showed a large, apparently malignant tumor of the antrum, which biopsy confirmed to be an antral carcinoma. Upon review of the initial study, it was clear that the films had been misinterpreted: a circumscriptive stenosis of the antrum was present which, if interpreted correctly at the time, would undoubtedly have led to gastroscopic examination (fig. 29).

The check of the records of the Regional Pathological Laboratory (group IV) revealed no additional malignancies.

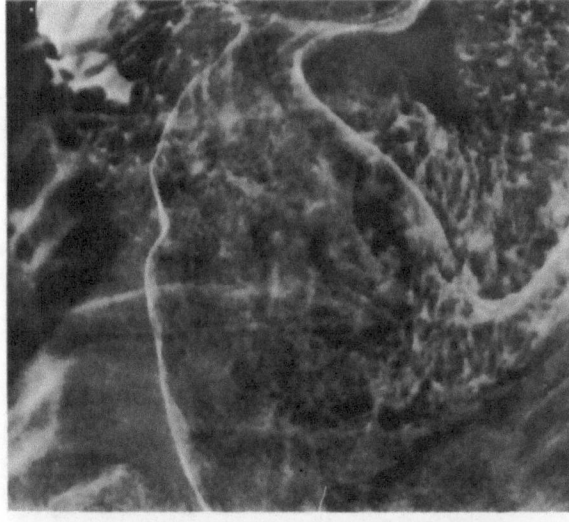

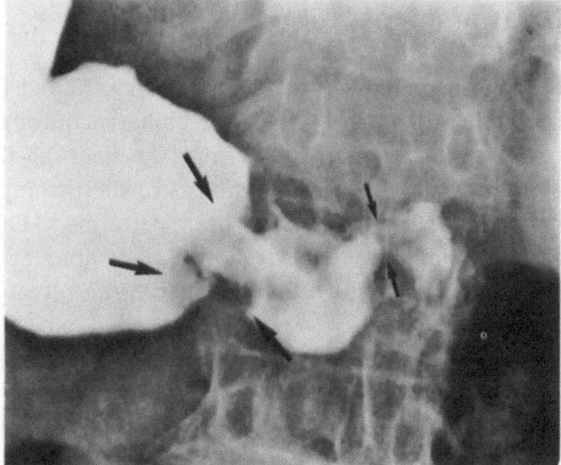

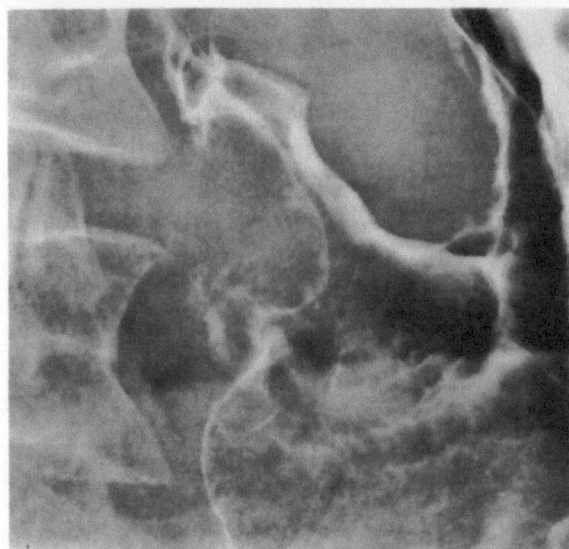

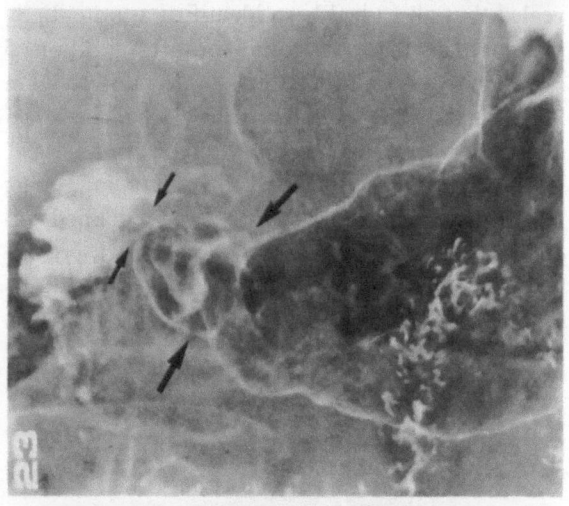

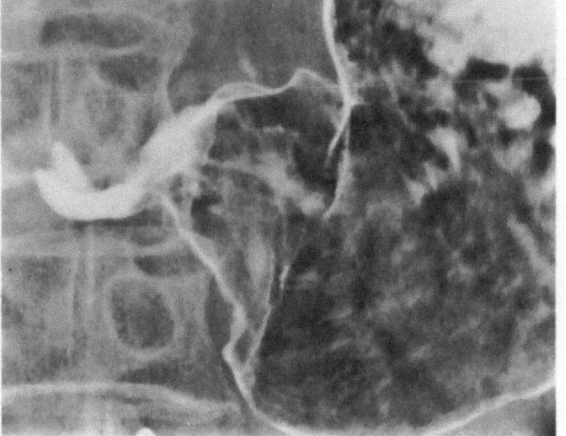

Fig. 28

a. DC study, supine position, LPO. No gross pathology was found, but a somewhat funnel-shaped antrum (as had been observed on previous examinations).

b. Same patient examined by the same technique, more than 3 months later. Now there is a large stenosing tumor in the antrum. Biopsy revealed a malignant non-Hodgkin lymphoma.

Fig. 29 →

a. PC study, prone position. Circumscriptive stenosis (large arrows) about $2\frac{1}{2}$ cm proximal to the pylorus (small arrows).

b. Same patient, DC study, supine position, LPO. Note the stenosis (large arrows) and the pylorus (small arrows). In this patient, PC studies are more diagnostic than the DC studies. The nature of the stenosis was not interpreted correctly – a human error of film reading, resulting in a false-negative radiological report.

c. Same patient, examined by the same technique as b above, more than 18 months later. DC study, supine position, LPO. Huge malignant tumor of the antrum. Biopsy: adenocarcinoma.

6.3. Summary

During the period between 1 September 1973 and 1 September 1976, 4,054 standard biphasic-contrast gastric series were carried out in 3560 patients aged 30 years and over, on whom no gastroenterostomy or partial gastrectomy had been performed. Of these, 776 underwent one or more gastroscopies between 1 September 1973 and 1 January 1977, revealing 57 carcinomas.

From study of the resected specimen, 12 of these could be classified as Early Gastric Cancer, i.e. 21 per cent of the total number of cases of diagnosed adenocarcinomas.* The radiological reports revealed that all 12 had been identified as potentially malignant at the first examination. In addition, 5 histologically confirmed malignant non-Hodgkin lymphomas were found, of which 3 had been detected as potentially malignant lesions. In one case, the radiological report had been misleading, being false-negative. In another, the error remained uncorrected, because of the progressive nature of the lesion and the relatively long time lag between radiological and endoscopic examinations. As far as

the radiological examination is concerned, both these cases dated to the early months of the investigation, when experience of the standard-biphasic method was still limited.

In the course of the follow-up study (1 September 1973 to 1 March 1978), an adenocarcinoma which had initially been missed radiologically, was detected at a subsequent radiological examination. This was an instance of misinterpretation; retrospectively, the carcinoma could be clearly defined in the films of the first series.

6.4. Conclusion

The radiological standard biphasic-contrast gastric series is a reliable screening method for the detection of potentially malignant lesions of the stomach – not least in respect to the extremely important group of Early Gastric Cancer – to determine which patients should be subjected to gastroscopy and biopsy.

---

* This percentage is high in comparison with other results recently obtained in the Western World (including Australia). A review of this literature yields percentages varying from 6.3 to 20 (65, 72, 89, 111, 156, 217, 229, 248). It even equals a Japanese report of 24 per cent (135), although it should be stressed that this particular series consisted of patients admitted to a surgical department and it probably does not represent the total group of patients in whom a diagnosis of adenocarcinoma was made. Another Japanese series (43) claimed a percentage of 40.5, but these results were obtained at a mass survey.

Part III

RADIOLOGICAL ATLAS
OF COMMON LESIONS OF THE STOMACH AND DUODENUM

Chapter 7

STOMACH

7.1. Normal and abnormal mucosal relief

7.1.1. NORMAL MUCOSAL RELIEF

In the stomach two kinds of mucosal relief can be distinguished, viz. those formed by the gastric folds or rugae, and those formed by the areae gastricae.

The gastric folds in the fundus and corpus of the stomach are anatomically preformed, but distal to the angulus there is no such anatomical arrangement. The thickness of the normal fold is said to be 4-5 mm. (76, 203). The normal fold disappears on compression and distension of the stomach; the use of hypotonic techniques nearly always effaces the antral folds.

The surface of the gastric mucosa consists of ovoid and polygonal elevations, each a few millimetres in diameter and separated by grooves. These elevations, which are more or less uniform in size and shape, are normal anatomical structures – the so-called areae gastricae. The maximal diameter of "normal" areae gastricae is 6 mm., and they are usually much smaller (41, 76, 157, 210). Success in demonstrating these structures largely depends on the radiological technique. Hypotonia improves visualization of the areae gastricae considerably; furthermore it is easier to demonstrate them by means of DC than with PC compression studies (fig. 5). The degree of visualization varies greatly with different kinds of barium suspension (142, 144, 145). Vielvoye (unpublished data), using a fresh cadaver specimen, demonstrated that the areae relief, which was not visible 30 minutes after an autopsy, could be visualized by treating the mucosa with a mucolytic agent. In addition to the areae relief, rimpling is sometimes demonstrated in the gastric antrum, which is attributed to contractions of the muscularis mucosae (236) (figs. 31, 32).

7.1.2. ABNORMAL MUCOSAL RELIEF

Abnormally coarse folds: Opinions differ about when a fold must be regarded as abnormally coarse. Some authors believe that any fold thicker than 10 mm. is abnormal, others state 5-8 mm. (77, 203, 211, 267). Also, thick folds often have irregular margins and are therefore of uneven width. Abnormal folds cannot be easily flattened under external pressure and are not effaced when the stomach is distended.

The radiologist encountering this picture can generally provide no more than a differential diagnosis. For a histological diagnosis, gastroscopy and biopsy are required.

The causes of coarse folds are:

1. "Hypertrophic gastritis"
2. Menetrier's disease
3. Zollinger-Ellison's syndrome
4. in association with peptic ulceration or varioliform erosions
5. pseudolymphoma
6. malignant lymphoma
7. carcinoma
8. granulomatous disease (syphilis, sarcoidosis, Crohn's disease, tuberculosis)
9. impaired renal function
10. acromegaly
11. varices
12. gastrointestinal edema in hepatic cirrhosis

(8, 25, 36, 134, 271).

Abnormally thin folds: In cases of chronic atrophic gastritis the folds are sometimes thin, and they may be absent on the greater curvature of the stomach. Absence of rugae on the greater curvature combined with distal tubular deformity and a bald fundus strongly suggests chronic atrophic gastritis (79, 137). Personal experience in cases of chronic atrophic gastritis indicates that the pylorus often remains patent following the intravenous injection of glucagon 0.5 mg – in contrast to the normal pylorus, which closes for some minutes after such premedication.

Abnormal areae relief: Recent advances in the gastric radiological examinaion ensure the areae gastricae are visualized far more frequently. So far only a few criteria have been defined for regarding areae gastricae relief as normal or abnormal. Frik (77) stated that irregular and uneven polygonal areae in the prepyloric region with a diameter of 3-5 mm. indicate a diffuse gastritis, in most cases a diffuse atrophic gastritis. Mackintosh and Kreel

(157) found a high incidence of duodenal ulceratio in patients in whom areae gastricae with a diameter of 4 mm. were well seen in the gastric antrum ("good coaters") and – using the same technique – a low incidence in patients in whom the areae were not visualized ("non-coaters"). Koga et al. (140), in studying magnification radiographs of resected gastric specimens, found that destruction of the areae gastricae and the grooves between them predominated in a carcinomatous mucosa. A similar pattern was encountered in only a few cases of non-carcinomatous mucosa with marked atrophy. Much work remains to be done in this field.

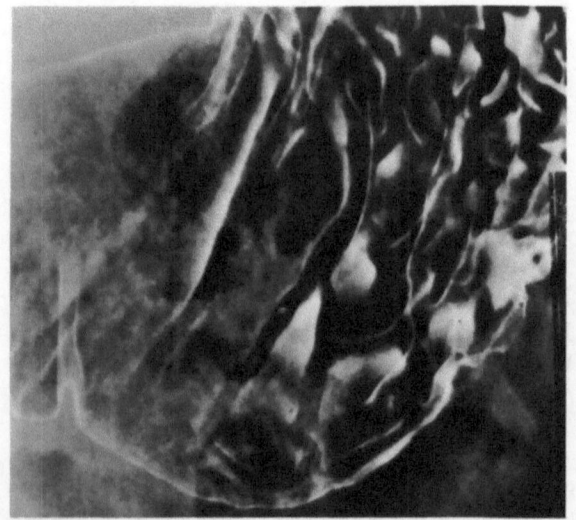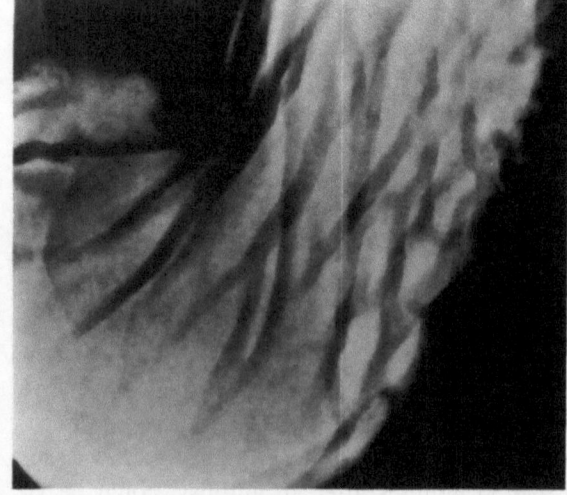

Fig. 30
a. DC study, supine position.
b. PC compression study, erect position. Normal gastric folds. The fold crossings in 30 b indicate that the folds in the anterior as well as the posterior wall are visualized. The endoscopist also regarded these folds as normal.

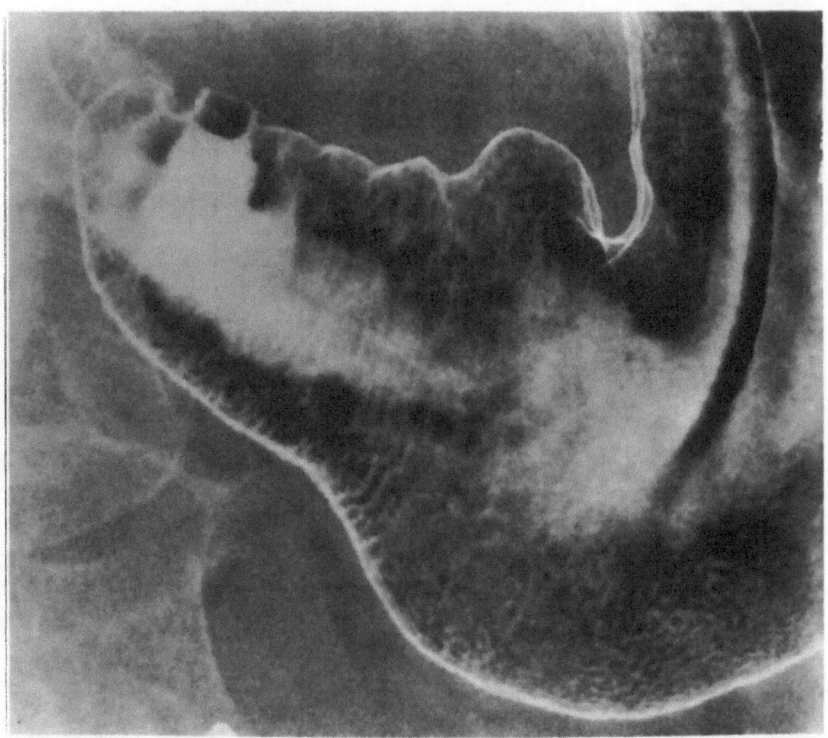

Fig. 31
DC study, supine position. Opposite the angulus a normal areae gastricae relief is visualized. In the pyloric region there is additional rimping probably caused by contraction of the muscularis mucosae.

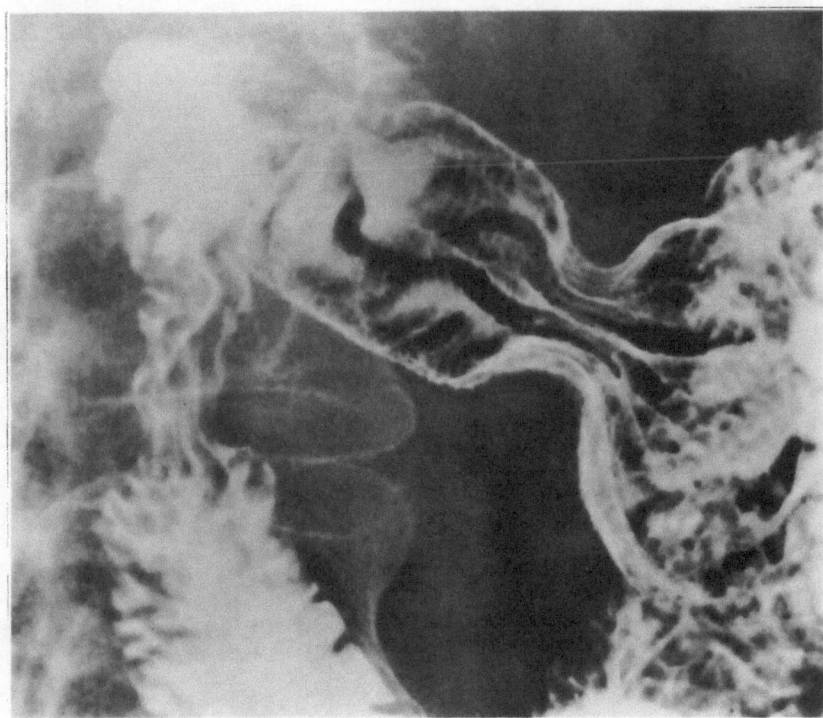

Fig. 32
Another example of rimpling in the pyloric region.

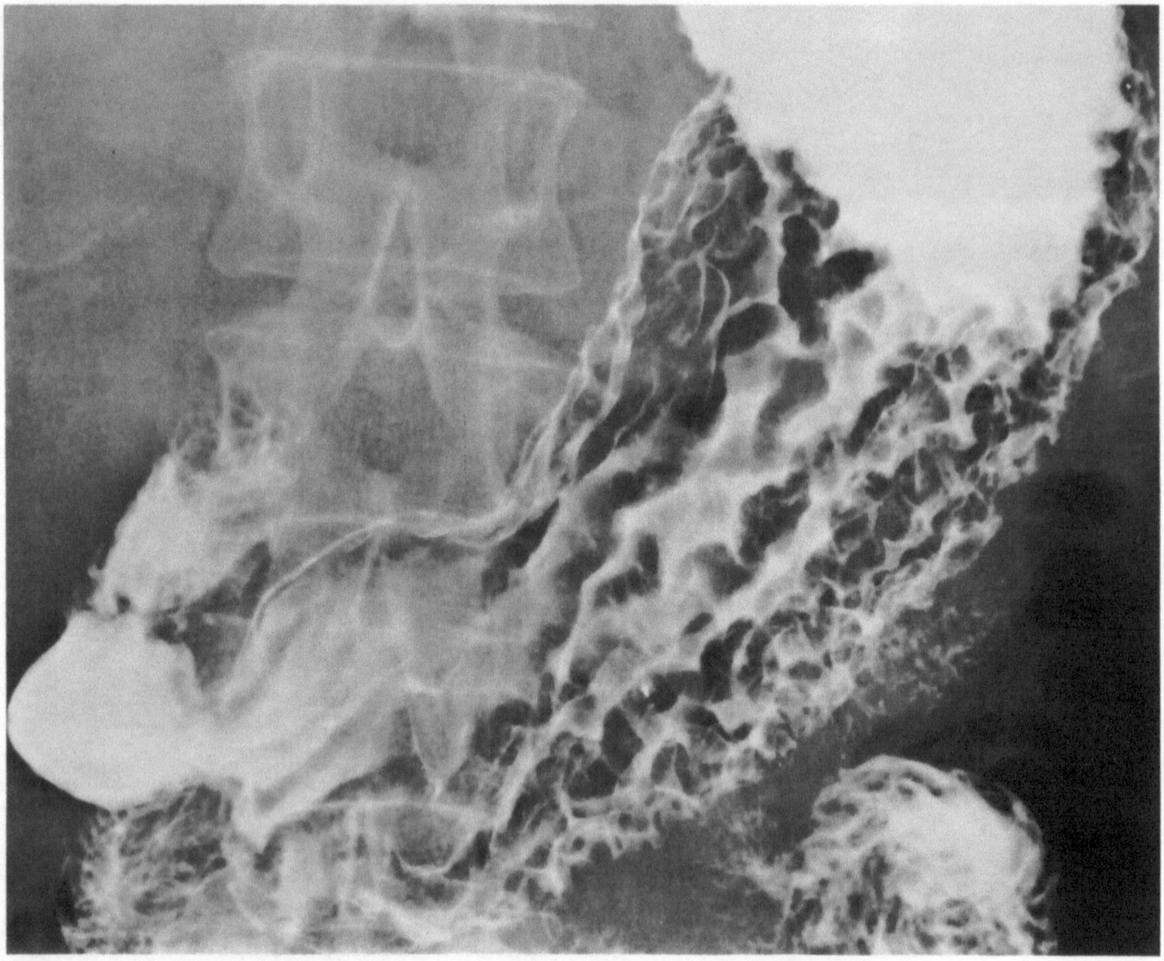

Fig. 33
DC study, supine position. The folds in the corpus are rather
coarse with unevenness in width. The endoscopist considered this
a case of hypertrophic gastritis. The biopsies were compatible
with gastritis.

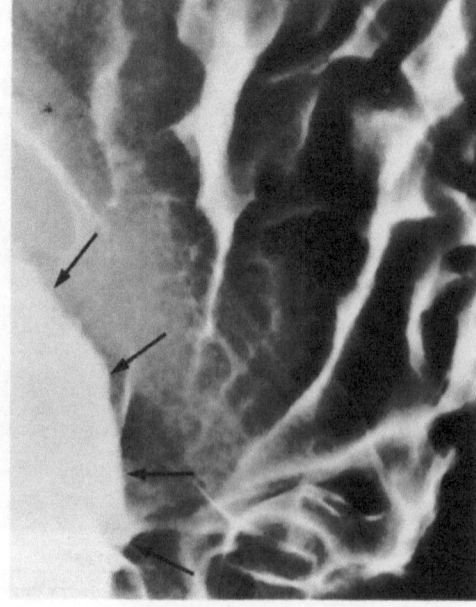

Fig. 35
DC study, supine position. Extremely coarse folds in association
with a peptic ulcer (arrows). Biopsies: no signs of malignancy.

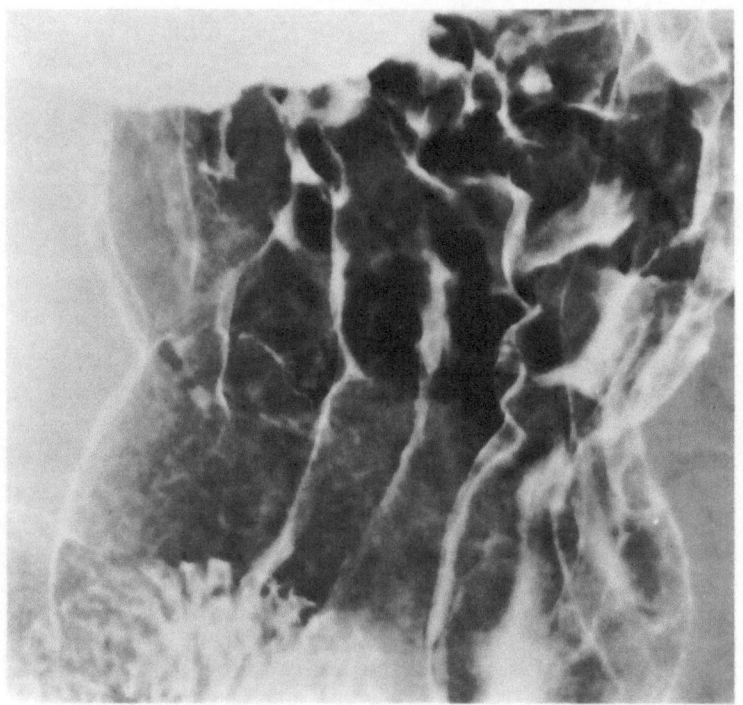

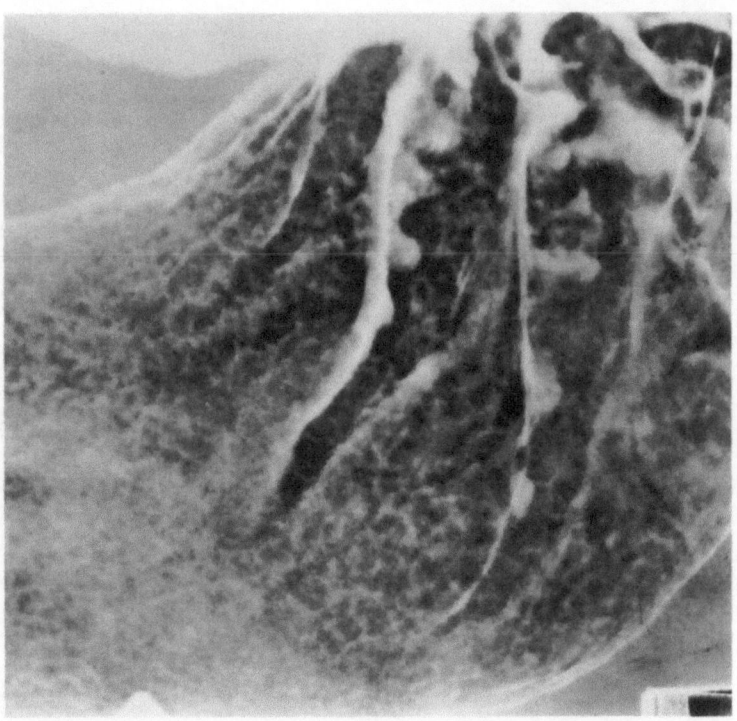

Fig. 34
a & b. DC studies, supine position. Very coarse folds in the corpus showing unevenness in width. Prominent areae gastricae relief in the region of the angulus.
Endoscopy: coarse edematous folds; Menetrier's disease was considered. The
biopsies, including a big particle biopsy, were practically normal. There was
neither important inflammation nor indications of Menetrier's disease.

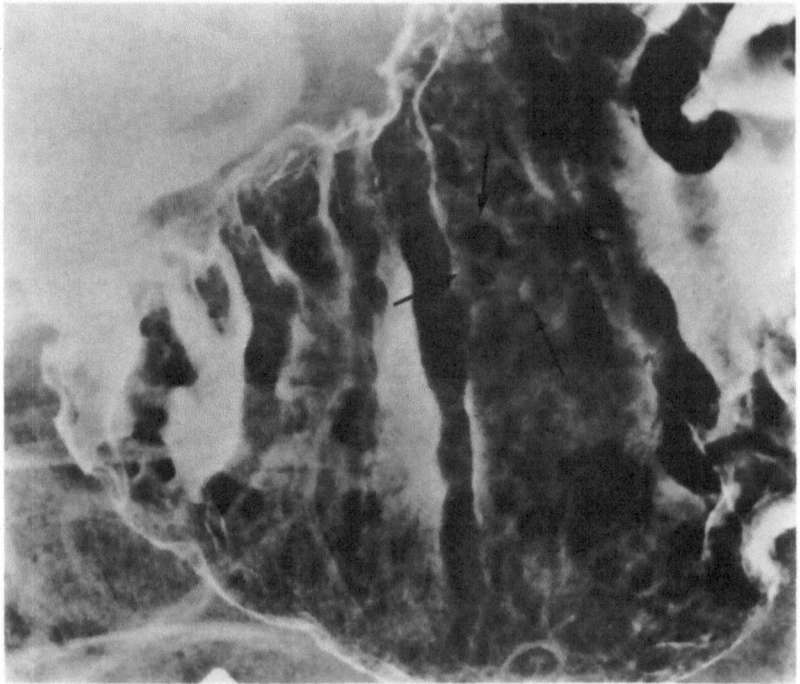

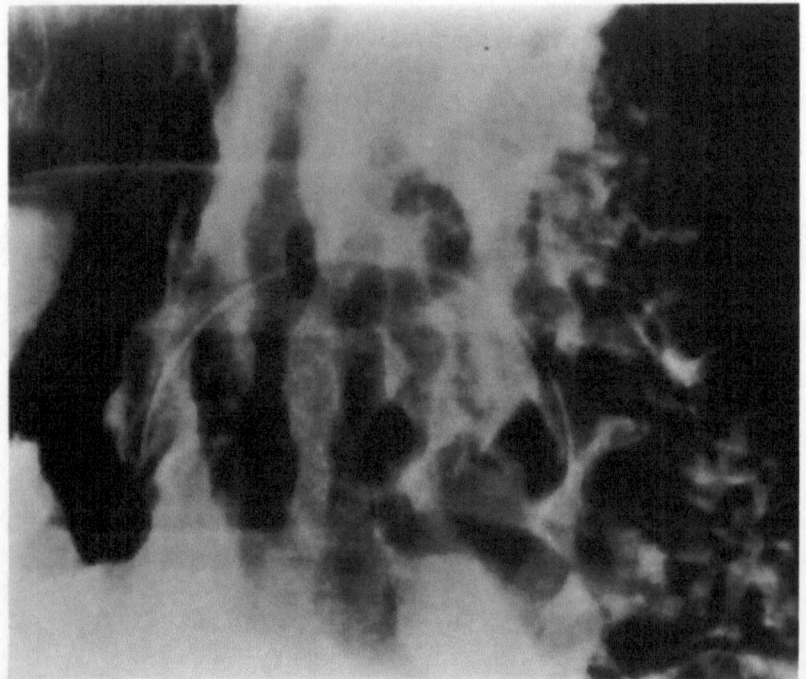

Fig. 36
a. DC study, supine position.
b. PC compression study, erect position. In the antrum coarse folds with local thickening.
   Thickened folds in the lower corpus. Several varioliform erosions are visualized (arrows).
   Endoscopy: erosive gastritis with thickened folds.
   Gastrobiopsy: gastritis and in the antrum intestinal metaplasia.

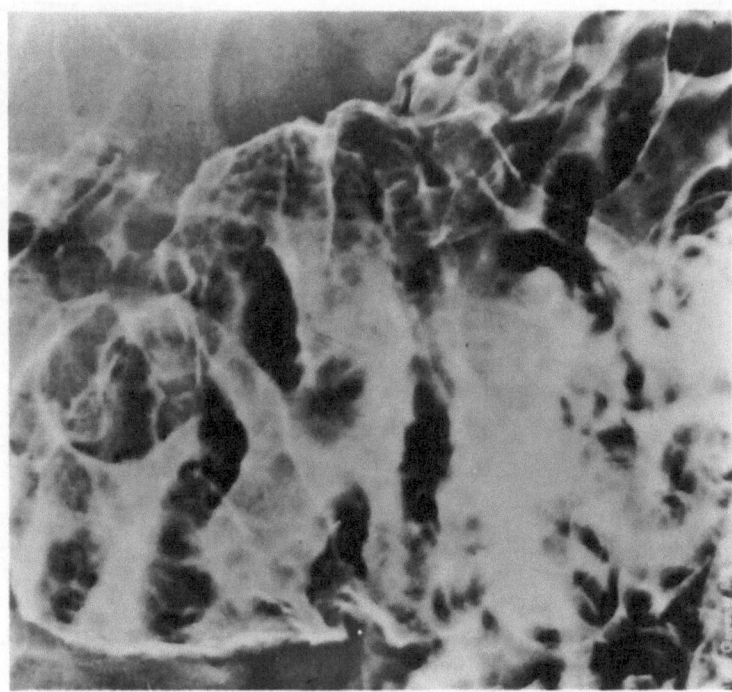

Fig. 37
DC study, supine position, LPO. Coarse folds with irregular margins in the antrum. The endoscopist considered "hypertrophic gastritis." Biopsies were compatible with a malignant lymphoma; those of the rectal mucosa were diagnostic of malignant lymphoma.

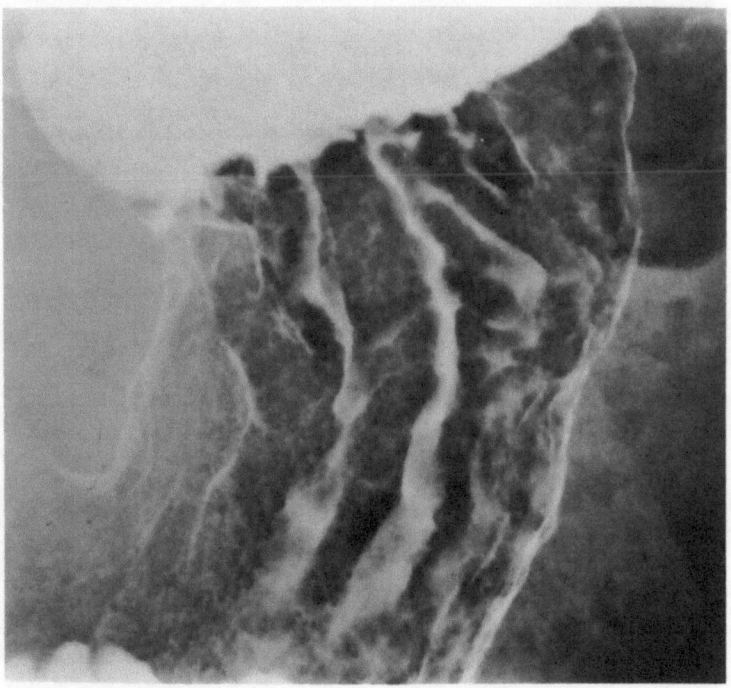

Fig. 38
DC study, supine position. Extremely coarse folds in the corpus in a patient with an adenocarcinoma (as proved by gastrobiopsy) extending from the lower esophagus to the lesser curvature of the antrum (same patient as shown in fig. 96).

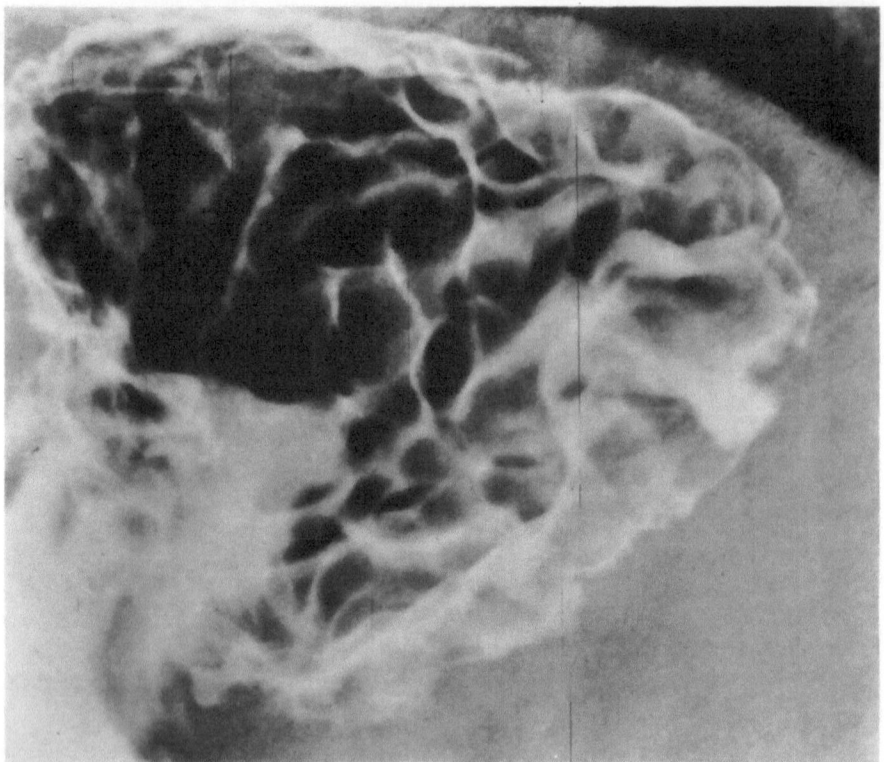

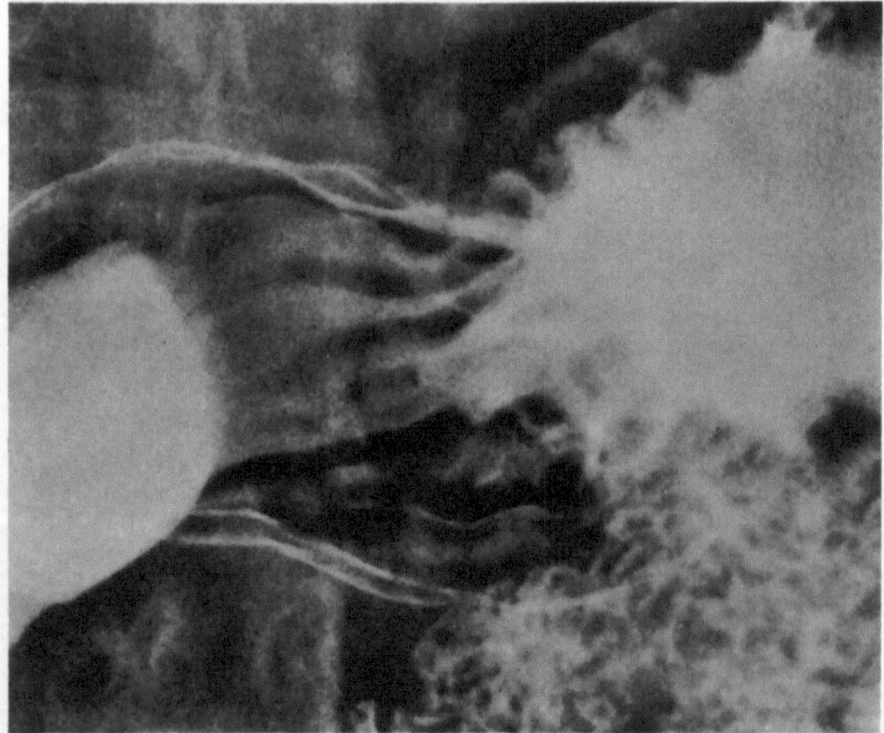

Fig. 39

a. DC study, supine position, RPO; table 30° anti-Trendelenburg. Prominent folds in the fundus.

b. DC study, supine position. Normal folds in the corpus. Endoscopy revealed varices in the gastric
   fundus but no esophageal varices. A further examination demonstrated an obstruction of the splenic
   vein.

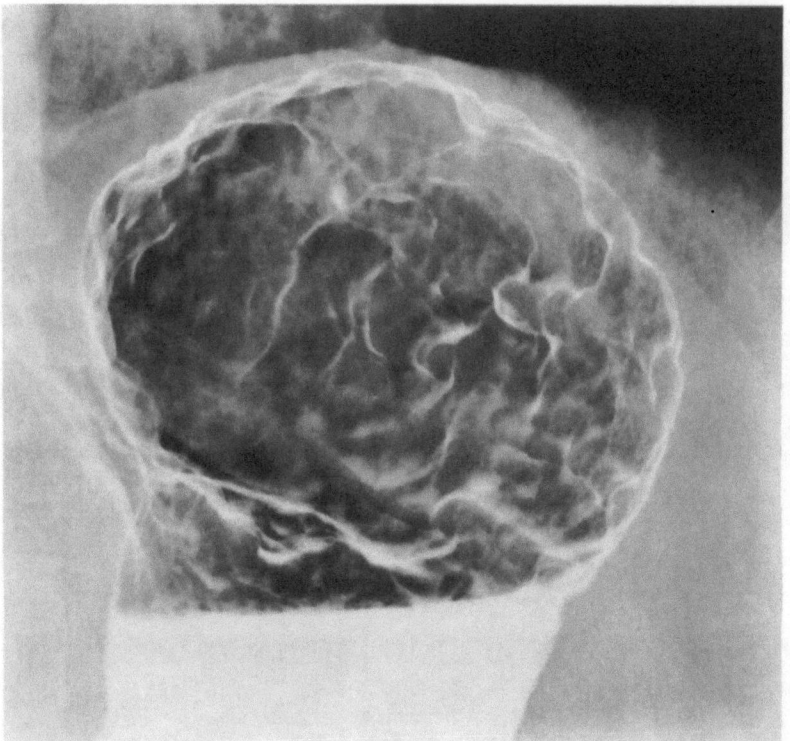

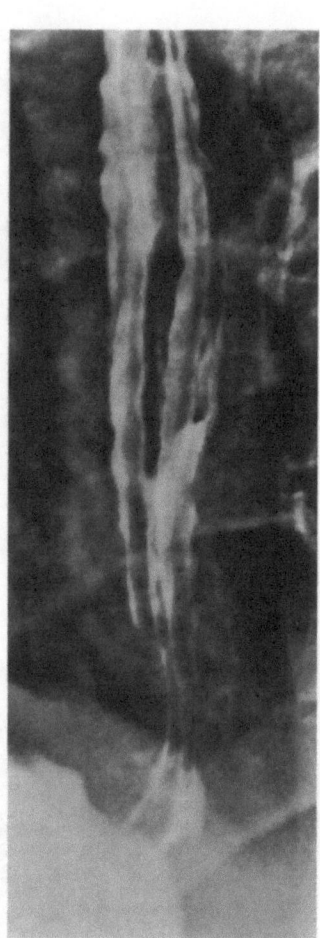

Fig. 40
a. DC study, erect position. Tortuous folds in the fundus.
b. Esophageal varices. The diagnosis of varices of the distal esophagus and the gastric fundus was endoscopically confirmed.

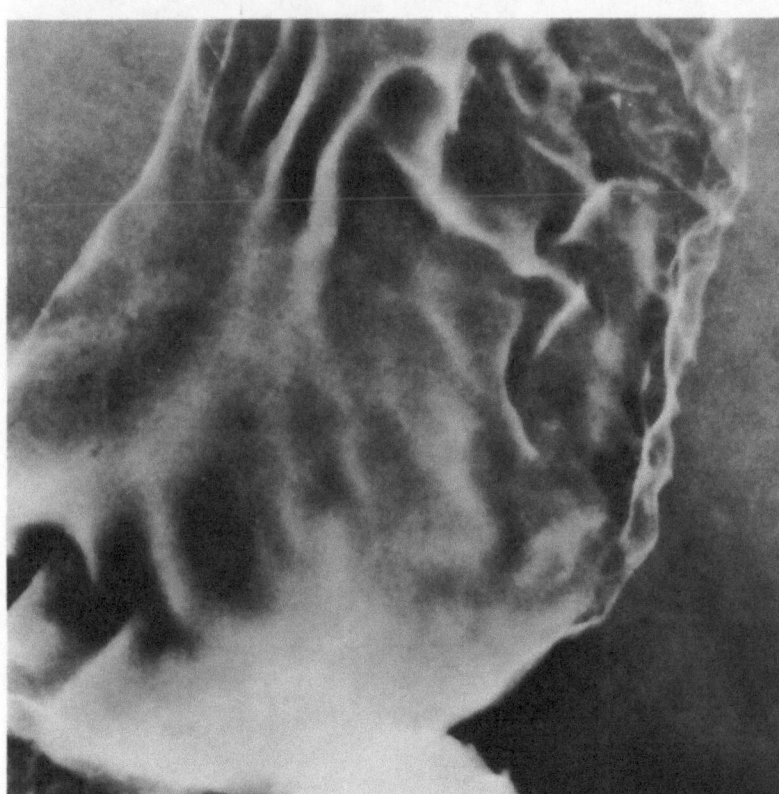

Fig. 41
DC study, supine position. Extremely swollen nearly effaced folds in a cirrhotic patient. Endoscopy demonstrated edema; the biopsies showed no signs of malignancy. Through several years, follow-up studies revealed a changing appearance of the folds which, however, remained thickened; furthermore varices of the fundus became obvious. The appearance of the folds was interpreted as being caused by gastric edema in hepatic cirrhosis.

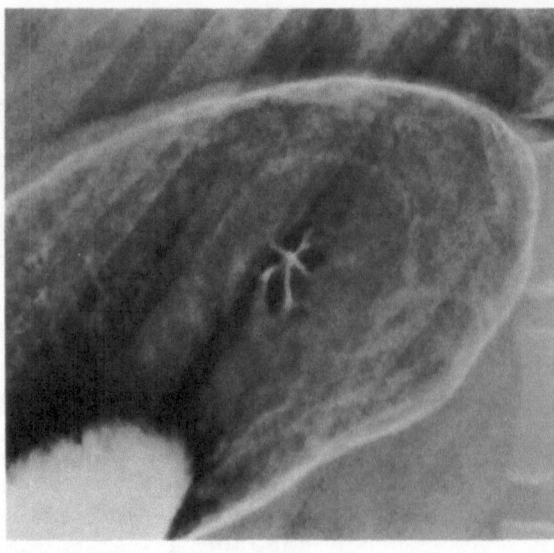

Fig. 42
DC study, supine position, RPO; table 40° anti-Trendelenburg.
Bald fundus, note the converging folds to the cardia in the centre
of the film. Endoscopy: diffuse atrophic gastritis. Biopsies:
chronic inflammation with atrophy.

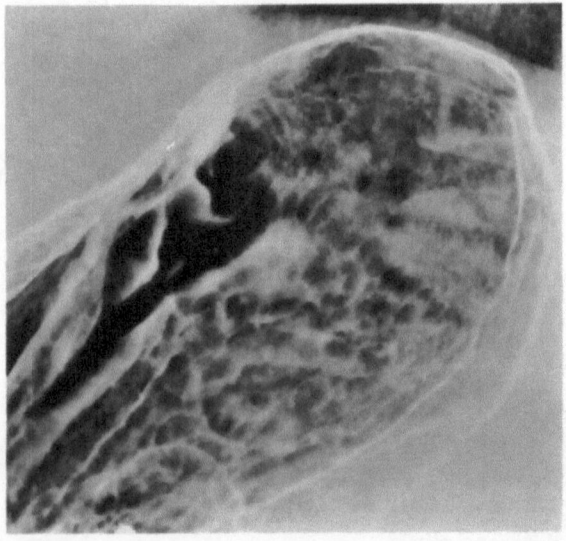
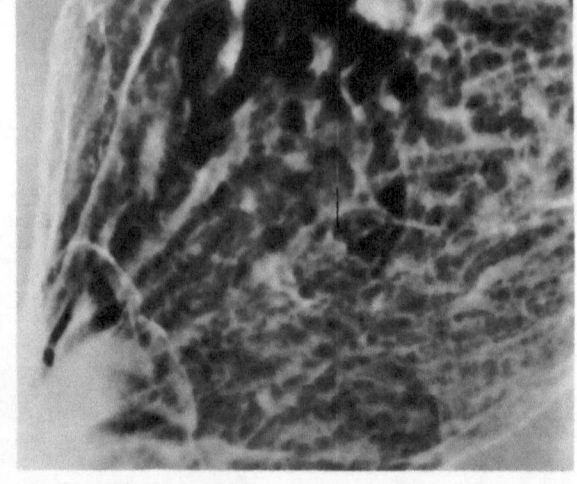

Fig. 43
a. DC study, supine position, RPO; table 40° anti-Trendelenburg.
b. DC study, supine position, partial RPO; table about 30° anti-
   Trendelenburg. Coarse irregular areae gastricae relief.
   Examination of the duodenál bulb revealed an ulcer. No
   endoscopy.

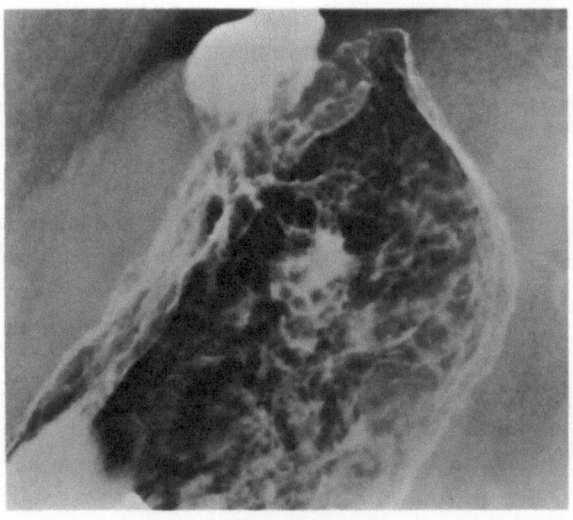

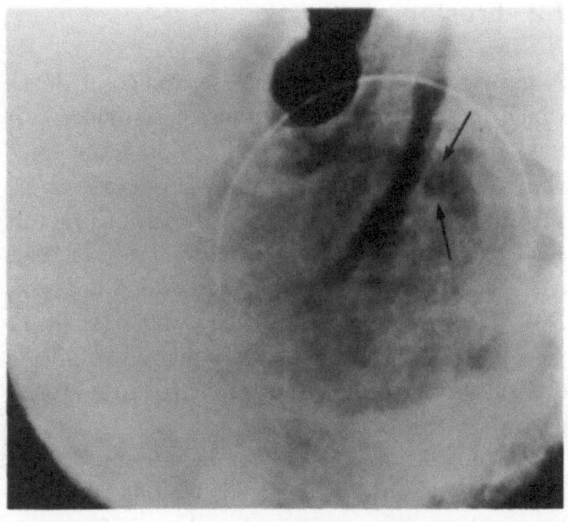

Fig. 44

a. DC study, supine position, RPO; table 30° anti-Trendelenburg. Very coarse irregular areae gastricae relief.

b. Compression study of the gastric angulus reveals at least one erosion (arrows). Autopsy demonstrated chronic gastritis with erosions.

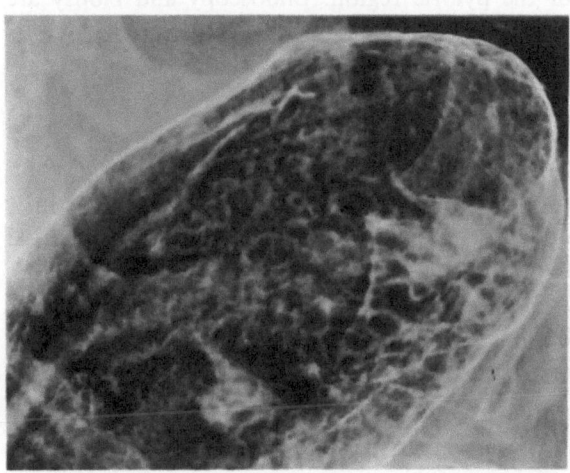

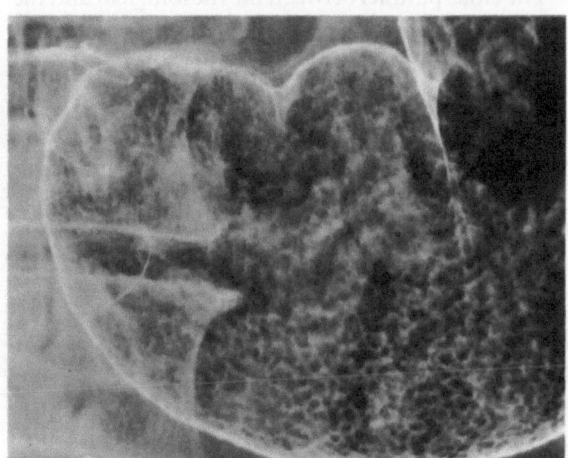

Fig. 45

a. DC study, supine position, RPO; table 40° anti-Trendelenburg.

b. DC study, supine position, LPO. Prominent areae gastricae relief in the fundus. The areae are coarse and irregular. Gastrobiopsy demonstrated a gastritis with local atrophy.

7.2. Erosions

A gastric erosion is defined as a mucosal defect which does not penetrate the muscularis mucosae. A flat erosion can be diagnosed radiologically only with great difficulty. However, many erosions are surrounded by walls produced by various factors such as contractions of the muscularis mucosae, edema, cellular infiltration or fibrosis (125, 255, 268, 269). If an erosion possesses such a wall, it is called a varioliform erosion. If there are many varioliform erosions, the condition is often referred to as erosive gastritis.

Varioliform erosions are common lesions. In the first three months of 1976, 500 biphasic gastric examinations were performed, and varioliform erosions were diagnosed in over 10 per cent and strongly suspected in a further 5 per cent. Previously a good correlation had been shown in this material between the endoscopic and the radiological diagnoses (194).

The close parallel between the radiological and the gastrophotographic findings was indicated as early as 1933 by Henning and Schatzki (109), but the definitive radiological publications are more recent (1, 75, 267). Numerous publications in the past 4 years have stressed the importance of the DC technique in the radiological visualization of varioliform erosions (87, 97, 143, 148, 149, 152, 202).

PC compression studies, also, are useful in the diagnosis of varioliform erosions (3, 20, 182, 194). They may even be mandatory, because elevated lesions with gently sloping edges situated on the anterior wall of the stomach may be missed without the use of compression (194) (fig. 53; see chapter 2).

Relation to duodenal and gastric ulceration: Varioliform erosions are often found in a stomach that is normal in other respects. They are usually confined to the antrum but may at times occur in the corpus. Antral varioliform erosions are frequently encountered with an ulcer of the duodenal bulb. Sometimes they accompany a gastric ulcer. It is still not clear whether a gastric erosion ever turns into a gastric ulcer (36, 125, 255).

Differential diagnosis: The diagnosis of multiple varioliform erosions usually presents no difficulties, although Crohn's disease is said to produce the same appearance (64, 149, 152, 216). A focal lesion with appearances of a solitary varioliform erosion may entail the following differential diagnosis: a sessile polyp with central ulceration, heterotopic pancreatic tissue, a neurogenic tumor, a metastasis or even a malignant erosion (131). It should be remembered that the site of predilection for heterotopic pancreatic tissue is the greater curvature of the antrum or the pyloric region. Endoscopy and biopsy are often advisable. Of course, the differential diagnosis between deep erosions and a shallow ulcer can only be completed by histological examination of a resected specimen.

Prognosis: Varioliform erosions may heal completely and disappear within a short time. Sometimes no improvement occurs. The lesion is also reported to recur through decades (269). Several authors (132, 268) maintain that varioliform erosions ultimately become polyps.

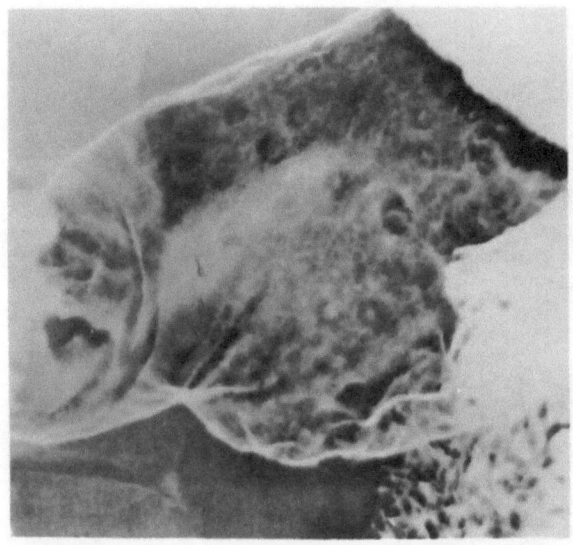
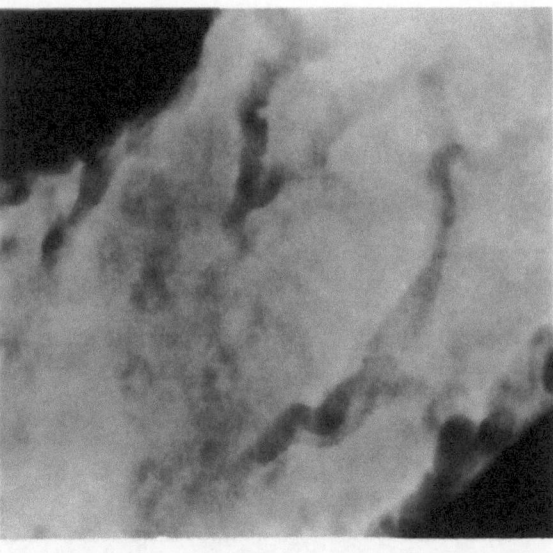

Fig. 46
a. DC study, supine position. Multiple varioliform erosions.

b. PC compression study, erect position. Thanks to the use of high kV and a medium-high density barium suspension, the erosions are well shown in this study.

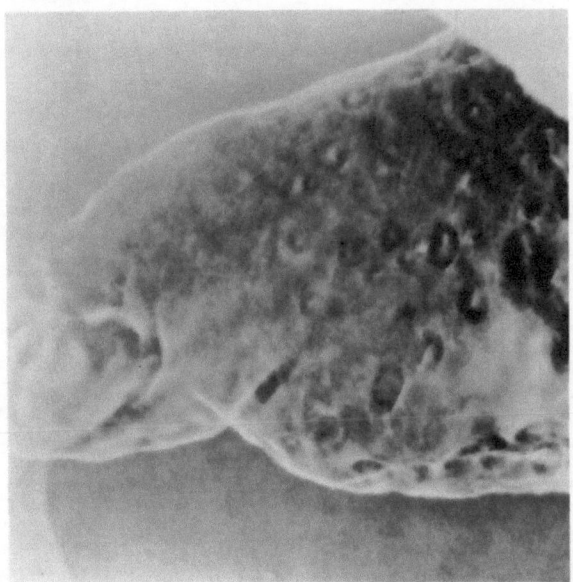

Fig. 47
DC study, supine position. Same patient 1 year after the examination as shown in fig. 46.

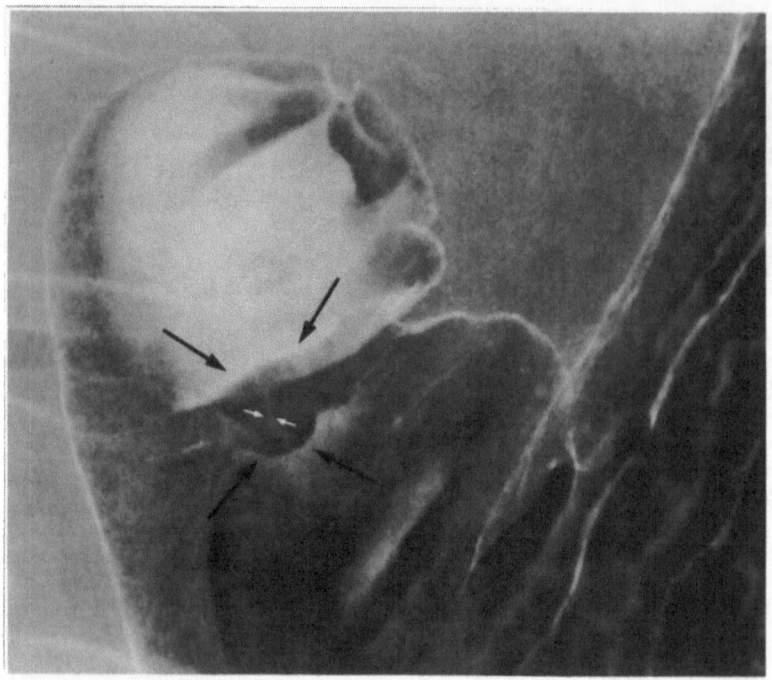

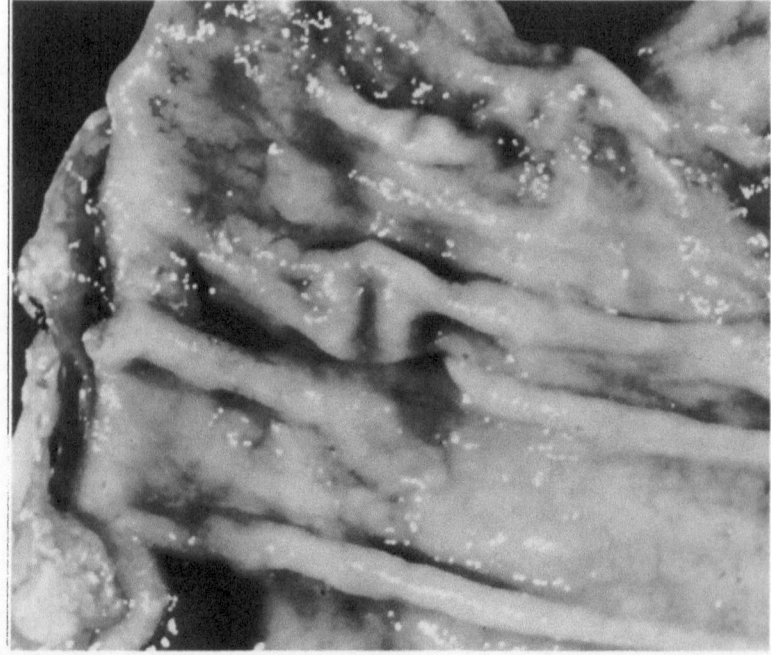

Fig. 48

a. DC study, supine position, LPO. Linear erosion (white arrows) on a thickened fold
(black arrows) of the posterior wall of the antrum.

b. Resected specimen. The patient was operated upon because biopsies suggested a malignant lesion. More distal to the linear erosion there is a smaller erosion on a thickened
fold, which can be identified retrospectively in fig. 48a. Histological examination revealed that the mucosa at the side of the linear erosion was interrupted as far as the
muscularis mucosae, which was still identifiable as such. Fibrosis and an inflammatory
infiltration were present, which extended nearly to the muscularis propria. No malignant lesion.

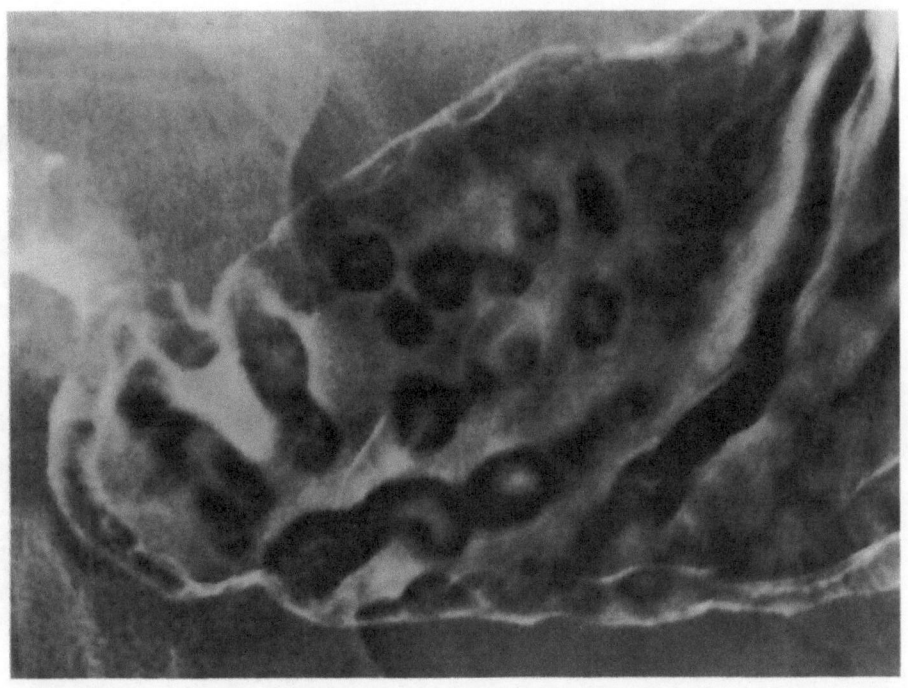

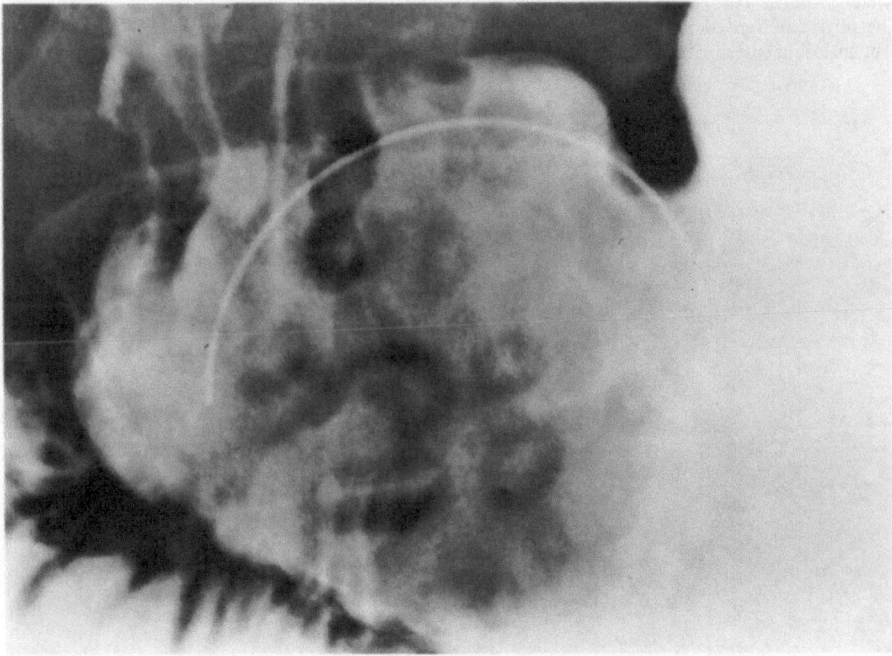

Fig. 49
a. DC study, supine position, partial LPO. Multiple varioliform erosions.
b. PC compression study, erect position. Thanks to the use of a barium suspension of medium-high
  density and high kV, the erosions can be well identified. The patient suffered from Crohn's disease of
  the small bowel. However, biopsy failed to reveal Crohn's disease of the stomach.

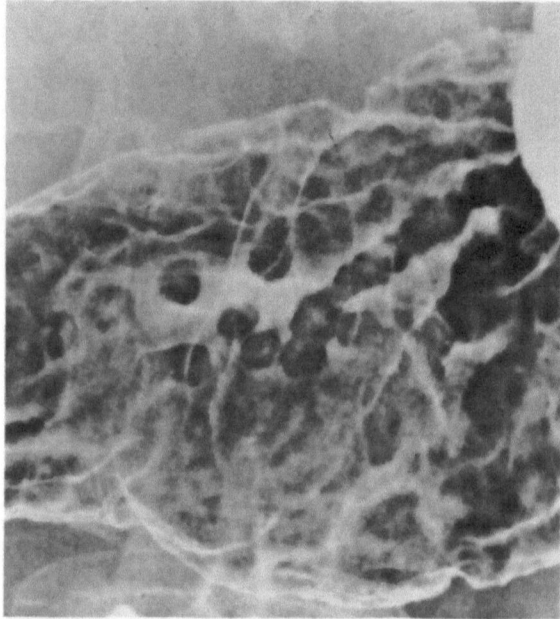

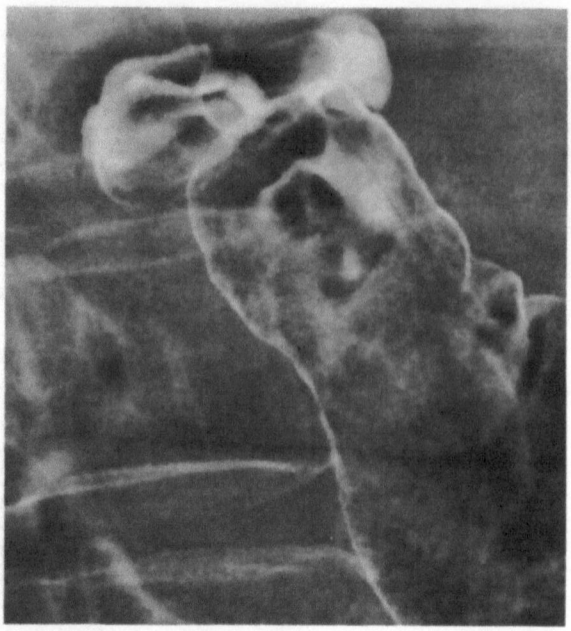

Fig. 50
DC study, supine position. Multiple varioliform erosions in a patient with a protein-losing gastroenteropathy. Gastroscopy confirmed the erosions. The erosions were coated with a thin fibrinous exudate. Histological examination: chronic inflammation. The physician viewed the gastric erosions as the cause of the protein-losing enteropathy (73).

Fig. 51
DC study, supine position, LPO. Two typical varioliform erosions are visible on the posterior wall of the prepyloric region. There is an ulcer niche in the base of the apical cap.

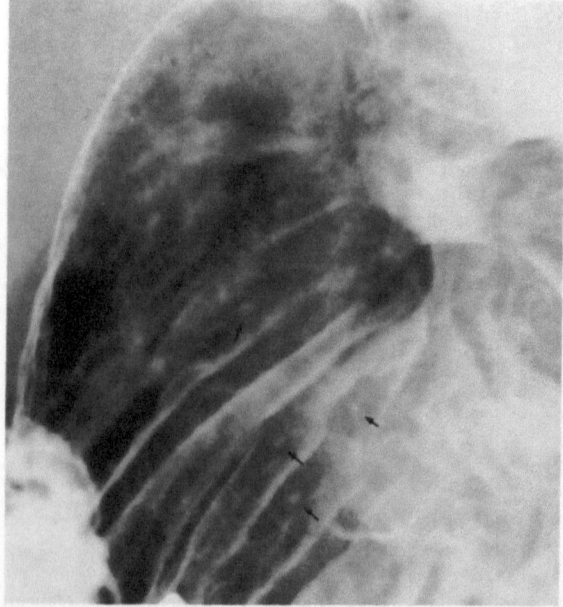

Fig. 52
DC study, supine position, RPO; table 20° anti-Trendelenburg. There is an ulcer niche on the posterior wall of the corpus of the stomach. Erosions (arrows) are present on converging folds distal to the ulcer. Endoscopic confirmation. (Reproduced by permission of Radiologia Clinica.)

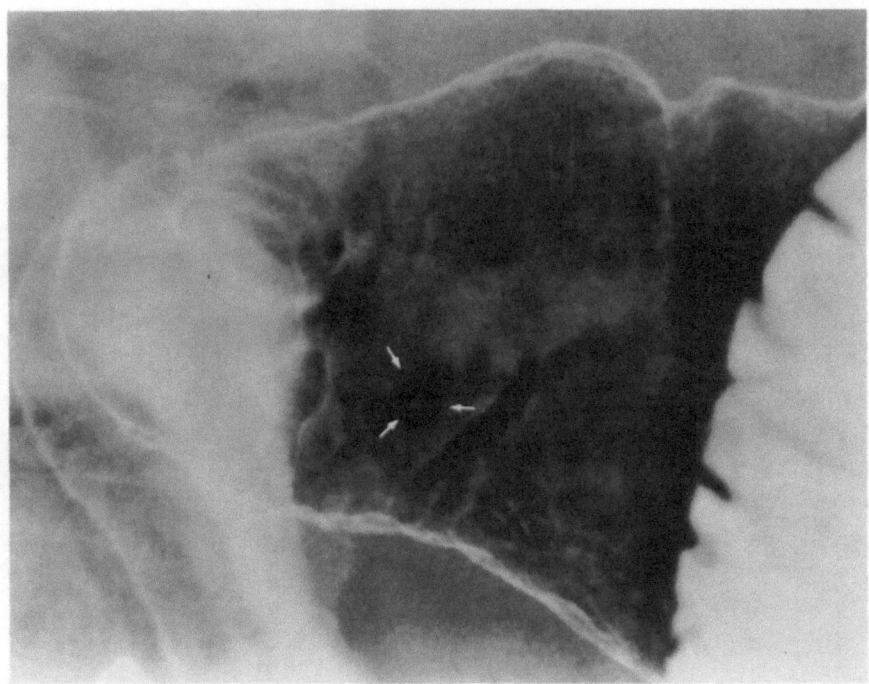

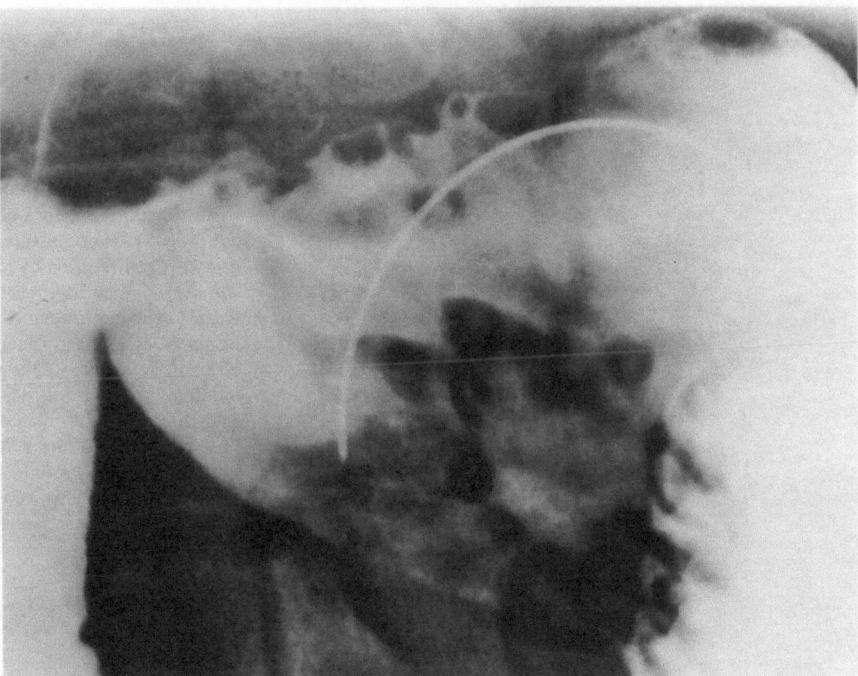

Fig. 53

a. DC study, supine position, LPO. There is a solitary varioliform erosion (arrows) on the posterior wall of the gastric antrum.

b. PC compression study, erect position, LPO. Multiple varioliform erosions are present. If these lesions are not visualized on the DC study, they are in all probability localized on the anterior wall of the antrum. PC compression studies are superior to DC studies in the case of elevated lesions with gently sloping edges on the anterior wall. This situation stresses the need for a biphasic gastric examination.

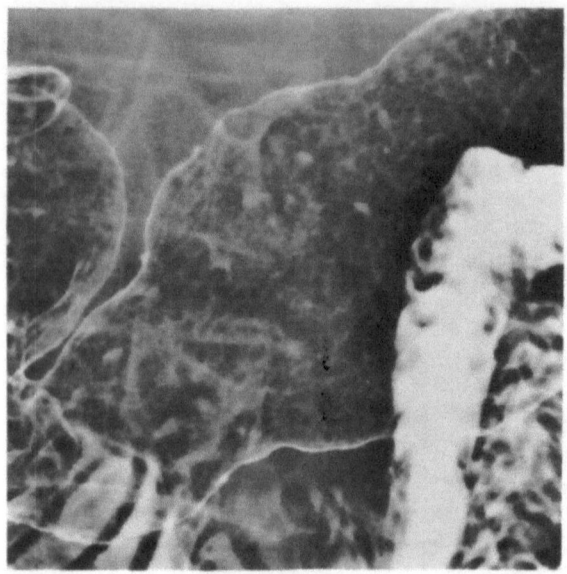

a

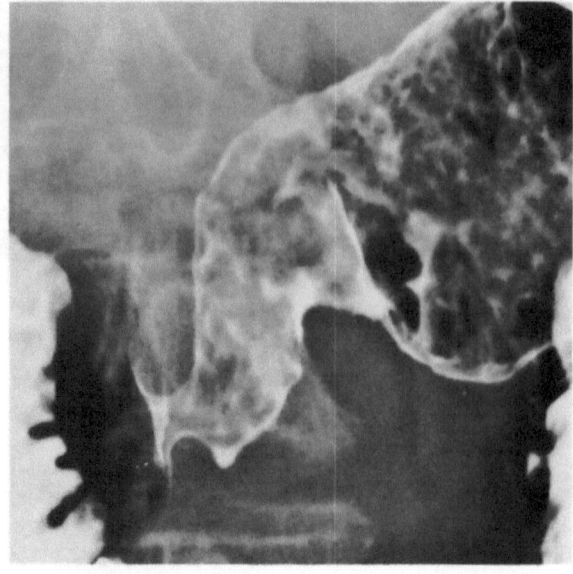

b

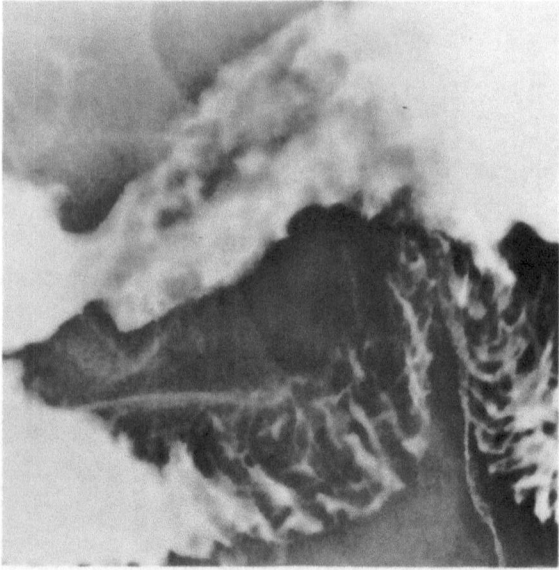

c

Fig. 54

a. DC study, supine position, LPO. There are numerous spots of barium on the posterior wall of the gastric antrum, representing either deep erosions or superficial ulcers, suspicious of Crohn's disease. Confirmation by gastroscopy. Biopsy revealed a nonspecific inflammatory reaction.

b. Repeat examination under identical conditions, 1 year later.

c. PC compression study, erect position. There are numerous ulcers and deformity of the gastric antrum. The patient died 2 months later. Autopsy showed multiple ulcers. Histological examination (which included the expert opinion of Dr B.C. Morson (The Pathology Department of St. Mark's Hospital, London, England) revealed no evidence of Crohn's disease or of an ischemic etiology of the ulceration.

7.3. Antral gastritis

The radiological diagnosis of gastritis is a controversial subject. Only erosive gastritis (see page 58), extensive chronic atrophic gastritis (see page 47, 48) and antral gastritis can be diagnosed reliably by the radiologist. The more classical descriptions of antral gastritis (11, 19, 92) include symptoms such as antral spasm, narrowing of the antral region, irregularity of peristalsis, polypoid lesions and varioliform erosions. More recently Turner et al. (262) have proved that crenulation of the antral mucosa, transient antral spasm and an absence of normal antral distention are reliable criteria for the diagnosis. These workers believe that an abnormal upper gastrointestinal series never assumes normal appearances upon hypotonic examination.

Personal experience has shown that drug-induced hypotonia greatly facilitates the diagnosis. In a series of endoscopically-verified cases of antral gastritis, hypotonia revealed an abruptly marginated, concentric narrowing in the antral area with folds that ran transversely and multiple nodular filling defects which either were varioliform erosions or contained no central excavation. Once the hypotonia subsides, the irregular peristalsis that then occurs generally rules out the diagnosis of antral carcinoma. Other lesions to consider in differential diagnosis include Crohn's disease, malignant lymphoma, corrosive gastritis and eosinophilic gastritis (270).

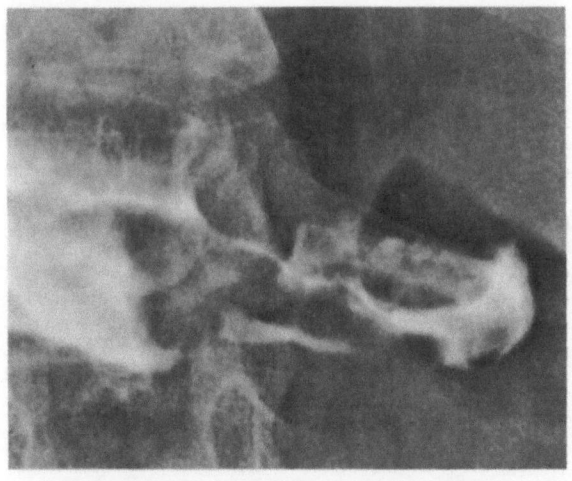

a

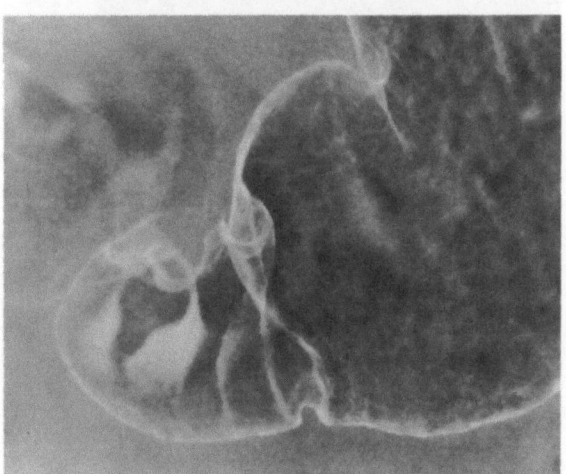

b

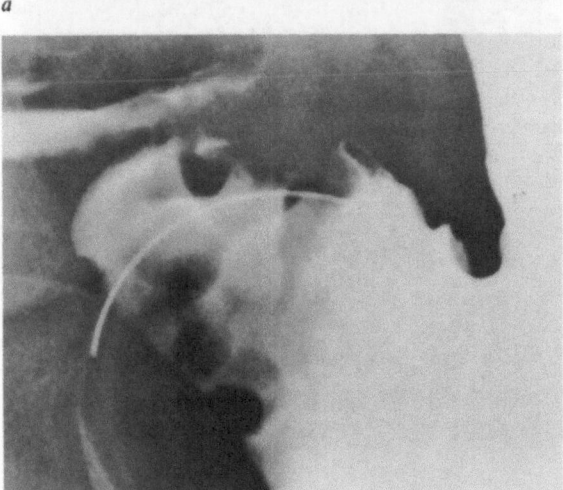

c

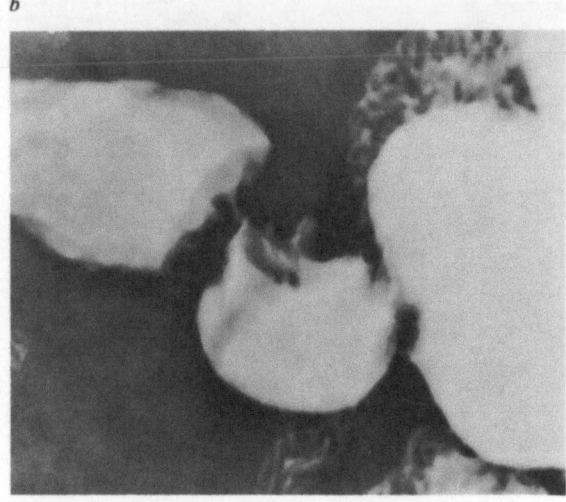

d

Fig. 55

a. PC mucosal relief study, prone position. Irregular filling defect in the prepyloric region.

b. DC study, supine position, LPO.

c. PC compression study, erect position, LPO. Abruptly marginated narrowing of the prepyloric region with transversely running thickened folds and nodularity.

d. Same examination, after the hypotonia subsided. Slightly irregular peristaltic waves. The radiological appearances are most suggestive of the diagnosis antral gastritis. Endoscopy showed thickened edematous folds with varioliform erosions. Biopsies revealed a non-specific inflammatory reaction.

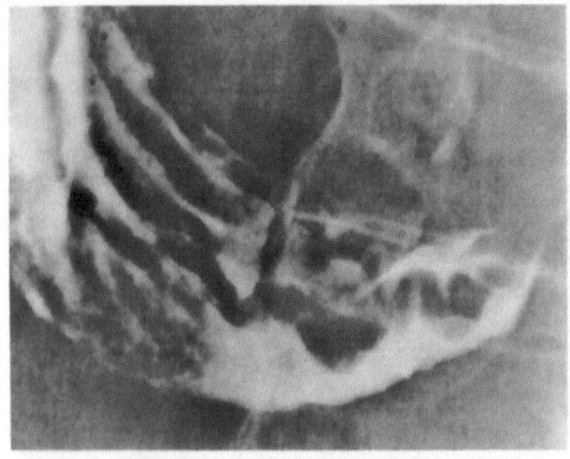

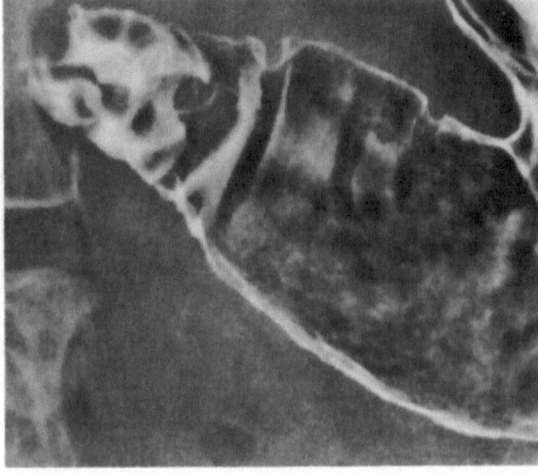

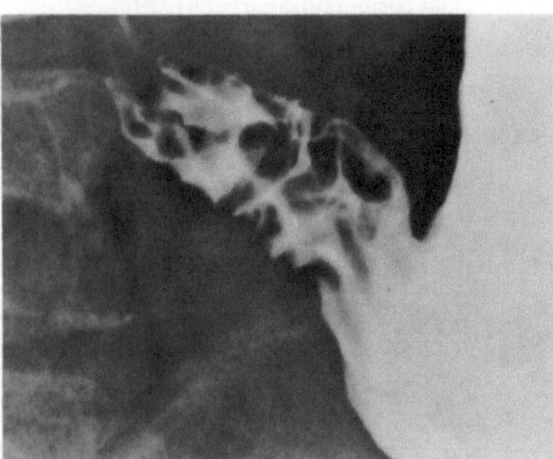

Fig. 56

a. PC mucosal relief study, prone position. Thickened folds in the prepyloric region.

b. DC study, supine position, LPO. Transversely running thickened folds and a nodular filling defect on the posterior wall.

c. PC compression study, erect position, LPO.

d & *e.* Same examination. PC compression studies after the hypotonia subsided. Peristalsis proved to be irregular but uninterrupted. The prepyloric distension is not altogether normal. Appearances of an antral gastritis. Endoscopy: thickened edematous folds and varioliform erosions. Biopsies: non-specific inflammatory reaction.

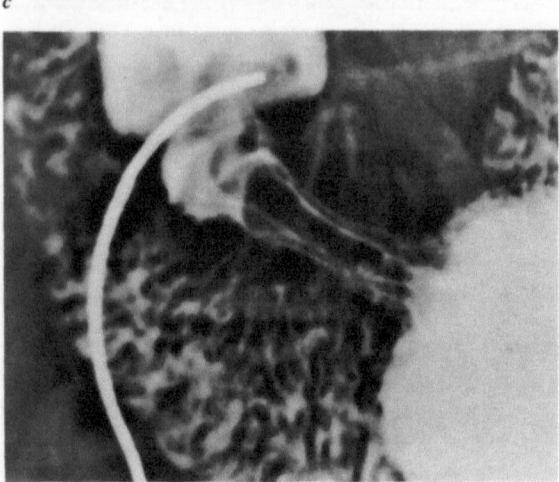

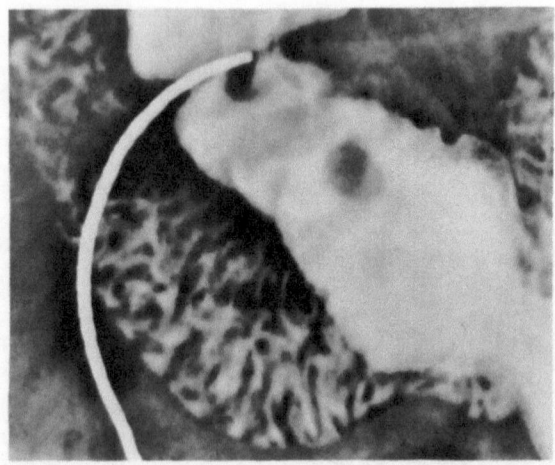

7.4. Ulcers

A gastric ulcer may be defined as a defect in the gastric wall extending through the muscularis mucosae. It may occur at any site in the stomach, but peptic ulcers predominate on the lesser curvature, especially in the region of the angulus. The posterior wall is more commonly involved than the anterior wall (93, 212, 246, 251). Although conventional concepts, based on PC techniques, suggest that most ulcers occur in the distal half of the stomach (212, 246, 252), modern experience with DC examination and endoscopy (251) indicates that ulcers can be demonstrated frequently in the proximal half of the stomach.

Whenever possible, an ulcer crater should be demonstrated by profile and en-face views, which is nearly always possible in the vertical part of the stomach. It is sometimes difficult to obtain both views in the antrum, but angulation of the tube using a remote controlled apparatus may be useful. The en-face view is more reliable than the profile view (fig. 58).

Any peptic ulcer may heal without leaving a visible scar. However, healing with scarring frequently occurs, resulting in a pattern of radiating folds, sometimes with a small central excavation (133, 213). Differentiation between an active ulcer and an excavated scar is impossible by radiological methods alone (fig. 25). Only the endoscopist may be able to judge if the epithelium at the base of an excavation is intact.

Malignant ulcers are to be divided into ulcer-carcinomas, in which the carcinoma has arisen on the basis of a chronic gastric ulcer, i.e. carcinoma is present in the edge of the ulcer, and ulcerating carcinomas, in which carcinoma is also found at the base of the ulcer (247). Dekker (32), in discussing the extensive literature on malignant degeneration in the edges of an originally benign ulcer, considers the subject a controversial one. He believes that malignant degeneration is likely to be a rare event – if it occurs at all.

The student may be justifiably confused or overwhelmed by the large number of publications dealing with the radiological features of malignancy in ulcerating gastric lesions (a.o. 18, 119, 186, 223, 224, 272, 273). On the one hand, Gutmann (102, 103) believes it impossible to decide, purely on the radiological appearances of a niche, if the ulcer is malignant or benign. On the other hand, there is strong evidence that there are several valid radiological indications (though none is absolute) of ulcer malignancy, viz. an indistinct nodular border of the crater, an irregular shape of the crater and an asymmetric crater (272). Two other features are that the folds, which are often deformed, end fairly far from the center of the crater (119, 126), and that the base of the crater projects within the contour of the stomach (224, 273).

Although endoscopy with biopsy has become established as the most reliable method of reaching a preoperative diagnosis of malignancy (35), it remains important for the radiologist to possess his own criteria of malignancy. This knowledge is necessary, not in order to attempt a definite histological diagnosis but to direct the work of endoscopists to ensure that they make biopsies and repeat the procedure if the biopsy findings are inconsistent with the radiological diagnosis.

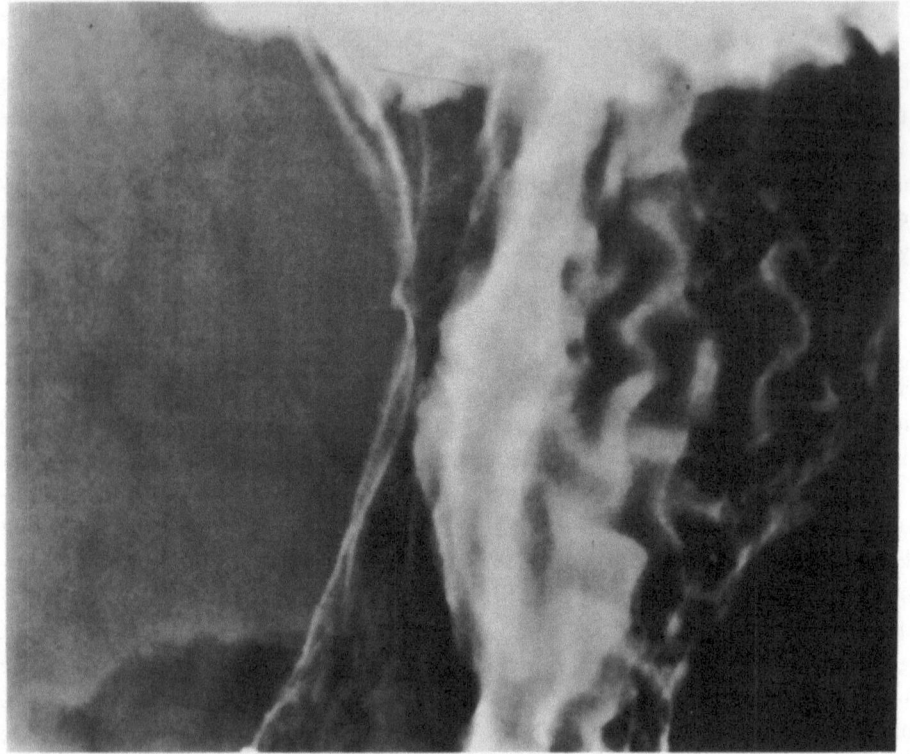

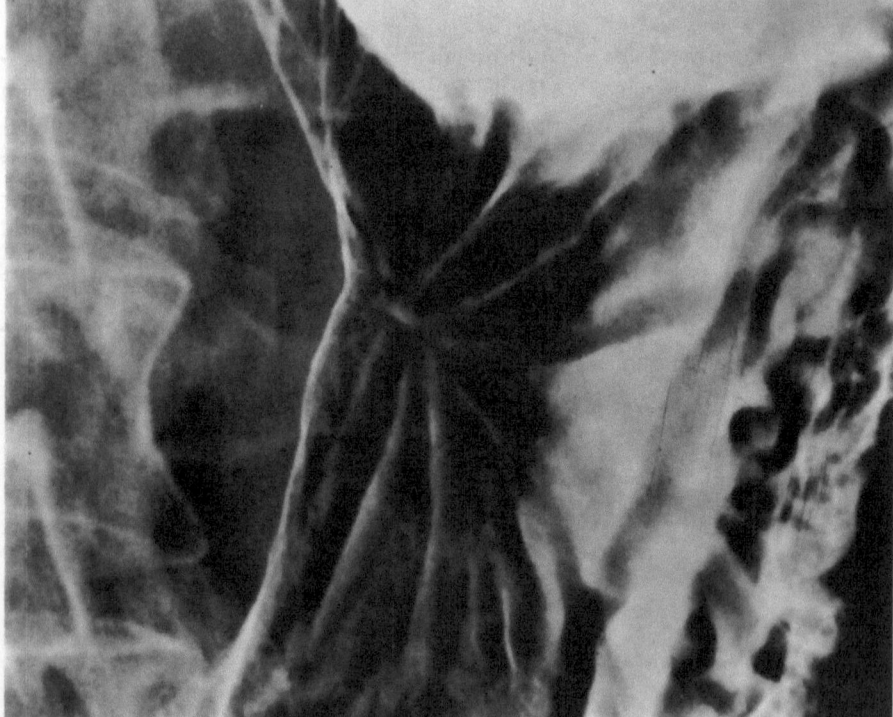

Fig. 57

a. DC study, supine position, LPO.

b. DC study, supine position. Ulcer niche on the posterior wall of the corpus demonstrated by a profile
and a en-face view. The latter gives the best information: the converging folds are visible in this
projection only.

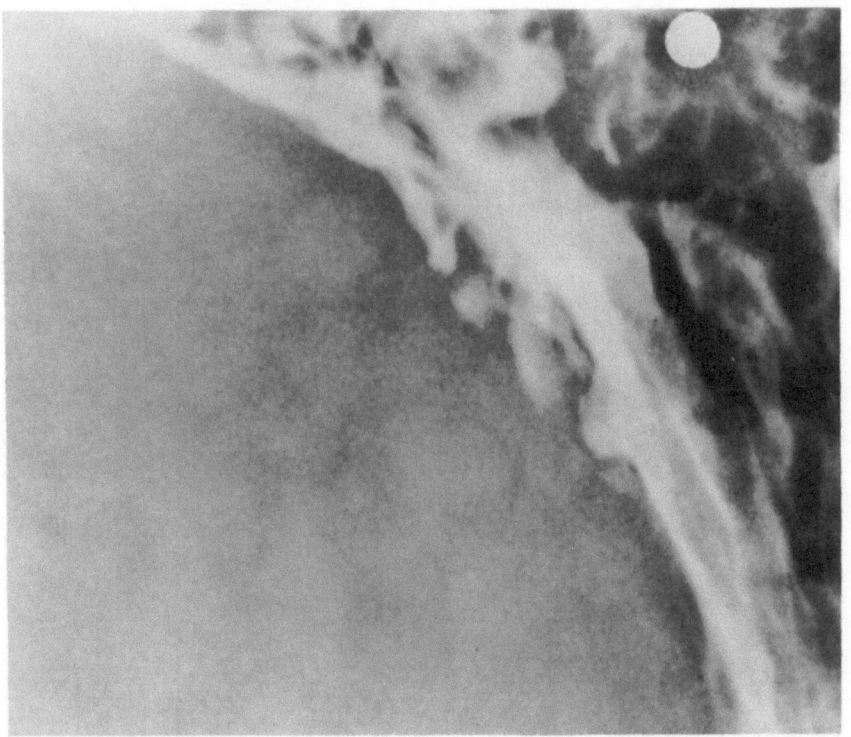

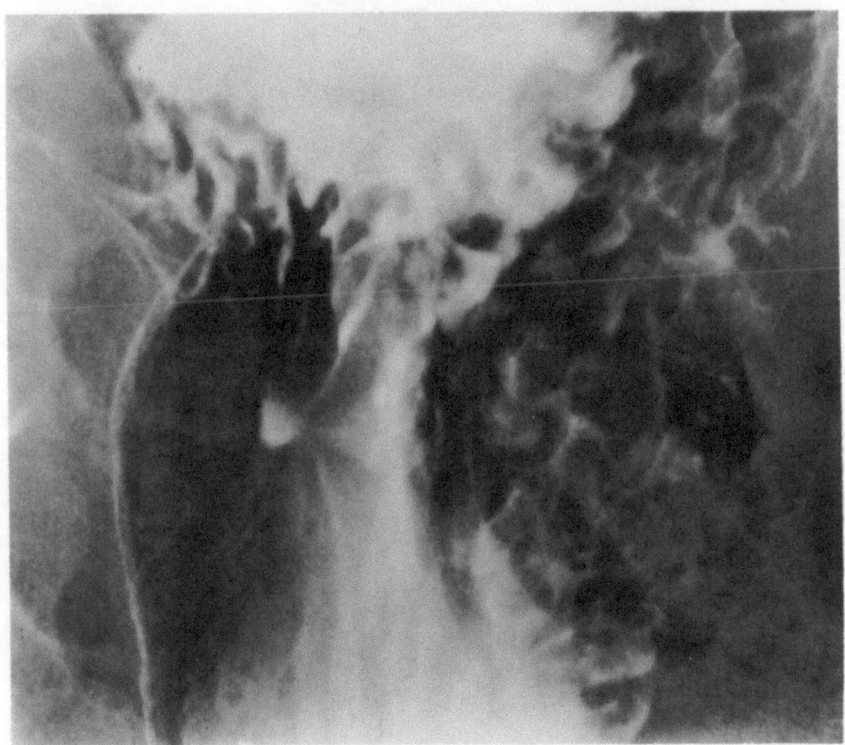

Fig. 58
a. Nearly erect position, LPO.
b. DC study, supine position. The profile view (58a) shows an irregular contour of the lesser curvature; appearance is suggestive of at least one ulcer niche which could only definitely be demonstrated in the en-face view. The en-face view is of more importance than the profile view.

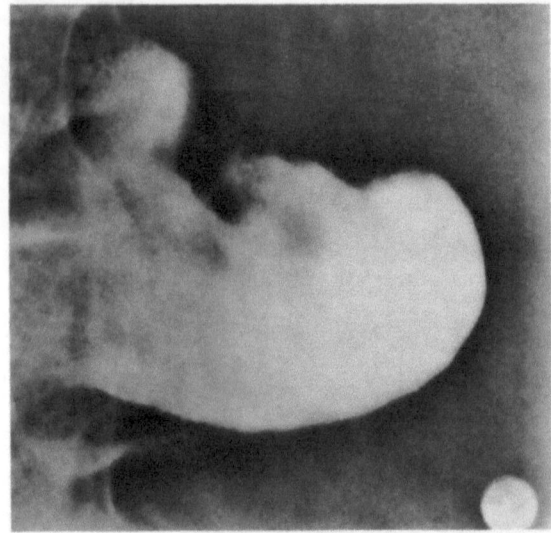

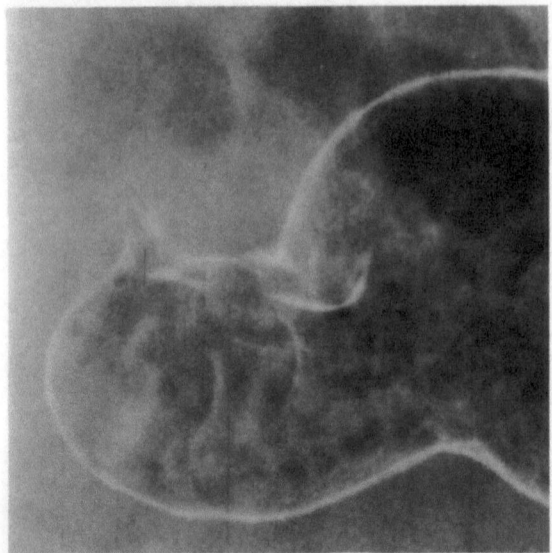

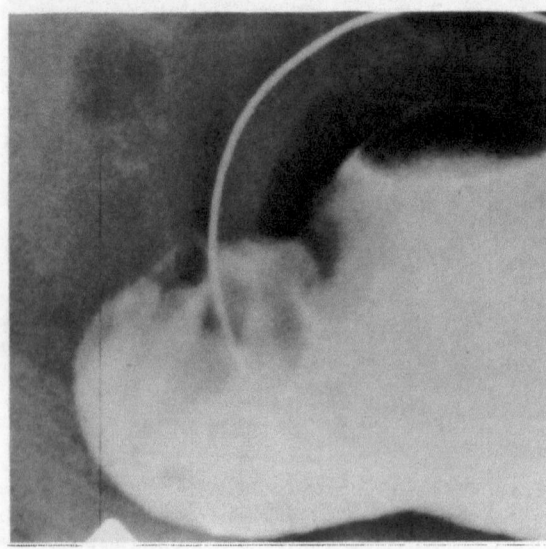

Fig. 59
a. PC mucosal relief study, prone position.
b. DC study, supine position, LPO.
c. PC compression study, erect position, LPO. The DC study shows
   a curved line shadow that represents the edge of an ulcer niche in
   the anterior wall. PC studies show the niche and its surroundings.
   This case stresses the need of a biphasic gastric examination.

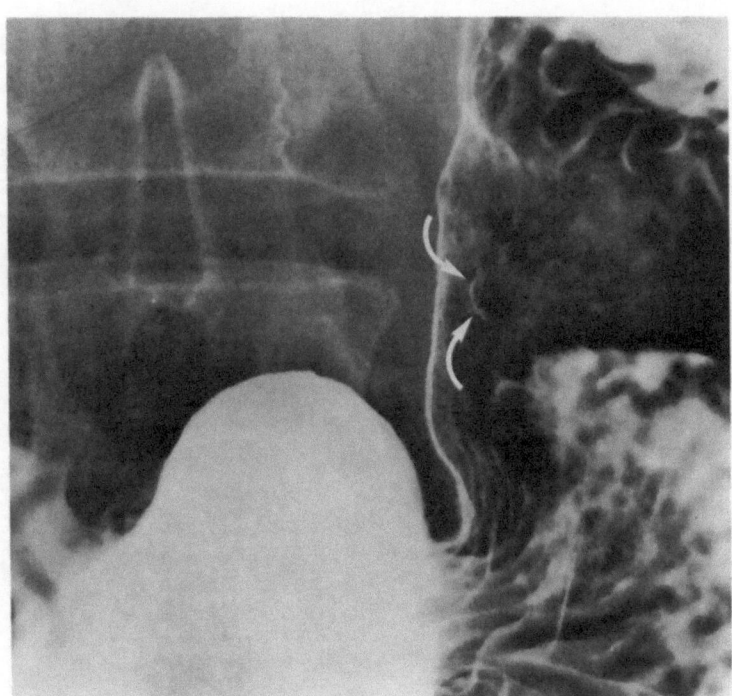

Fig. 60
DC study, supine position. Curved line shadow (arrows) highly suspicious of an ulcer niche in the anterior wall. Confirmation by gastroscopy. Biopsies demonstrated benignancy.

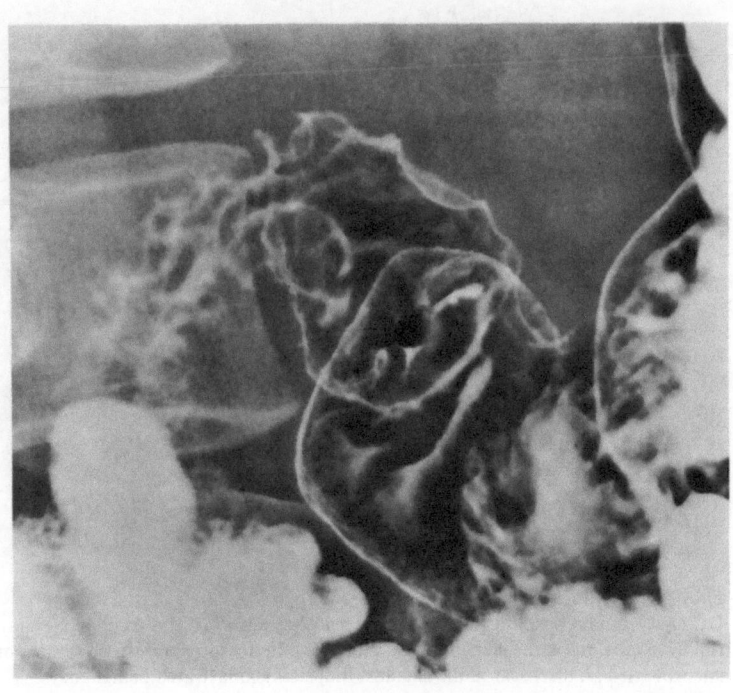

Fig. 61
DC study, supine position, LPO. Linear niche in the posterior wall of the prepyloric region. Note the open pylorus. Endoscopic confirmation.

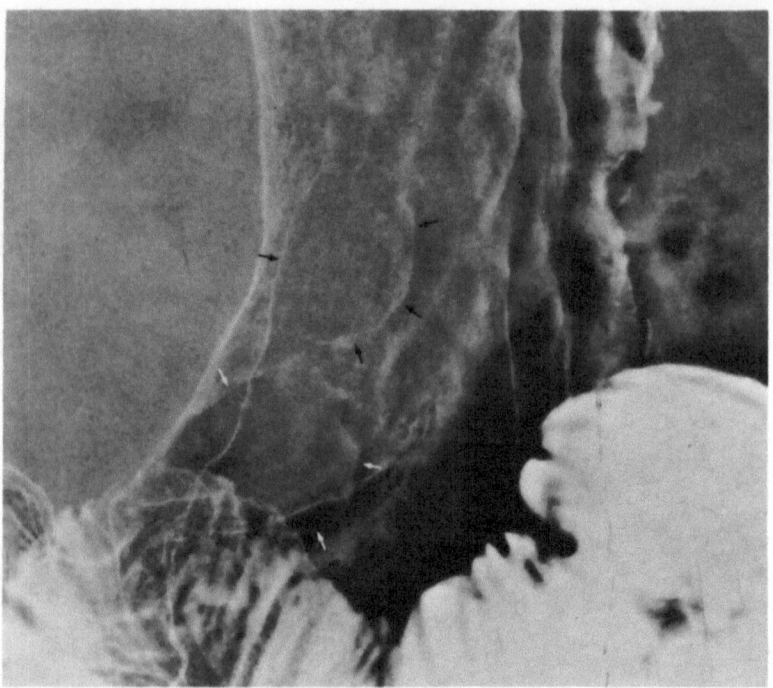

Fig. 62
DC study, supine position. Difficult examination because the patient was in a very bad shape. Only supine films were made; PC compression studies were not possible. Two coin-like configurations on the lesser curvature of the lower part of the corpus (arrows), which could not be explained at the time of the examination. The patient died shortly afterwards. Autopsy showed two coin-like very shallow benign ulcers.

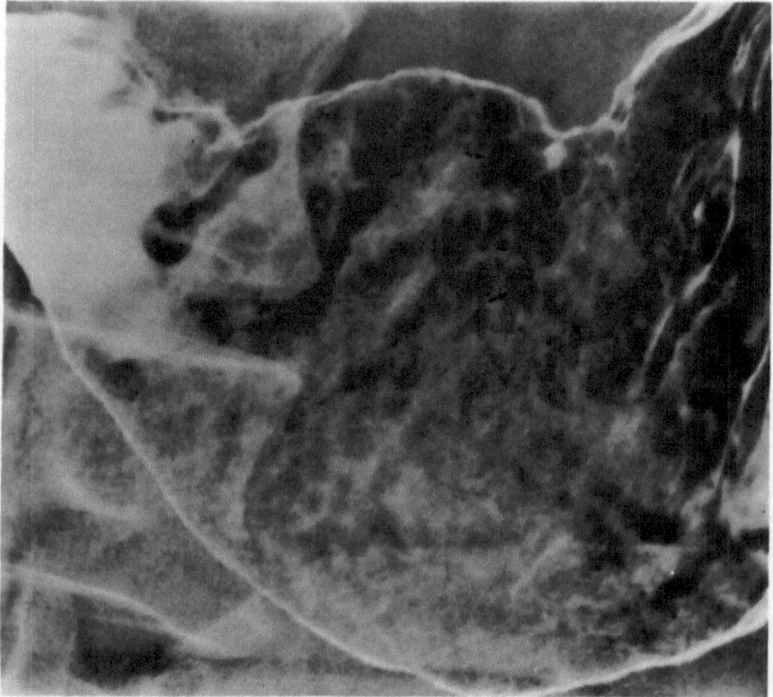

Fig. 63
DC study supine position, LPO. Tiny ulcer in the region of the angulus. Several varioliform erosions in the neighbourhood (arrows). Endoscopy performed some months later revealed an ulcer scar in the angulus. Biopsies demonstrated benignancy.

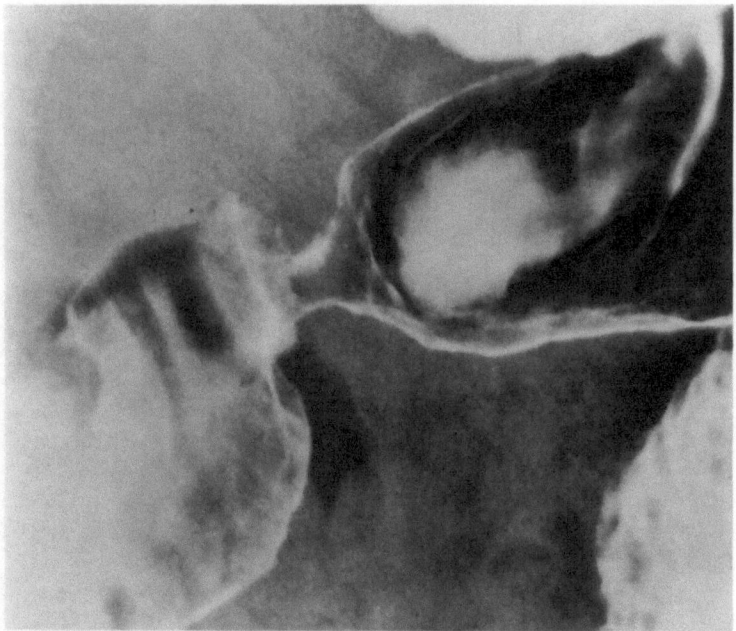

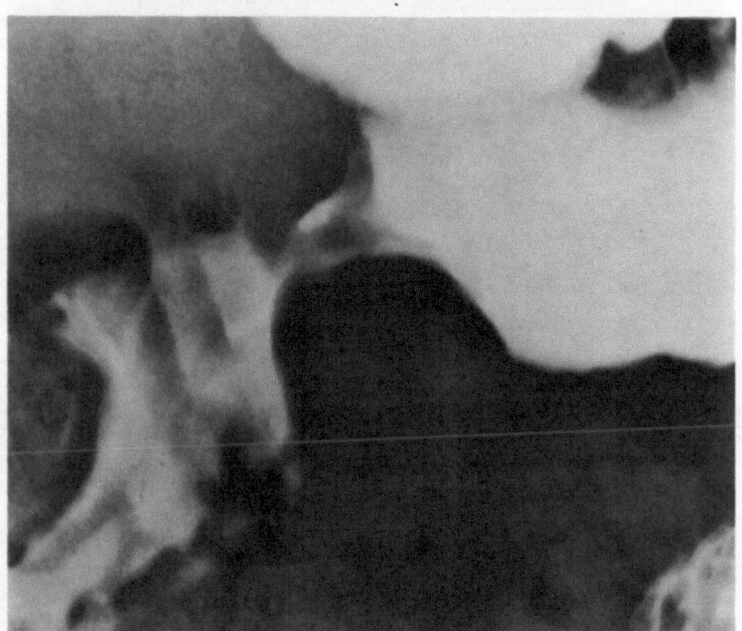

Fig. 64
a. DC study supine position, LPO.
b. PC compression study, erect position, LPO. Ulcer niche on the lesser curvature of the pylorus. Endoscopic confirmation. Biopsies: benign.

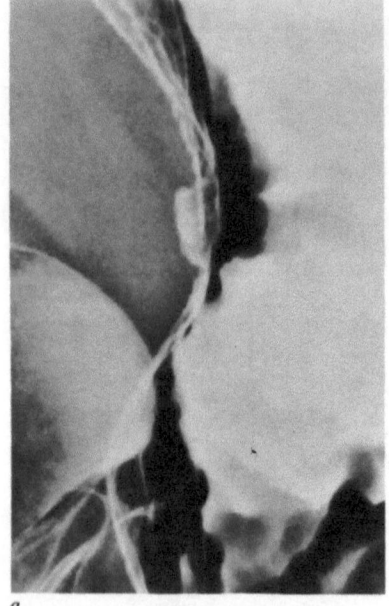

a

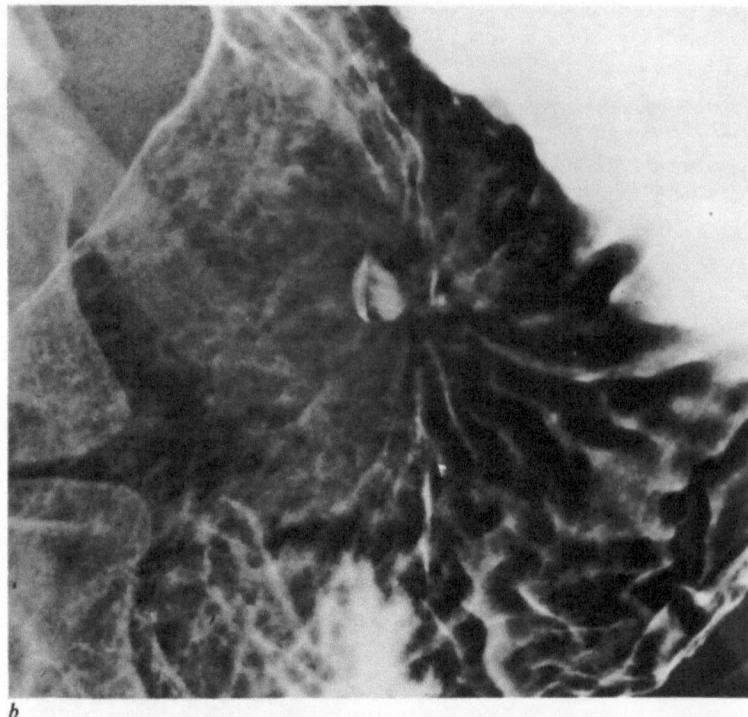

b

Fig. 65

a. DC study, supine position, LPO.

b. DC study, supine position, partial LPO. Demonstration of an ulcer niche. The converging folds and the surroundings of the ulcer are best visualized in the en-face view.

c. Repeat examination after 2 months under the same conditions as in 65 a and b. The ulcer crater has disappeared. Radiating fold pattern, typical ulcer scar.

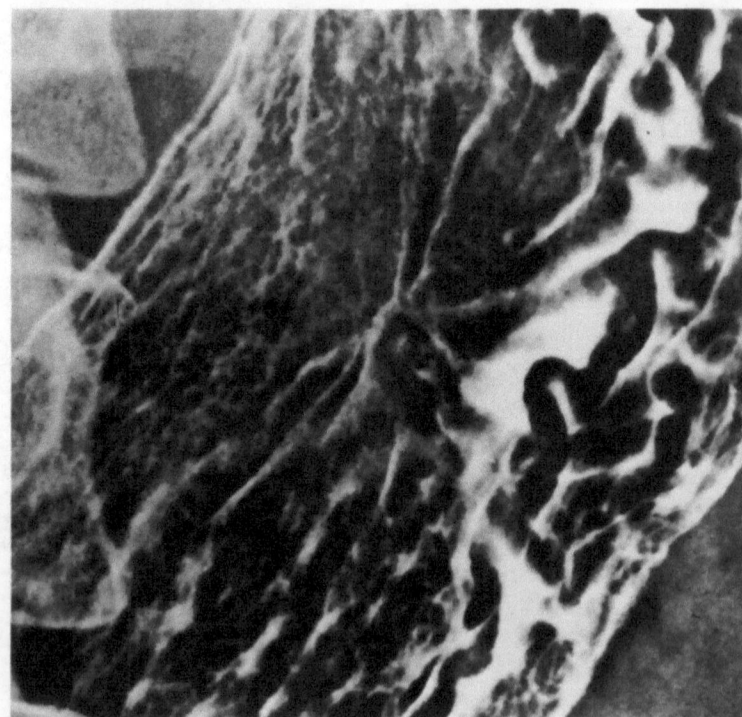

c

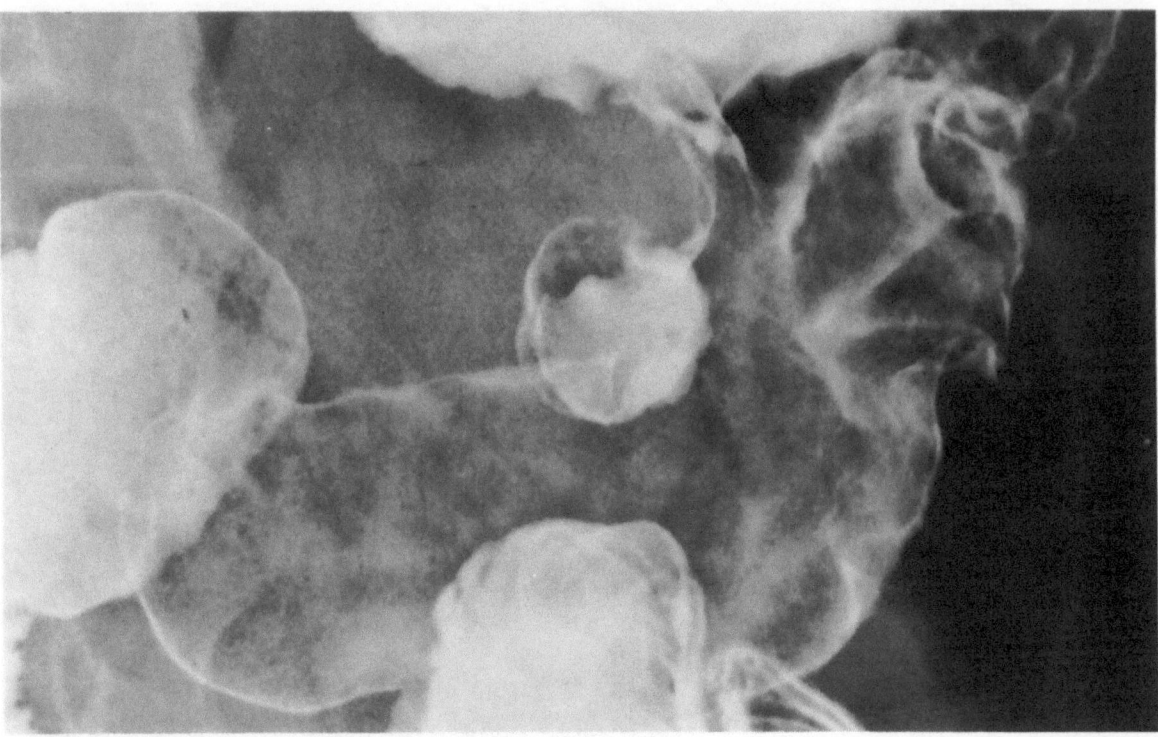

a

Fig. 66

a. DC study, supine position. Large ulcer niche in the angulus.

b. DC study, supine position, after 3½ weeks' treatment. The ulcer niche has diminished in size.

c. DC study, supine position, after an additional treatment of 2 months. The ulcer niche has completely disappeared. Converging folds and irregular areae gastricae relief indicate scarring. Endoscopy confirmed these findings. Several series of biopsies demonstrated benignancy.

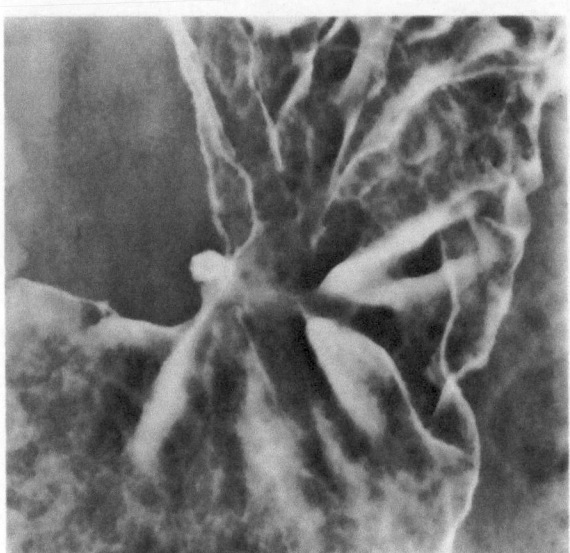

b

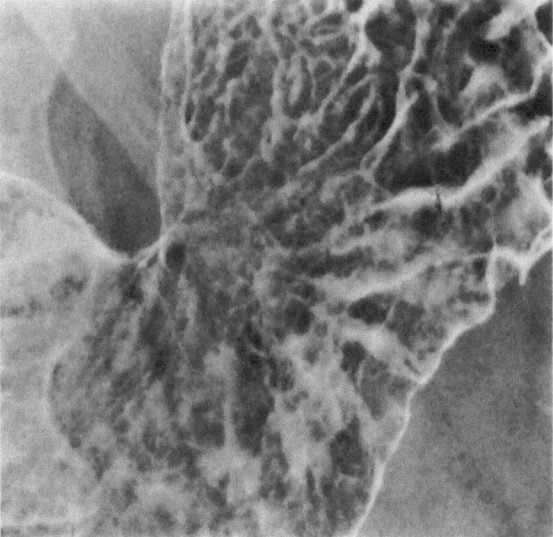

c

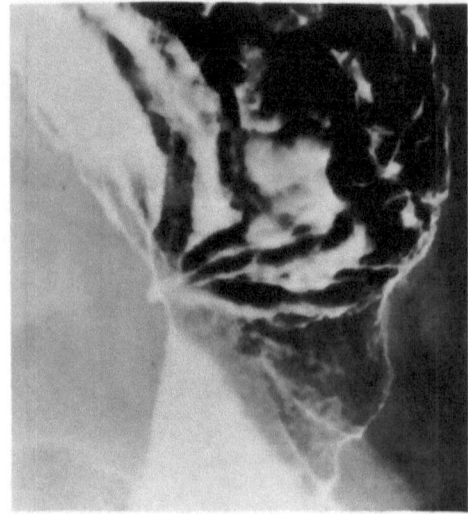

a

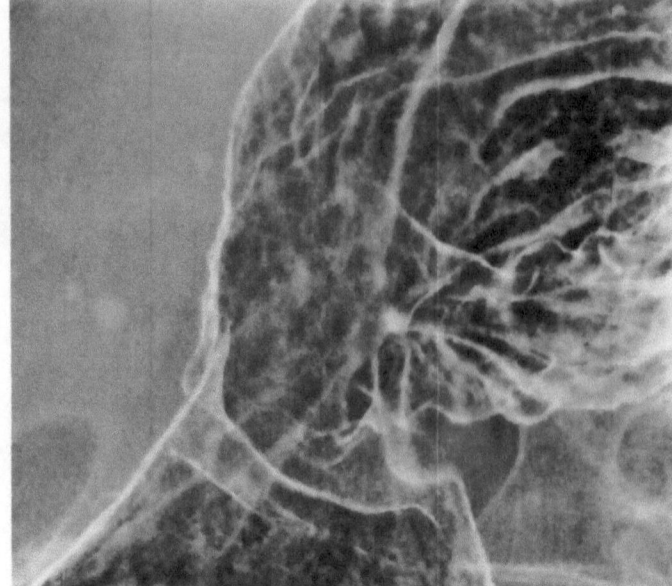

b

Fig. 67

a. DC study, supine position, LPO; table 40° anti-Trendelenburg.

b. DC study, supine position, RPO; table about 30° anti-Trendelenburg. There is an ulcer niche rather high on the lesser curvature.

c. Repeat examination under identical conditions one year later. Only a tiny niche is left. Radiologically it is impossible to distinguish between an excavated ulcer scar and a tiny active ulcer. Endoscopy has not been performed (cf. fig. 25).

c

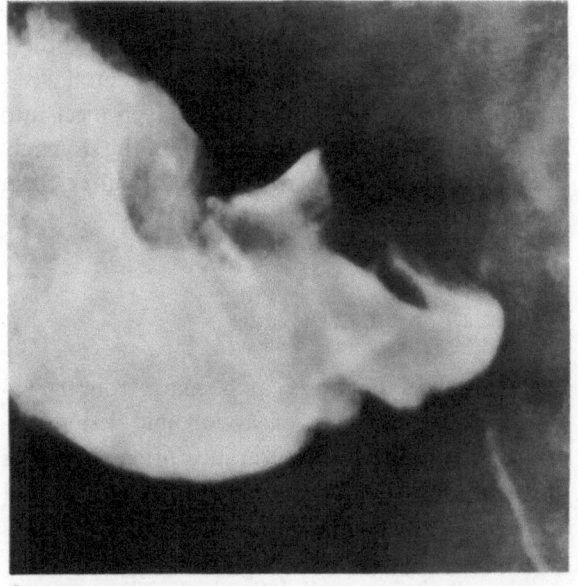

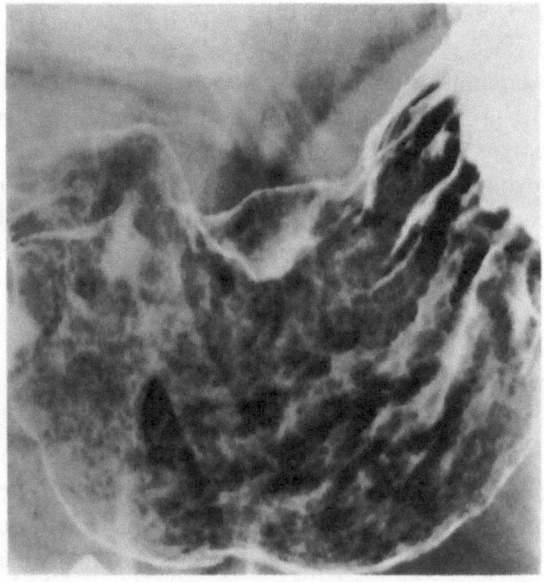

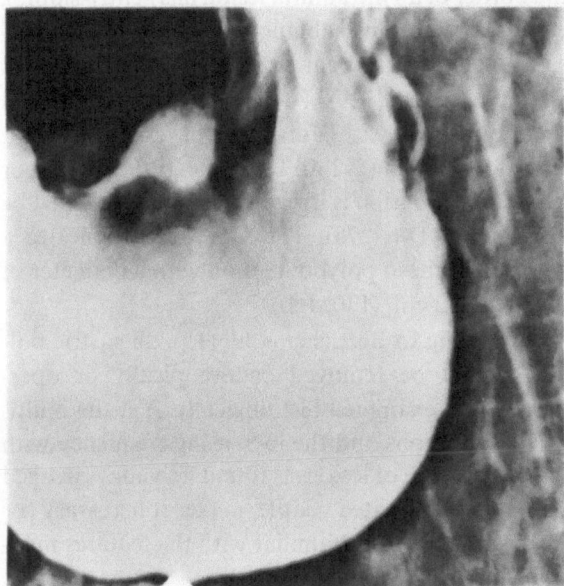

Fig. 68

a. PC mucosal relief study, prone position.

b. DC study, supine position.

c. PC compression study, erect position. Although the DC study demonstrates a definite lesion, the typical Kirklin complex is only visualized in the PC studies. Although such a complex is considered to be highly suspicious of malignancy, a series of biopsies showed benignancy. After 1 month's treatment the ulcer niche has completely disappeared (cf. fig. 89).

7.5. Benign tumors

Common benign tumors of the stomach belong to two groups, viz. those of epithelial origin, i.e. gastric polyps and those of muscular origin, i.e. leiomyomas. Elevated lesions in the stomach forming part of the picture of diffuse gastrointestinal polyposis are not included in this chapter because such entities are rare.

7.5.1. GASTRIC POLYPS

A gastric polyp may be defined as a lesion which projects from the mucosal surface into the lumen of the stomach (174). The most common varieties of benign epithelial polyp encountered are the hyperplastic polyp and the adenoma (181).

Hyperplastic polyps: These lesions are composed of hyperplastic but in other respects normal glandular epithelium, and only rarely turn malignant (2, 160, 181). They are often multiple, sessile or pedunculated and have a smooth surface. Their size varies from a few mm. to 2 cm. in diameter. Although the reported incidence is under 1 per cent (160, 181), personal and other workers' experience with modern radiological techniques indicate that they are far commoner.

Adenoma: This lesion is a true neoplasm. It is composed of dysplastic glands and often turns malignant (2, 181). It is usually single and may be sessile or pedunculated. Generally an adenoma is larger than a hyperplastic polyp and often has a lobulated or papillary surface.

A stomach containing a polyp of either variety often harbors a coexisting carcinoma. The high incidence of carcinoma is probably connected with the high incidence of atrophic gastritis in these cases, particularly those with adenoma (181).

7.5.2. LEIOMYOMA

Leiomyomas are benign tumors originating from the muscular tissue in the gastric wall. If small leiomyomas are included, they probably represent the commonest tumors of the stomach (178). Although the mucosa on the tumor may be intact, central ulceration often occurs. Leiomyomas may project into the lumen or onto the serosal aspect of the stomach. Macroscopically the tumor does not differ from leiomyosarcoma.

7.5.3. RADIOLOGICAL FEATURES

No histological diagnosis can be made from the radiological appearances of a polypoid lesion, although the naked-eye appearance often permits a judgment on its epithelial or intramural origin and if it is benign or malignant.

Epithelial lesions with a diameter greater than 1 cm., usually have a well-defined edge. By contrast, the border of an intramural lesion has gently-sloping edges, reflecting its submucosal origin. In small lesions, i.e. less than 1 cm. in diameter, this difference is not obvious (129). A smooth, sharply-defined polypoid lesion with a diameter of less than 2 cm., is usually benign (2, 130, 160, 275). If the surface or border of the lesion is irregular, malignancy must be considered (181, 275). The same rule applies to a smooth-surfaced polypoid lesion with a diameter of more than 2 cm. (130, 160).

According to Bötticher et al. (15), all gastric polyps should be removed endoscopically or operatively and examined histologically. Yet the multiplicity of lesions and the increasing frequency with which this type of lesions is found nowadays in aged and often debilitated people, makes it necessary for the radiologist to be familiar with the features mentioned above.

No radiological differential diagnosis between a sessile polyp with central ulceration and a solitary varioliform erosion is possible. Heterotopic pancreatic tissue is usually found on the greater curvature of the gastric antrum or pyloric region. It is also impossible to differentiate between multiple hyperplastic polyps with gently-sloping edges and healed varioliform erosions without the typical central excavation.

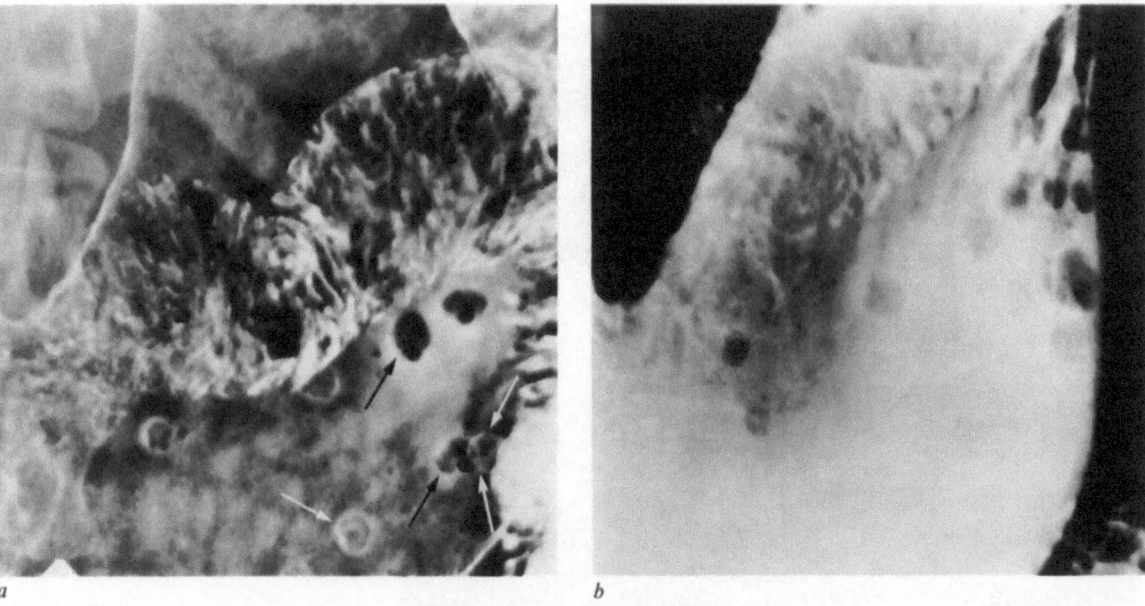

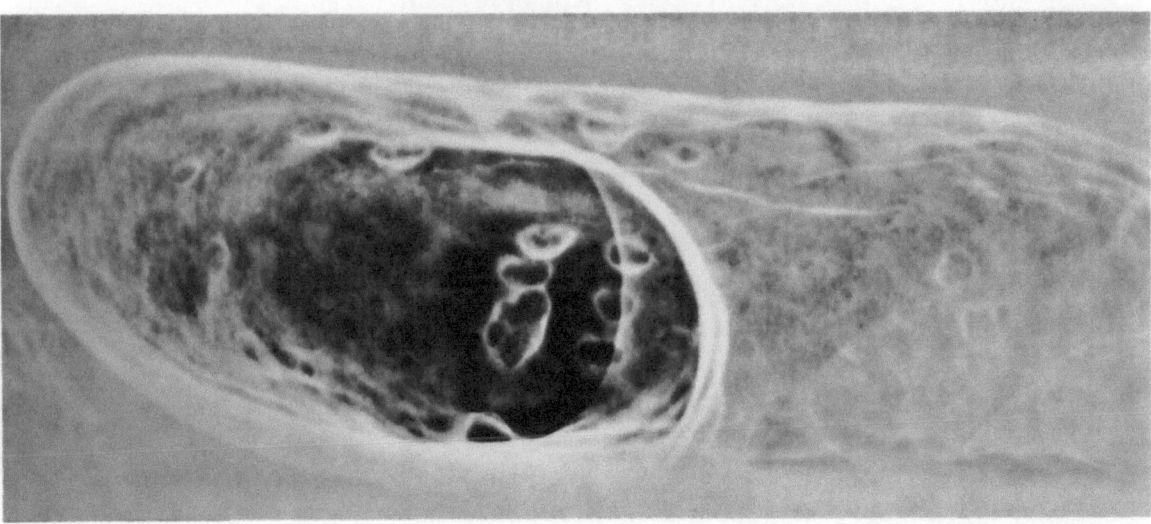

Fig. 69

a. DC study, supine position, LPO.

b. PC compression study, erect position.

c. DC study, supine position, horizontal beam projection. Multiple slightly irregularly marginated polypoid lesions. In fig. a. it is possible to distinguish between lesions on the posterior wall (black arrows) and on the anterior wall (white arows). Cf. fig. 14. Endoscopical confirmation. Biopsies: hyperplastic polyps.

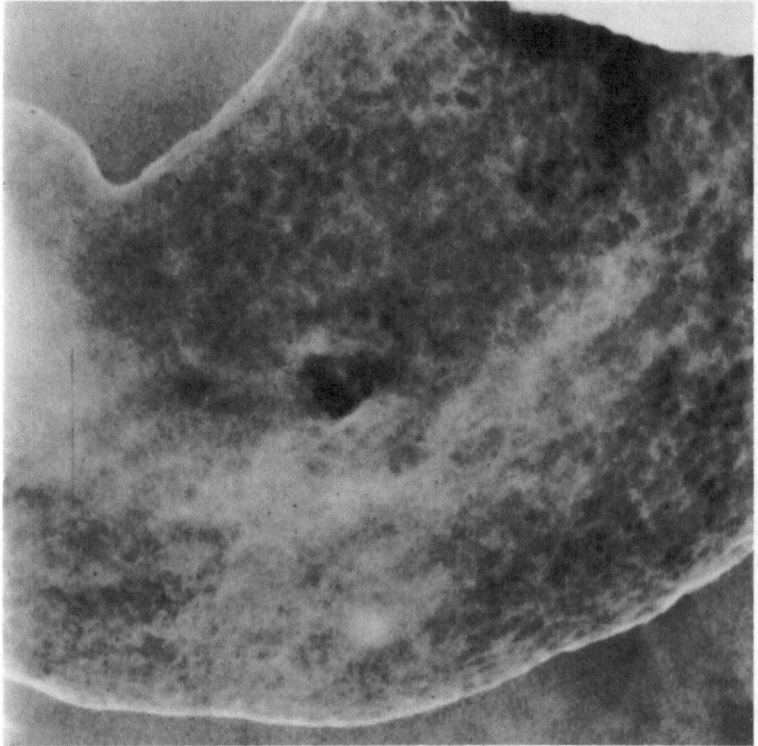

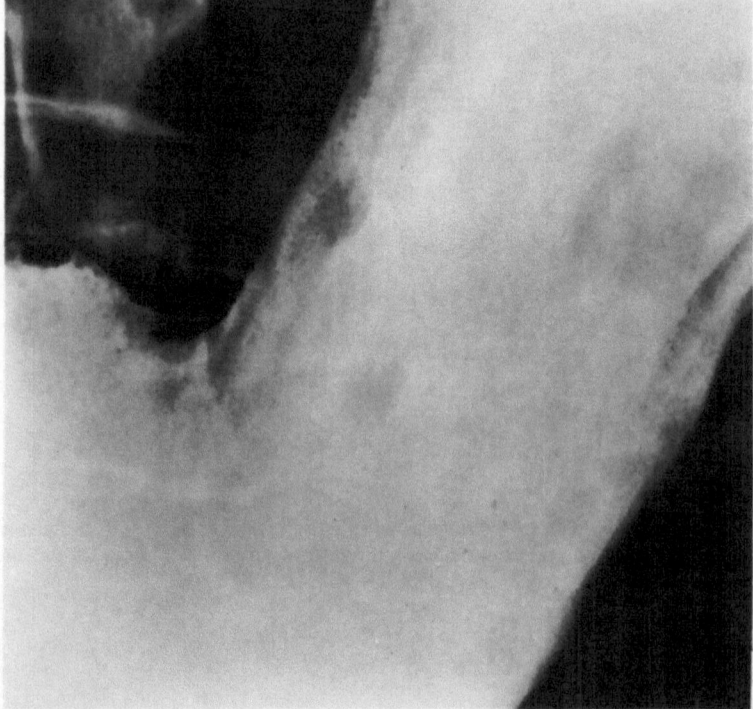

Fig. 70
a. DC study, supine position. Protrusion with gently sloping edges on the posterior wall.
b. PC compression study, erect position. This study reveals a second filling defect which
    has to be a polypoid lesion with gently sloping edges on the anterior wall of the lesser
    curvature. Gastroscopy: two polypoid lesions; one situated on the anterior wall and
    one on the posterior wall (cf. fig. 17). Biopsies: hyperplastic polyps. Need of a biphasic-
    contrast gastric examination.

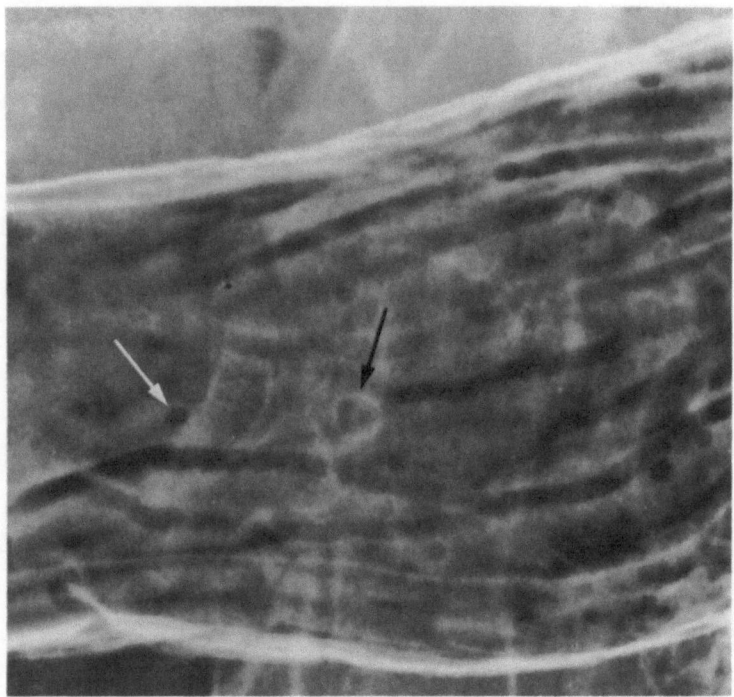

Fig. 71
DC study, supine position. Multiple small polypoid lesions situated on the anterior wall (black arrow) and the posterior wall (white arrow) of the corpus. Endoscopical confirmation. Biopsies: no definite diagnosis.

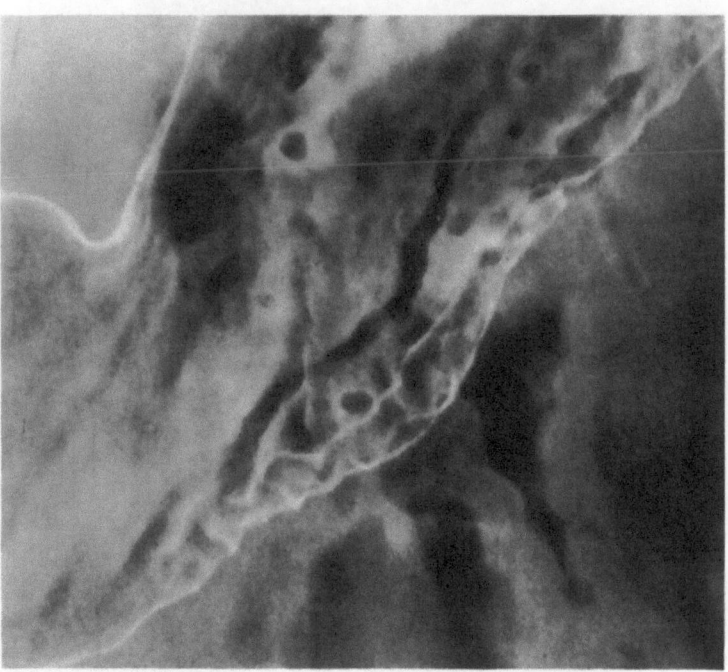

Fig. 72.
DC study, supine position. Multiple small polypoid lesions in a patient suffering from pernicious anemia. Endoscopy: atrophy of the mucosa; multiple small polyps. Biopsies: hyperplastic polyps.

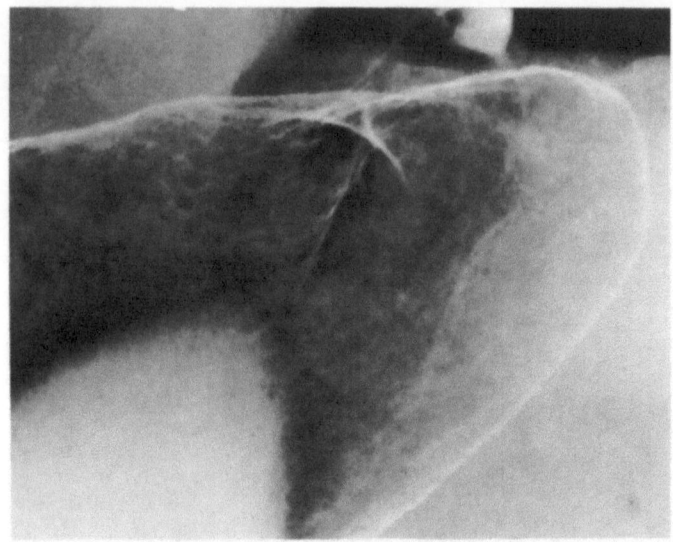

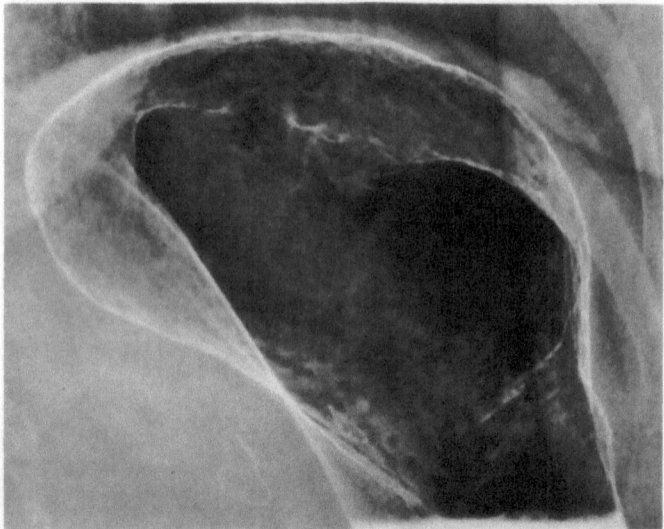

Fig. 73
a. DC study, supine position, RPO; table 40° anti-Trendelenburg.
b. DC study, erect position, horizontal beam projection. Multiple tiny polypoid lesions on the wall of the fundus. Endoscopy: atrophic gastritis; multiple small polypoid lesions. Biopsies: atrophic mucosa; hyperplastic polyps.

Fig. 74
DC study, supine position, RPO; table 40° anti-Trendelenburg. Multiple polypoid lesions in the fundus. Endoscopy revealed atrophic gastritis and confirmed the multiple polyps. Biopsies: hyperplastic polyps.

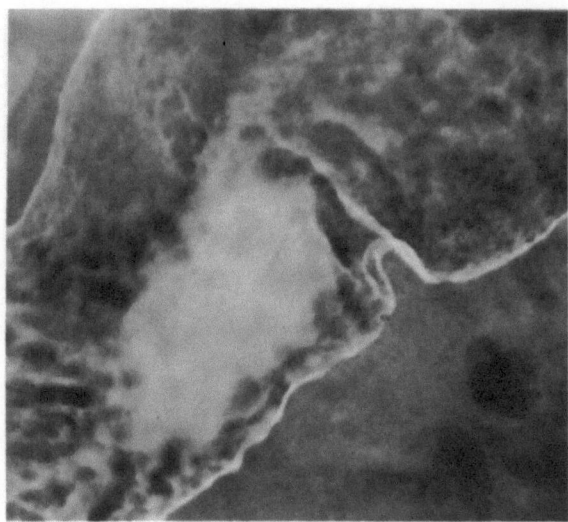

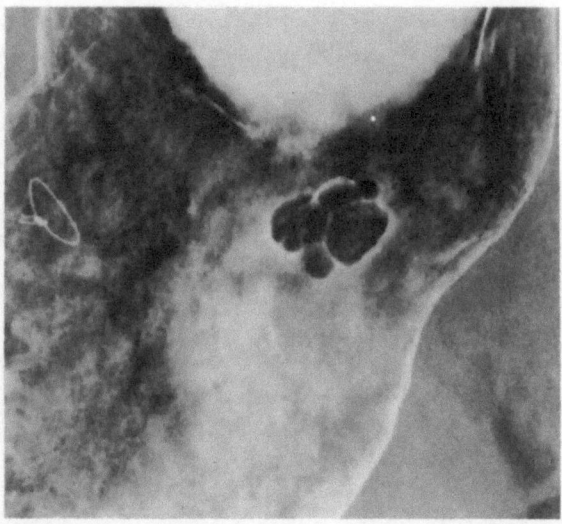

Fig. 75
DC study, supine position. Irregular polypoid lesion on the posterior wall in the region of the angulus and probably an atrophic gastritis. Endoscopy: atrophy of the mucosa in the corpus; protrusion in the region of the angulus, which may fit EGC. There were no signs of malignancy in the biopsy specimens.

Fig. 76
DC study, supine position. Large lobulated filling defect on the posterior wall; atrophic mucosa. Endoscopical confirmation. Histological report: gastric adenoma.

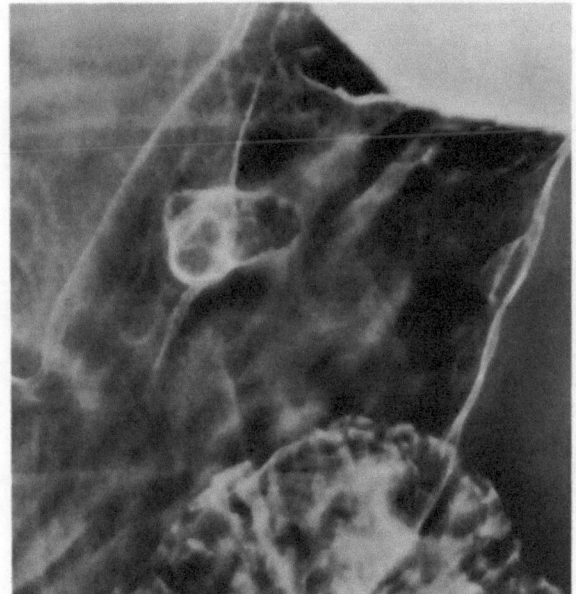

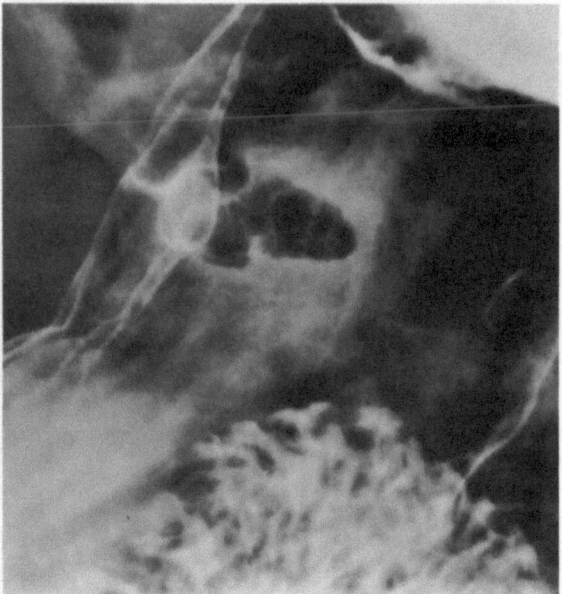

Fig. 77
Same patient as shown in fig. 74.
a. DC study, supine position.
b. DC study, supine position, partial RPO. Lobulated filling defect on the lesser curvature; smooth filling defect on the greater

curvature. Endoscopical confirmation. Histological examination (Pathology Department, Hospital of the University of Amsterdam) of the polypoid lesion on the lesser curvature: gastric adenoma.

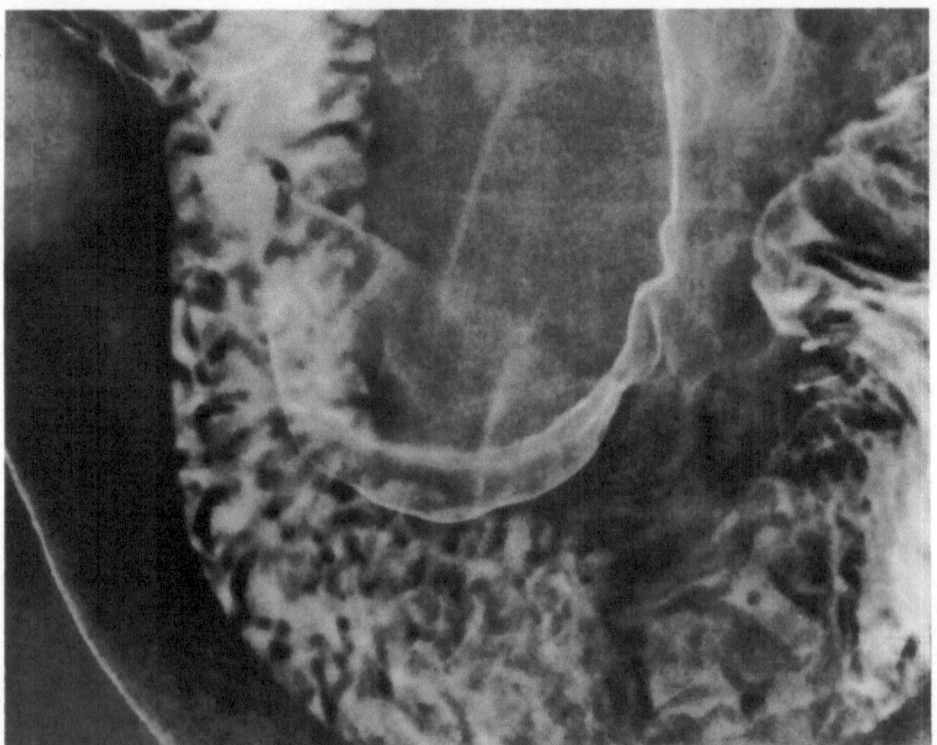

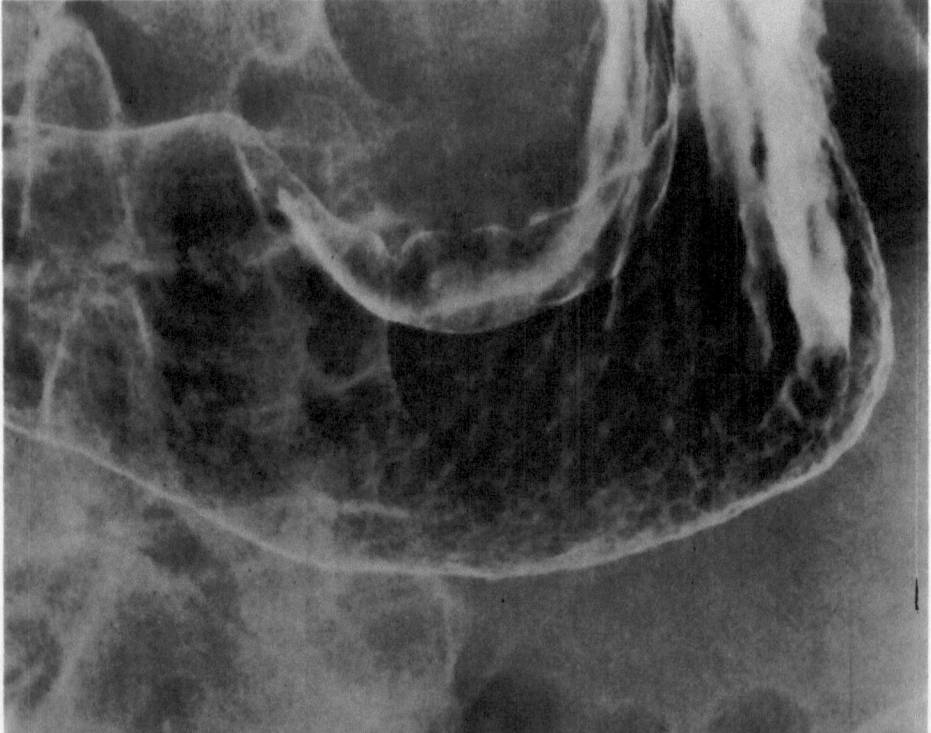

Fig. 78

a & b.DC studies, supine position. Filling defect with gently sloping edges with a diameter of more than one cm. on the lesser curvature of the antrum, either a submucosal lesion or an indentation. Endoscopy revealed a shallow central ulceration which is strongly in favour of the diagnosis leiomyoma or leiomyosarcoma. No operation.

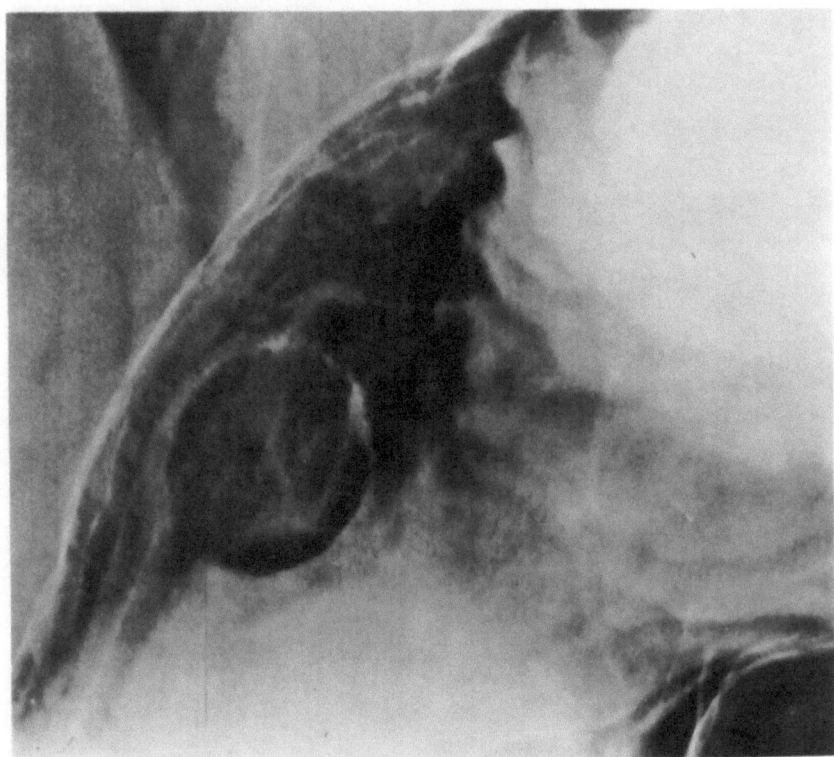

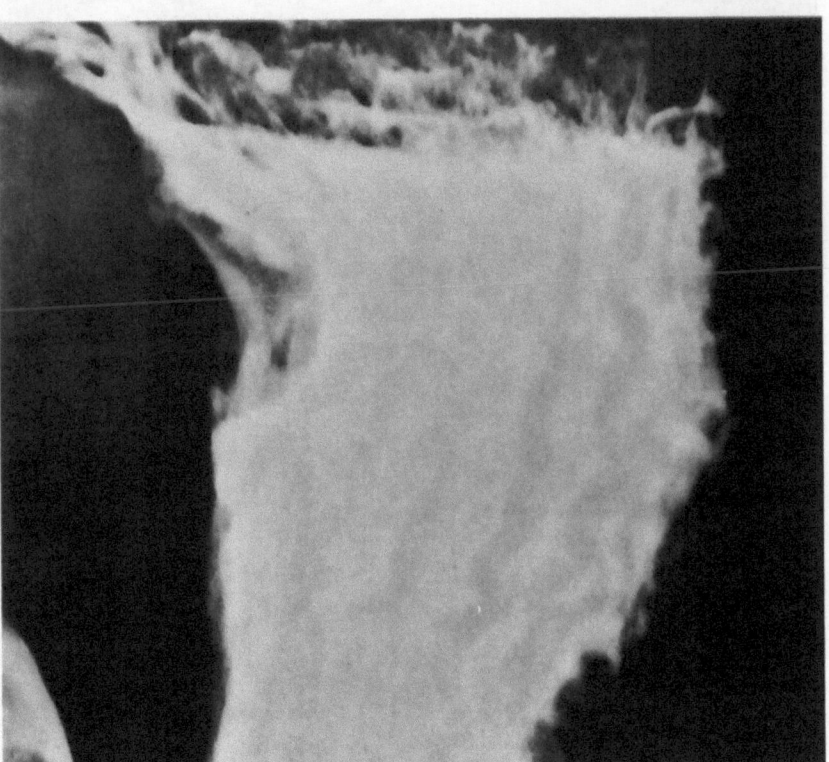

Fig. 79
a. DC study, supine position, RPO.
b. PC study, erect position, LPO. Filling defect with gently sloping edges with a diameter of more
   than 1 cm., probably a submucosal lesion. Histological examination of the resected specimen
   proved a leiomyoma.

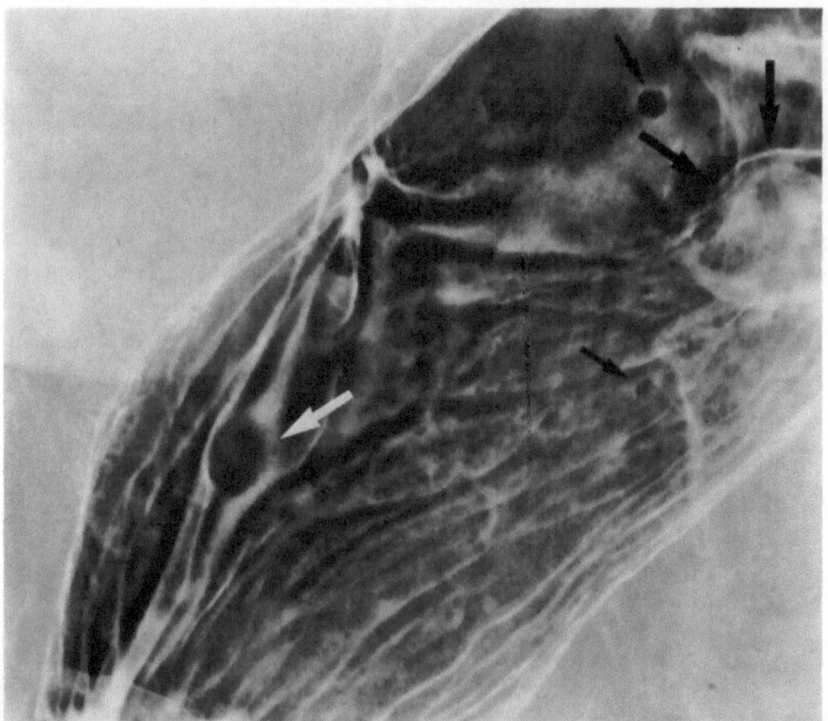

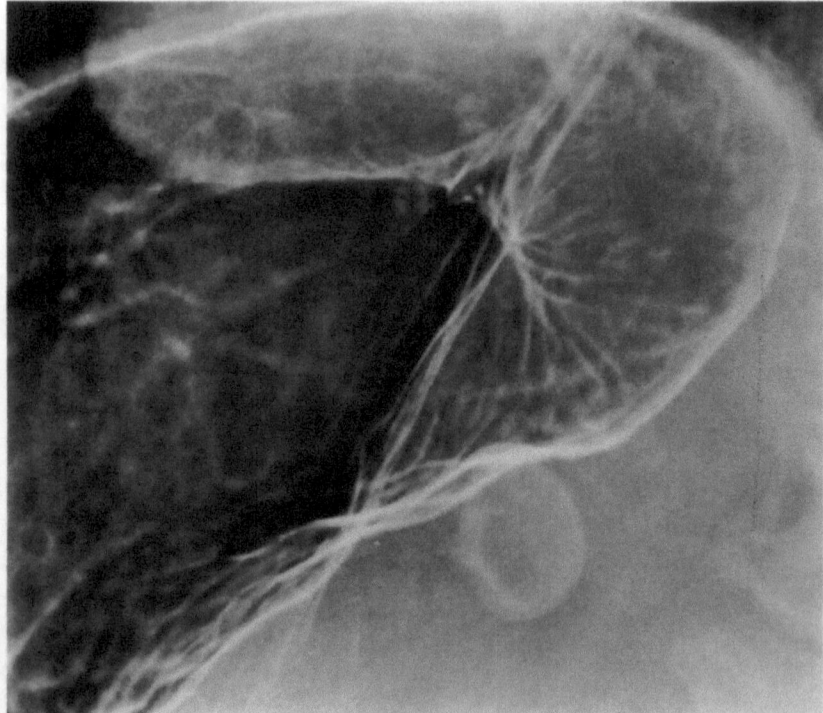

Fig. 80

a. DC study, supine position, RPO; table 40° anti-Trendelenburg.

b. DC study, supine position; nearly right lateral; table 40° anti-Trendelenburg. The large black arrows point to an indentation caused by an aneurysm of the splenic artery. The small arrows point to polypoid lesions with abruptly marginated edges. The large white arrow points to a polypoid lesion with a gently sloping margin on the lateral side and an abrupt margin on the medial side. Autopsy revealed that the small lesions were hyperplastic polyps and the large protrusion was a leiomyoma.

7.6. Carcinomas (including Early Gastric Cancer)

The prognosis of a patient with a gastric carcinoma which is nearly always an adenocarcinoma (177) – is usually poor at the time of the diagnosis and the 5-year survival rate is about 10 per cent (30).

At the Annual Meeting of the Japan Gastroenterological Endoscopic Society in 1962 and of the Japan Research Society for Gastric Cancer in 1963, the Early Gastric Carcinoma (EGC) was defined as a carcinoma of the stomach whose invasion is limited to the mucosa and the submucosa. Neither the size of the carcinoma nor the presence of metastases influences this definition. Only the depth of tissue infiltration matters.

EGC has a favorable prognosis. Takasugi et al. (253) analysed 732 cases of EGC with a single lesion operated on at the National Cancer Hospital in Tokyo, and found that the 5-year survival rate was 97.7 per cent and the 10-year survival 96.4 per cent.

In 1962 the Japan Gastroenterological Endoscopy Society proposed a classification of EGC which has been adopted all over the world (fig. 81). This classification, proposing protruded, flat and excavated

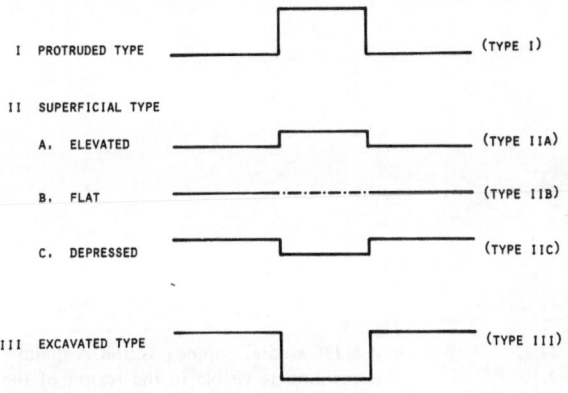

Fig. 81
Macroscopic classification of Early Gastric Cancer.

lesions, can also be applied to carcinomas penetrating deeper than the submucosa (advanced carcinoma). The diffusely infiltrative type of carcinoma (linitis plastica) does not fit comfortably into this classification. In this type of carcinoma there is extensive infiltration of the tumor along the gastric wall causing it to thicken and stiffen. The mucosal surface of the stomach may be slightly nodular and necrotic in some areas and macroscopically intact in

others (176). There is infiltration of the muscularis propria layer.

The author believes that the important rôle of the radiologist in diagnosing gastric carcinoma is to detect potentially malignant lesions. Each gastric ulcer must be regarded as such, even in the absence of any of the numerous more or less reliable signs of malignancy. Furthermore, any irregularity or destruction of the normal mucosal relief and any polypoid lesion – especially those with a diameter larger than 2 cm. or exhibiting surface irregularity – has to be viewed as a potentially malignant lesion. The same rule holds true if a part of the stomach fails to distend under the forces of gravity or palpation, or if stiffness of the gastric wall is noted during fluoroscopic study of peristaltic movements. The converse should also be stated, namely that normal distension, pliability and peristalsis in the presence of an otherwise suspicious lesion do not exclude malignancy (fig. 83). Unless there is an absolute contraindication, all patients showing such lesions, should be submitted to endoscopy.

In order to achieve the highest diagnostic accuracy, several – actually, more than 10 – endoscopically directed biopsy specimens should be taken after painstaking endoscopic inspection of the gastric mucosa (33). When all biopsy specimens are negative in spite of radiological and/or endoscopic doubts, a second gastroscopy must be performed in order to make even more biopsies. In cases of radiological and/or endoscopic evidence of linitis plastica, it should be borne in mind that biopsy is less reliable than in other types of malignancy, because the neoplastic infiltration may be submucosal and the mucosa may remain intact (fig. 92).

This diagnostic approach in most cases permits a preoperative diagnosis of adenocarcinoma. It is only the pathologist who, when determining the depth of carcinomatous infiltration in the resected specimen, is competent to classify a carcinoma as EGC.

Although an extensive description of symptoms is beyond the scope of this chapter, the radiologist should be aware that the symptom pattern of EGC is vague and quite different from the classical symptoms of gastric carcinoma. Some patients do not complain at all. Often longstanding and atypical abdominal symptoms are reported. Hematemesis and melena are infrequent (21, 33, 38, 166). Persistent and vague abdominal complaints in a patient over 30 years of age are an indication for radiological examination. Since carcinomas may arise at any site in the stomach (175), and since EGC is not infrequently located and diagnosed on the anterior wall (63, 239), the examination has to include views of the anterior gastric wall. The standard biphasic-contrast examination fits this purpose well. Then, if even the slightest radiological suspicion is raised or if the patient's symptoms persist in spite of negative radiological findings, gastroscopic examination should follow.

(For further information the reader is referred to the following texts: 98, 183 and 237).

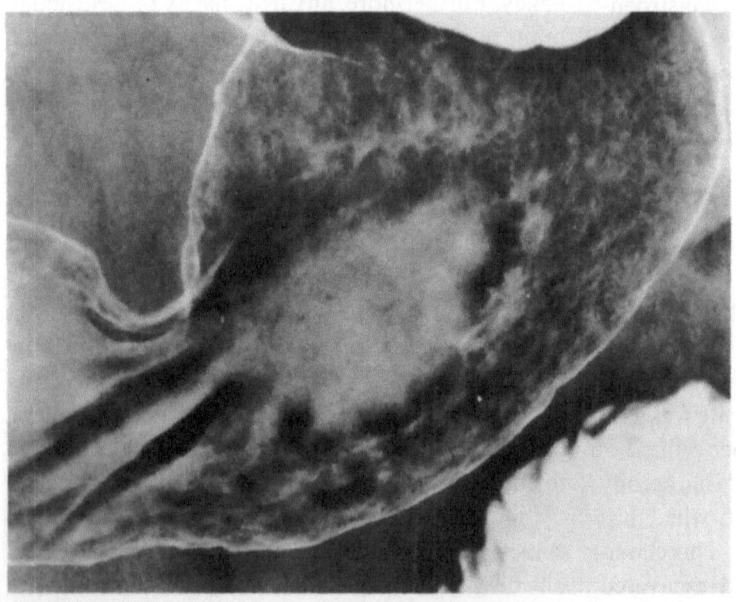

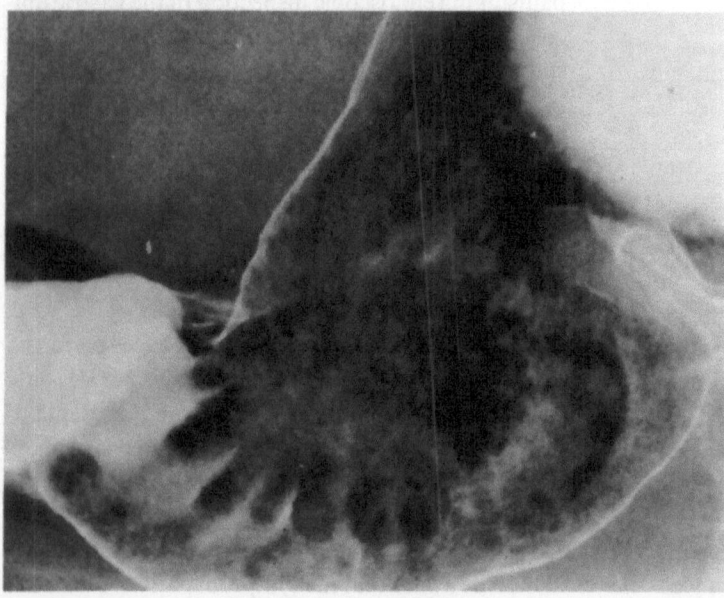

Fig. 83

a & b. DC studies, supine position. A shallow excavation is visible in the region of the angulus on the posterior wall. The folds end far from the center of the lesion. All 15 biopsies taken at gastroscopy showed no other changes than intestinal metaplasia. Three out of 20 biopsy specimens taken at repeat examination showed adenocarcinoma.

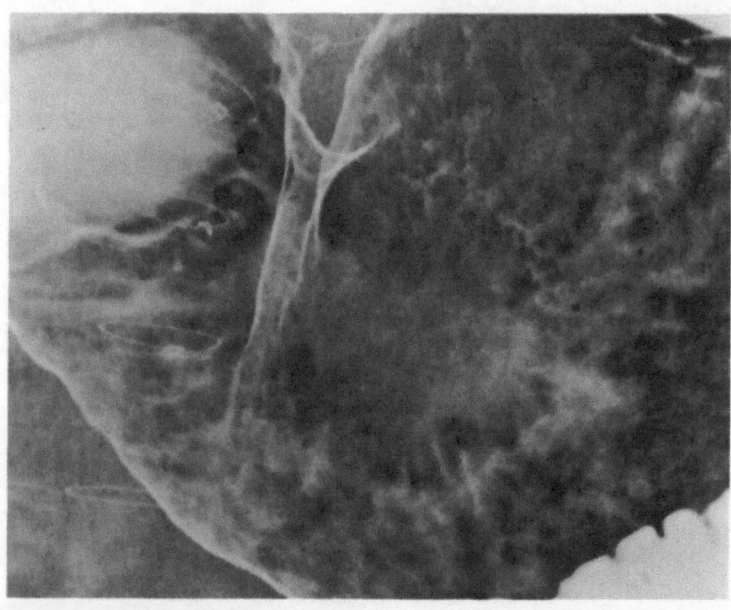

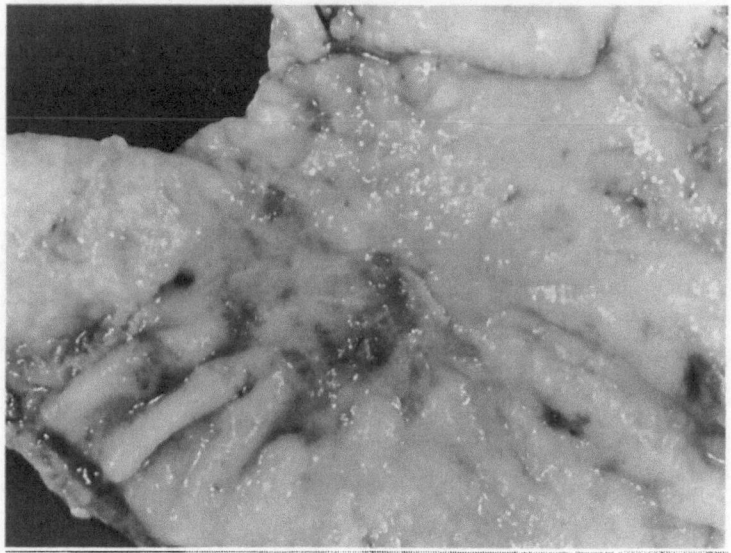

c. DC study made 6 months later. Although the patient had been operated upon, the stomach had not been resected due to unexpected additional difficulties. At both radiological examinations, peristalsis proved to be uninterrupted in the area of the lesion.

d. Resected specimen. Histological examination proved the adenocarcinoma to be restricted to the mucosa (EGC, type IIC). (Reproduced by permission of Radiologia Clinica.)

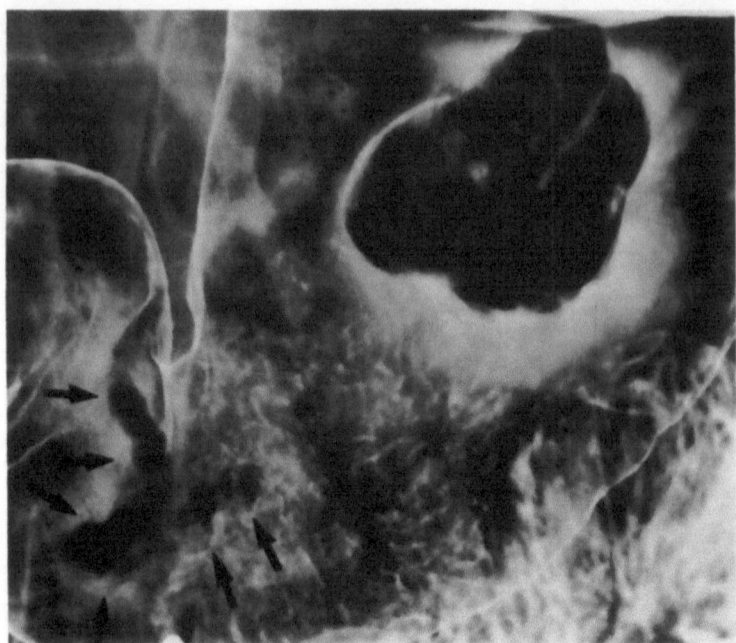

Fig. 82
DC study, supine position. Atrophic mucosal contours of the stomach are visible. There is an irregular polypoid tumor on the posterior wall of the gastric corpus. In the area of the angulus there is a slightly irregular, garland-like elevation (arrows). Biopsy made during endoscopy showed adenocarcinoma. Operation: when the patient was operated, the antral tumor could only be identified with great difficulty. It was shown in the resected specimen that both carcinomas were confined to the submucosa. The lesion in the corpus was of type I; the lesion in the angulus of type IIA. (Reproduced by permission of Radiologia Clinica.)

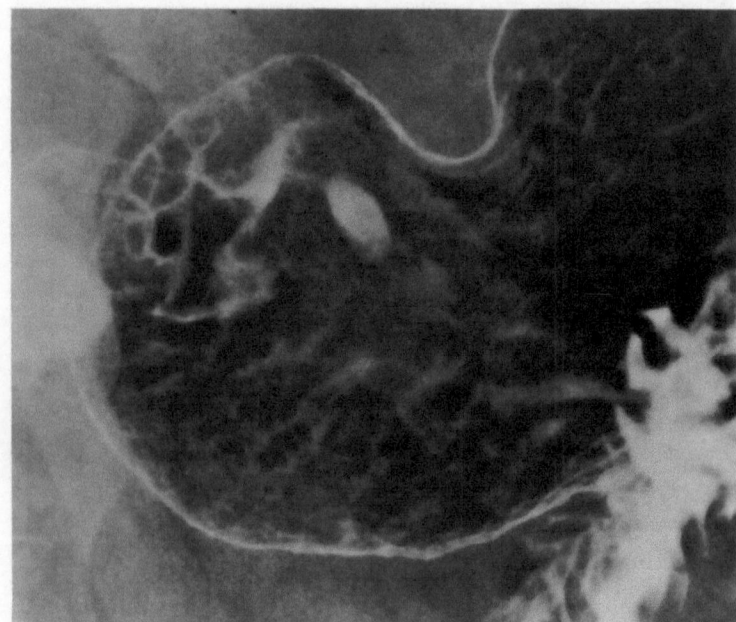

Fig. 84
DC study, supine position, LPO. There is an ulcer niche on the posterior wall of the antrum. The folds end fairly far from the center of this ulcer and they are deformed. Two out of 12 biopsies revealed adenocarcinoma. In the resected specimen the carcinoma was shown to involve the muscularis mucosae (EGC, type III). (Reproduced by permission of Radiologia Clinica.)

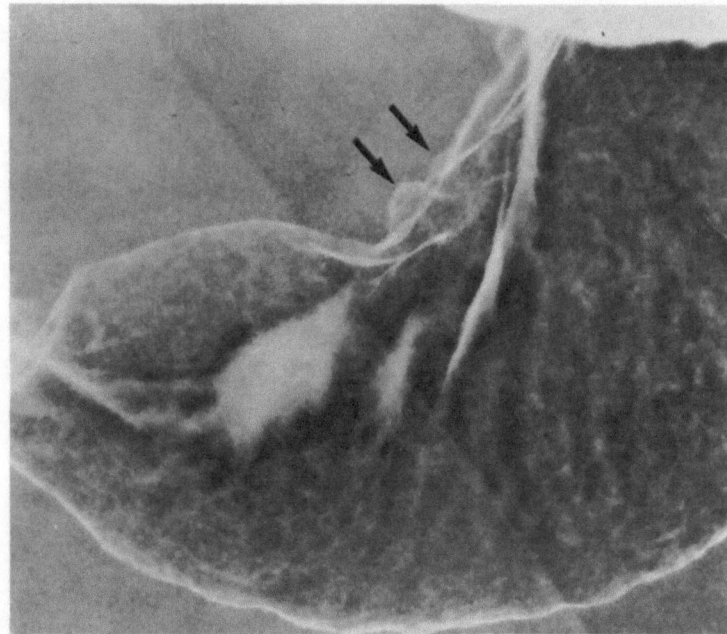

Fig. 85
DC study supine position, LPO. An elevated lesion in the angulus with two ulcer niches (arrows). The appearances are most suggestive of malignancy. Histological report on the 15 biopsies: carcinoma in situ, infiltrative growth cannot be excluded. The resected specimen proved an adenocarcinoma retricted to the mucosa (EGC of a mixed type).

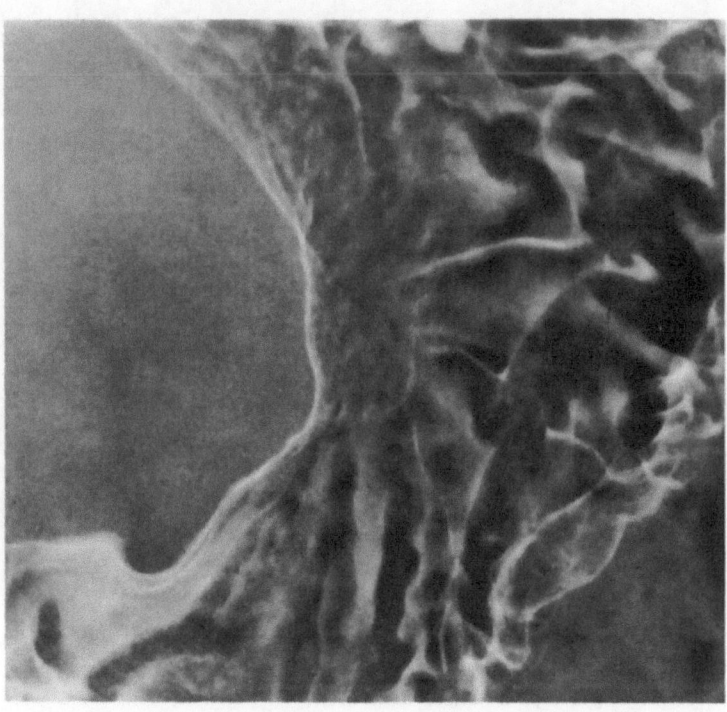

Fig. 86
DC study, supine position. Irregular mucosa is present in the vicinity of the angulus. The radiological appearances suggested that a diagnosis of scarring after a benign gastric ulcer might not be correct, and malignancy could not be excluded. Gastroscopy showed an inflammatory reaction of the mucosa with small erosions in the region of the angulus. There were no signs of malignancy in the biopsy specimens.

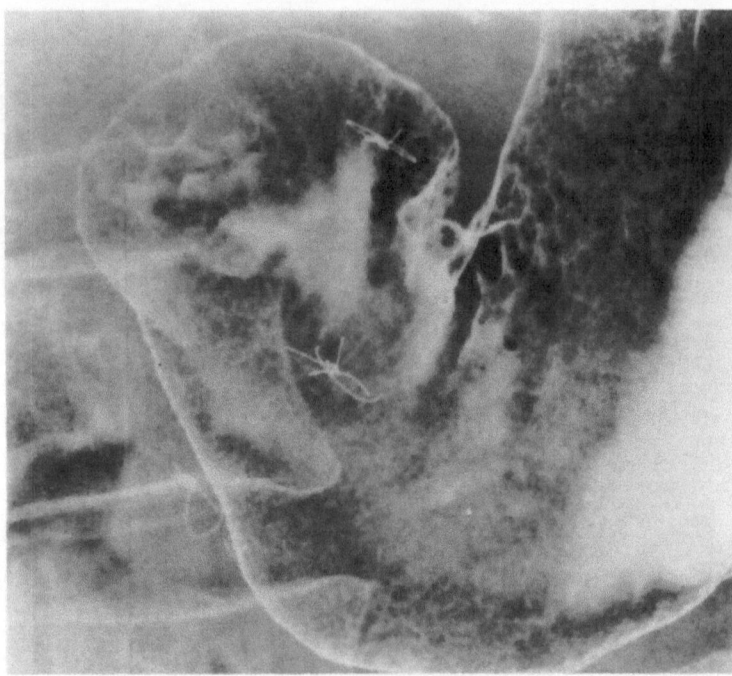

Fig. 87
DC study, supine position, LPO. Several irregular elevated lesions are present in the region of the angulus. The radiologist's report raised the possibility of EGC. Gastroscopy showed only a slightly irregular benign-looking angulus. Biopsies revealed a non-specific inflammation with epithelial atypia.

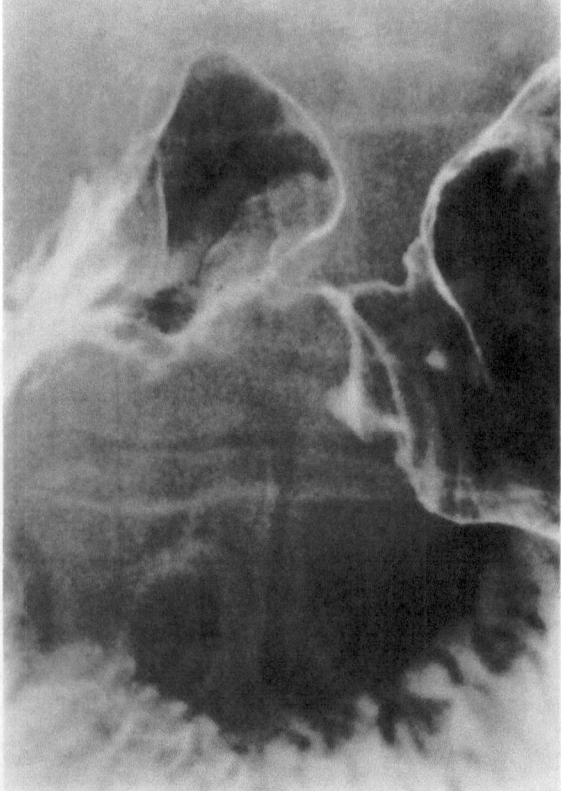

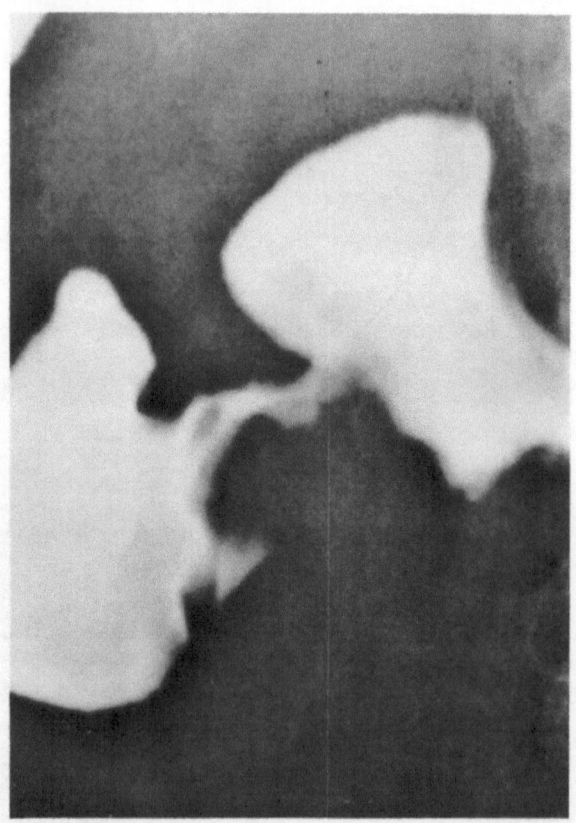

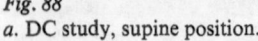

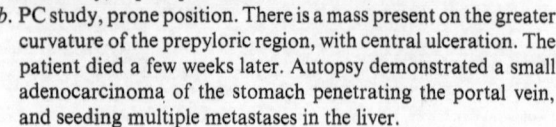

Fig. 88
a. DC study, supine position.
b. PC study, prone position. There is a mass present on the greater curvature of the prepyloric region, with central ulceration. The patient died a few weeks later. Autopsy demonstrated a small adenocarcinoma of the stomach penetrating the portal vein, and seeding multiple metastases in the liver.

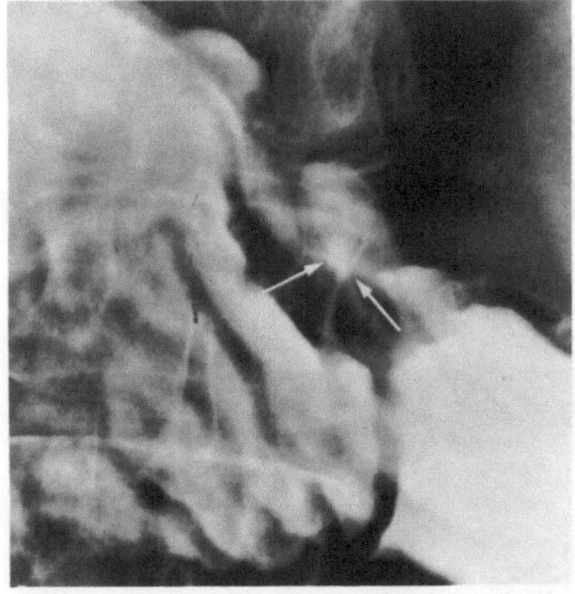

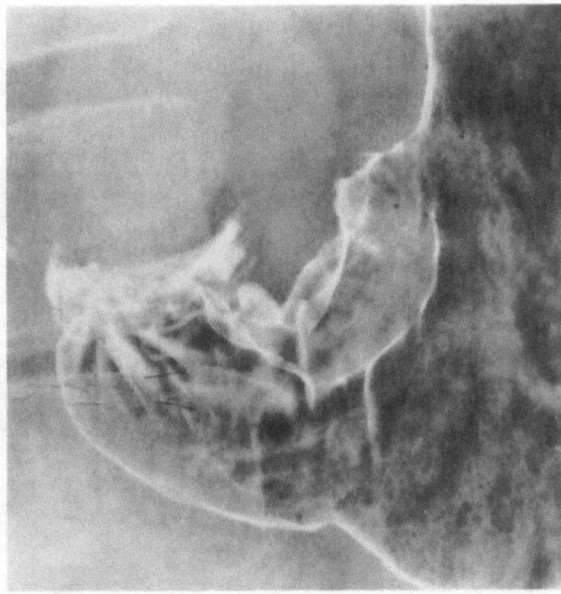

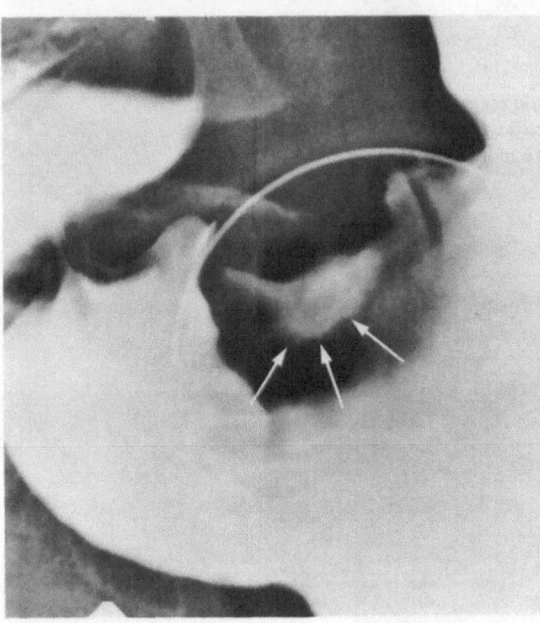

Fig. 89

a. PC study, prone position.

b. DC study, supine position, LPO.

c. PC compression study, erect position, LPO. Typical Kirklin complex consisting of Carman's meniscus sign (arrows), trapped barium collection being convex towards the lumen of the stomach, and an elevated ridge (186, 188). All the barium lies within the line of the normal gastric wall. This complex is most suspicious of a disc-shaped carcinoma with central ulceration. Biopsies: adenocarcinoma. Resected specimen: infiltration of the muscularis propria by malignant cells.

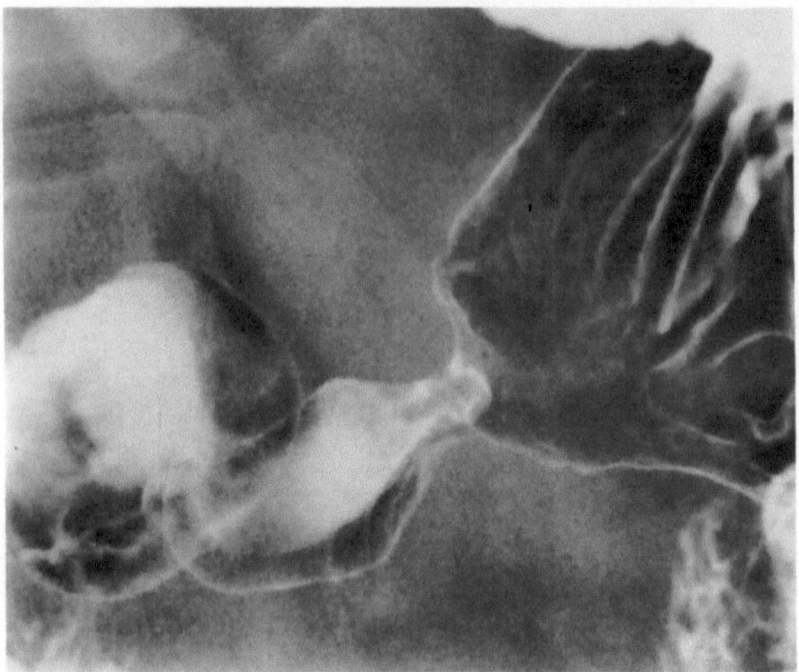

Fig. 90
DC study, supine position, LPO. There is a stricture of the prepyloric region which has
appearances suggesting linitis plastica. Biopsy: adenocarcinoma. Resected specimen: adenocarcinoma with infiltration of all layers of the gastric wall and the surrounding fatty tissue,
linitis plastica.

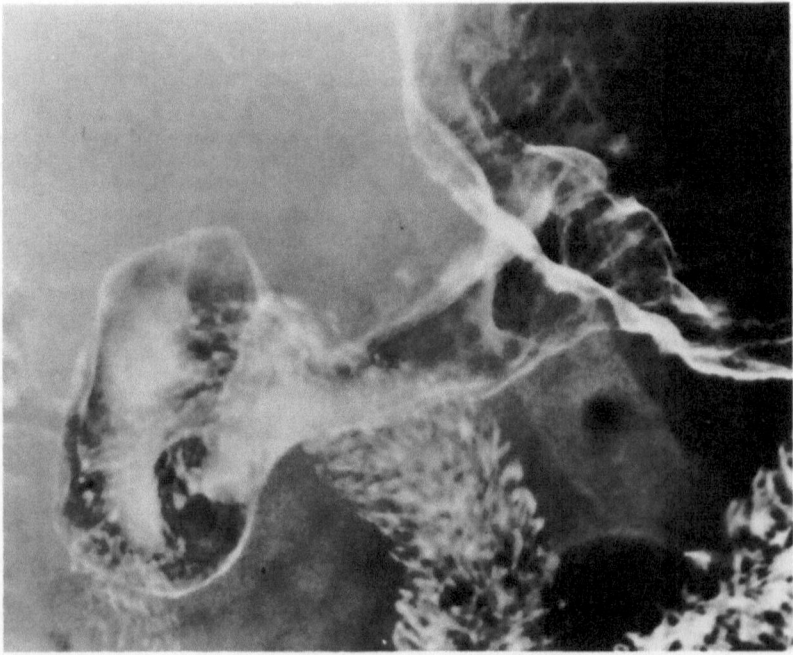

Fig. 91
DC study, supine position, LPO. There is an abruptly marginated stricture extending from
the angulus to within several centimeters of the pylorus. The prepyloric region distends well.
Biopsy: adenocarcinoma. Resected specimen: adenocarcinoma with infiltration of all layers
of the gastric wall and the surrounding fatty tissue.

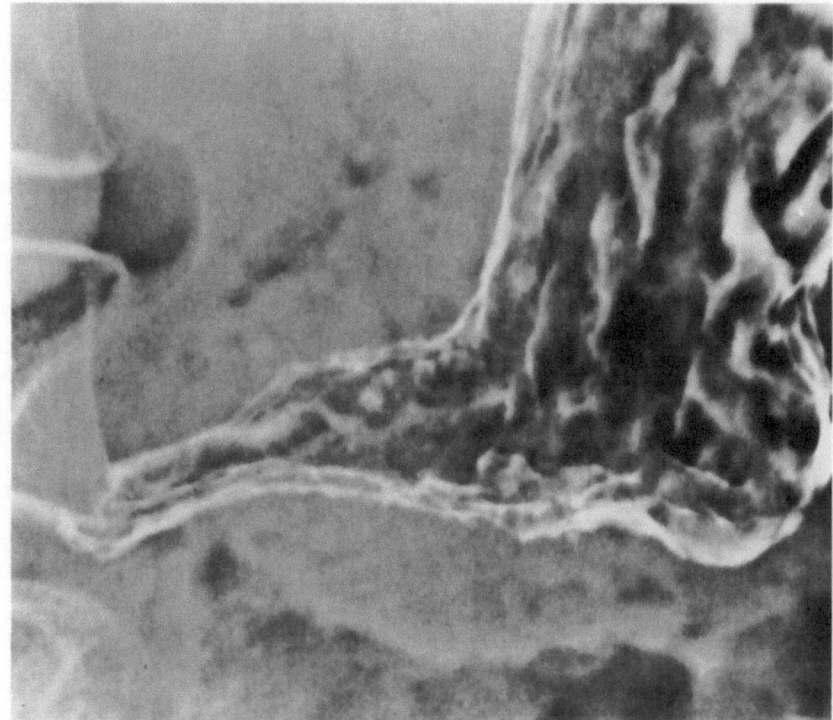

Fig. 92
DC study, supine position, LPO. There is narrowing of the antrum, appearances most suspicious of a linitis plastica. No peristaltic waves passed through the antrum. Gastroscopy: erosive gastritis in the region of the angulus; narrowing of the antrum, no peristalsis; appearances suspicious of a linitis plastica. Biopsies: chronic inflammation. At a second gastroscopy 2 large particle biopsies were taken, which again revealed chronic inflammation and no signs of malignancy. Resected specimen: linitis plastica with infiltration of the surrounding fatty tissue.

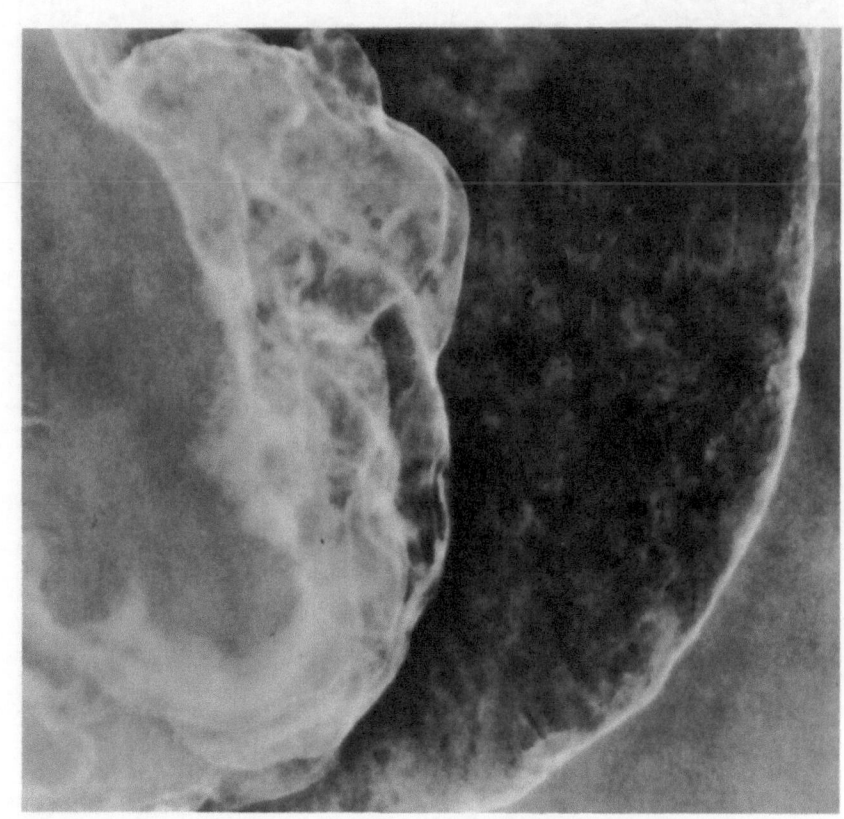

Fig. 93
DC study, supine position, LPO. There is a polypoid malignant tumor on the lesser curvature of the lower part of the corpus and the antrum. Gastroscopy: polypoid malignant tumor; atrophic gastric mucosa. Laparoscopy: histologically-confirmed metastases in the omentum. No operation.

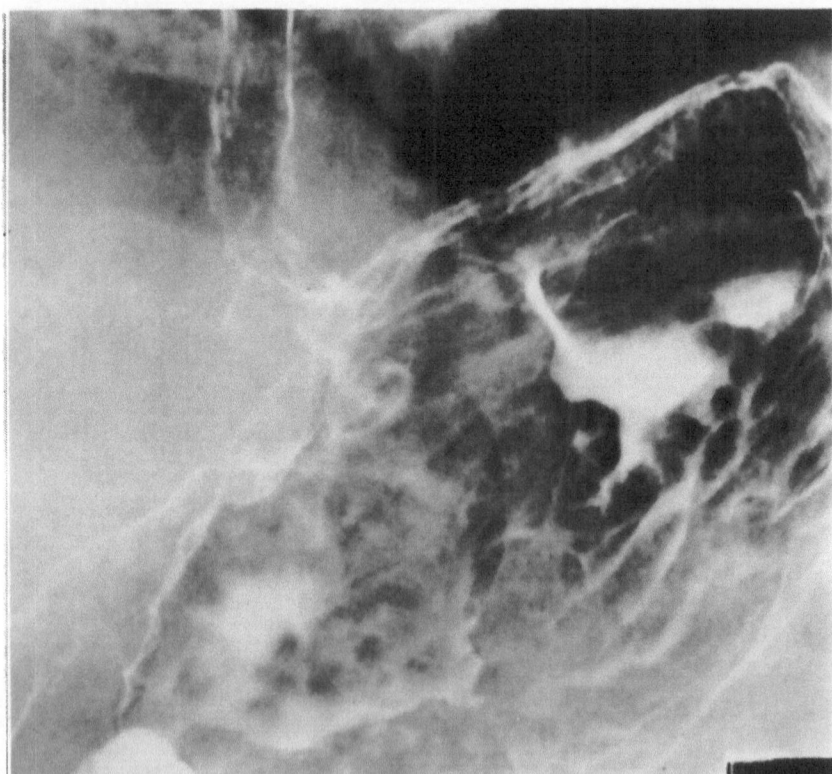

Fig. 94
DC study, supine position, LPO: table 40° anti-Trendelenburg. There is a large irregular filling defect in the fundus which extends into the lower esophagus. Gastroscopy: malignancy of the cardia fundus and upper part of the corpus. Gastrobiopsy: adenocarcinoma. The tumor was considered unresectable. A biopsy taken from the liver at laparoscopy revealed a metastasis in the liver.

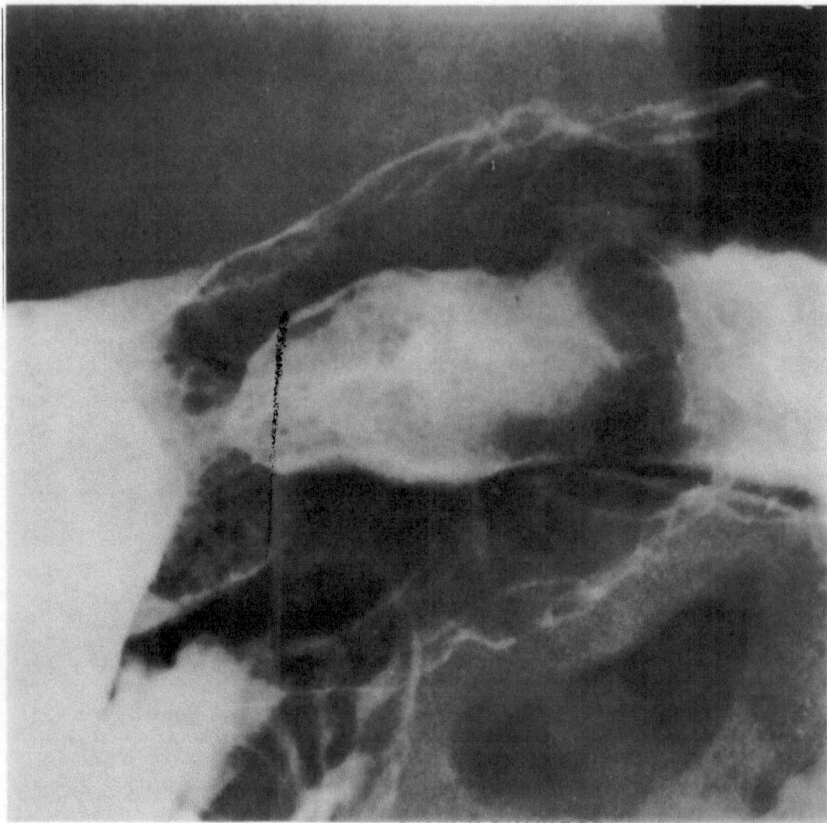

Fig. 95
DC study, supine position, LPO: table 40° anti-Trendelenburg. There is a large, flat irregularly-marginated ulcer niche in the upper corpus, with appearances suspicious of malignancy. Two series of biopsies failed to confirm malignancy. Biopsies taken at operation proved adenocarcinoma. The tumor was considered unresectable.

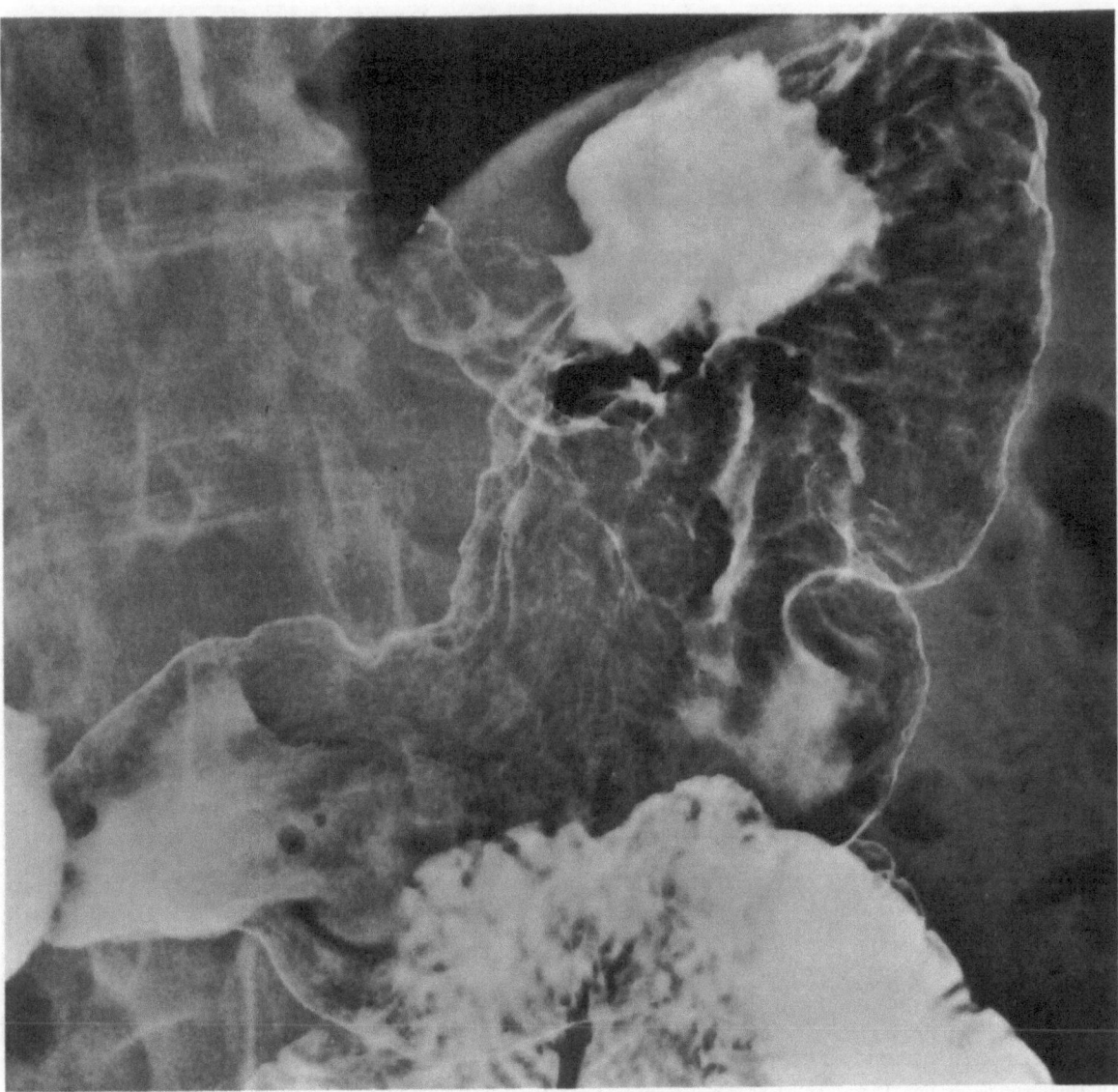

Fig. 96
DC study, supine position. There is an extensive and irregular malignant lesion extending from the lower esophagus to the lesser curvature of the antrum. Gastrobiopsy: adenocarcinoma. The tumor was considered unresectable.

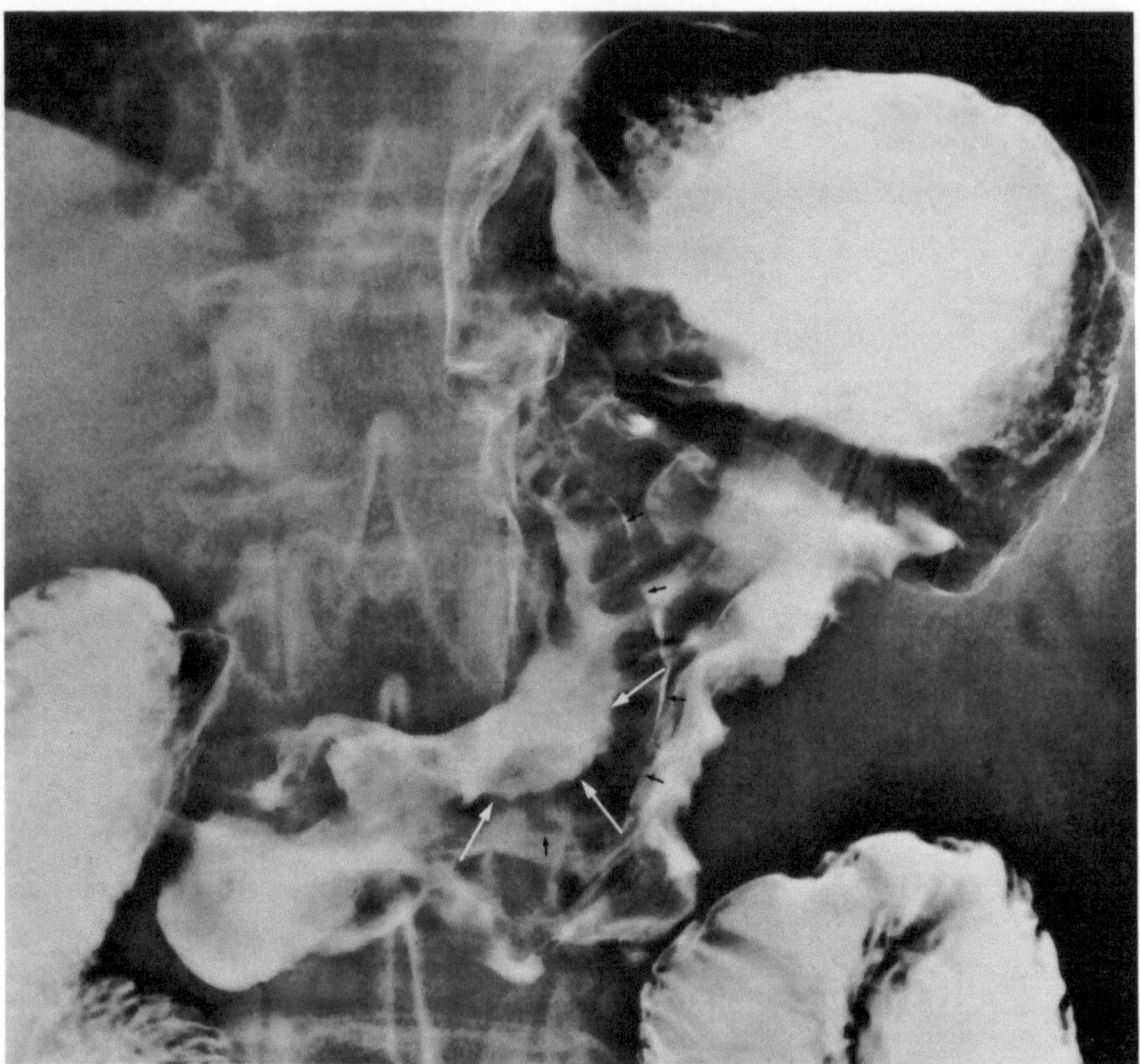

Fig. 97
DC study, supine position. There is an extensive malignant process extending from the fundus to the prepyloric region. A typical Kirklin complex is present in the region of the angulus (arrows); note the nodular elevated edge of the niche. Gastrobiopsy: adenocarcinoma. Resected specimen: infiltration of the muscularis propria by tumor cells.

7.7. Malignant tumors other than carcinomas

The most frequently encountered malignant neoplasm of the stomach after carcinoma is malignant lymphoma. An incidence of between 0.4 and 9 per cent of all neoplasms is reported (112, 172, 185). Hodgkin's disease itself is rare – 4-21 per cent of malignant lymphomas (180, 185). Other sarcomas are less frequently found, the most common one being leiomyosarcoma. The remaining non-carcinomatous tumors are clinical curiosities (112).

7.7.1. MALIGNANT LYMPHOMA

Malignant lymphoma develops in the gastric mucosa, from which the tumor cells infiltrate into the submucosa and muscular layers (179). This mode of spread is similar to that of carcinoma. Malignant gastric lymphoma may be either limited to the stomach or part of a disseminated disease.

Several authors (163, 184) have studied and described the radiological pattern in lymphomas. The majority of patients have large abnormal folds, often involving a long segment of the stomach. Diffuse infiltration produces a pattern of concentric pathological folds without significantly narrowing the lumen. None of these naked-eye features of lymphoma is pathognomonic. Lymphoma and carcinoma may be confused at operation (112) or upon inspection of the gross specimen (179). Malignant lymphoma located within the gastric antrum tends to involve the duodenal bulb by transpyloric submucosal extension (164). Since this also occurs in carcinoma, this mode of extension is not diagnostic of malignant lymphoma (139) (figs. 101, 102). As in gastric carcinoma, the radiologist's task is to determine whether the lesion he identifies may be malignant. Only gastroscopy permits a preoperative histological diagnosis.

7.7.2. LEIOMYOSARCOMA

Leiomyosarcoma resembles leiomyoma macroscopically, and no radiological differential diagnosis is possible. The overlying mucosa is often ulcerated. As in leiomyoma, the submucosal origin of leiomyosarcoma can easily be recognized in tumors with a diameter of more than 1 cm. (see chapter 7, section 5). Biopsy is often false-negative, due to the extraepithelial origin of the tumor.

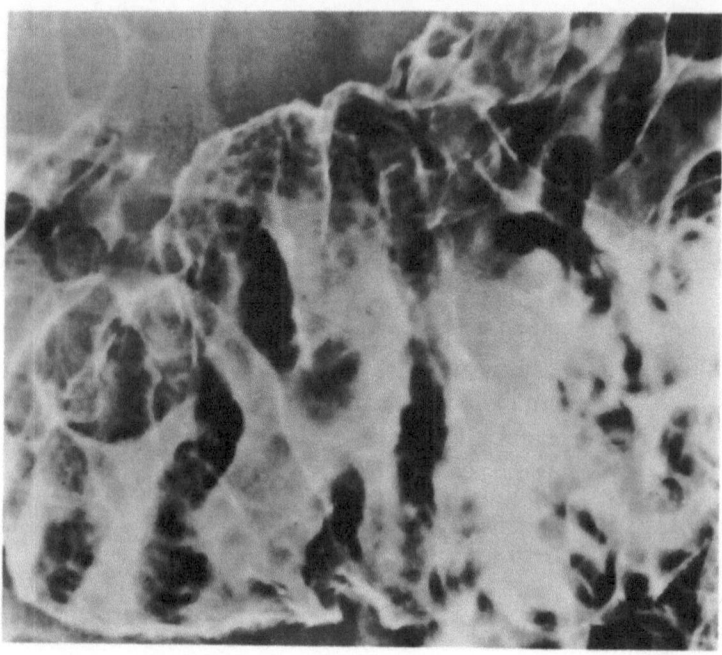

Fig. 98
DC study, supine position, LPO. Coarse folds
with irregular margins in the antrum. The endoscopist considered "hypertrophic gastritis." Biopsies were compatible with malignant lymphoma; those of the rectal mucosa
were diagnostic of malignant lymphoma.

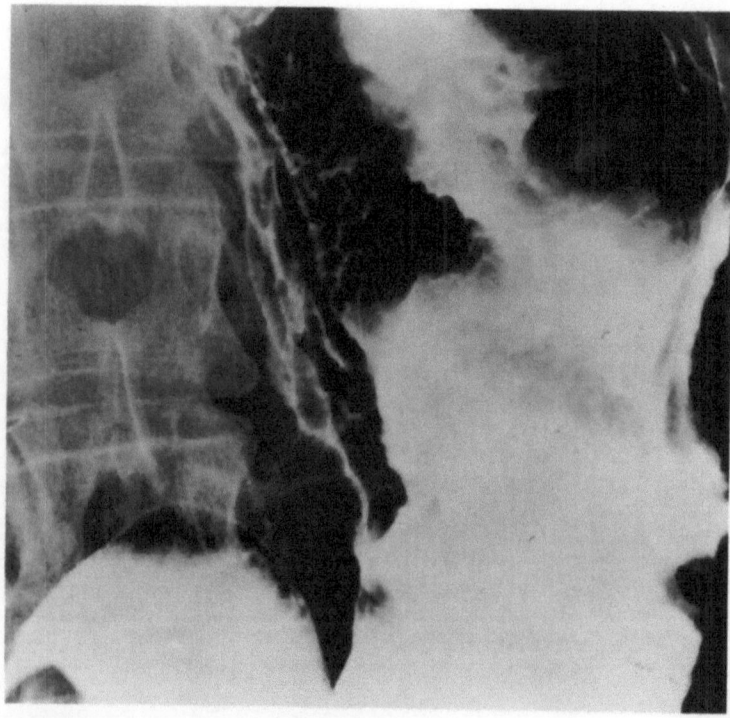

Fig. 99
DC study, supine position. Irregular mucosa
with very coarse areae gastricae in the vicinity
of the lesser curvature of the corpus. Two
years before a wedge resection for an ulcer of
the lesser curvature was performed. This was a
benign ulcer as proved by the histological
examination of the resected specimen. The appearance of the lesser curvature, however, is
most suspicious of a malignant lesion. Biopsies proved a malignant non-Hodgkin lymphoma.

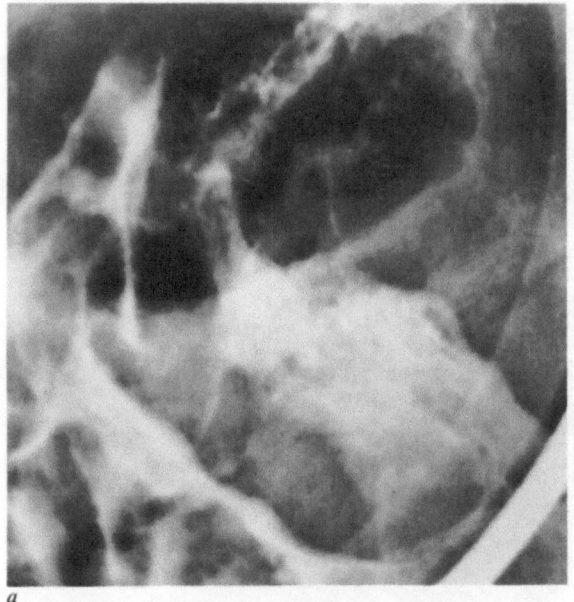

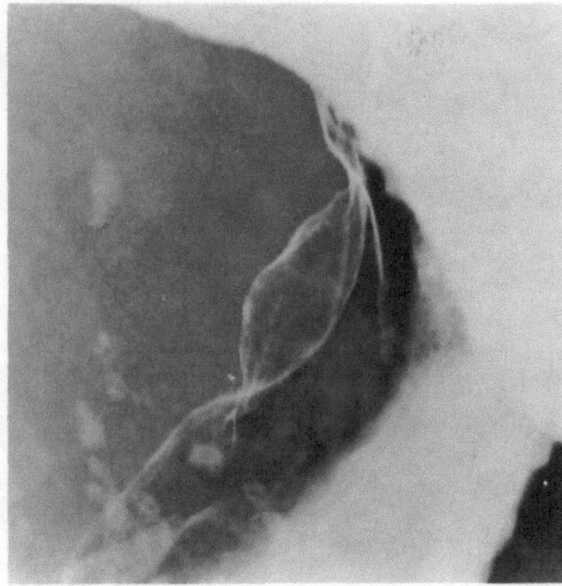

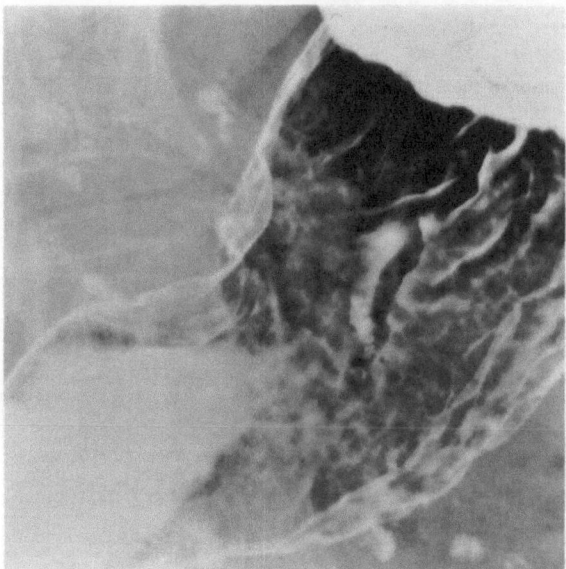

Fig. 100
a. Mucosal relief study, prone position.
b. DC study, supine position, LPO. This patient was previously
   irradiated for Hodgkin's disease. Large ulcer niche in the region of the angulus. The base of the crater lies in the line of the
   normal gastric wall. Kirklin complex. Appearance most suspicious of a malignant lesion. The biopsies proved malignant
   lymphoma; further histological differentiation was impossible.
c. Repeat examination under identical conditions after a 4 months'
   treatment with cytostatics showing some improvement.

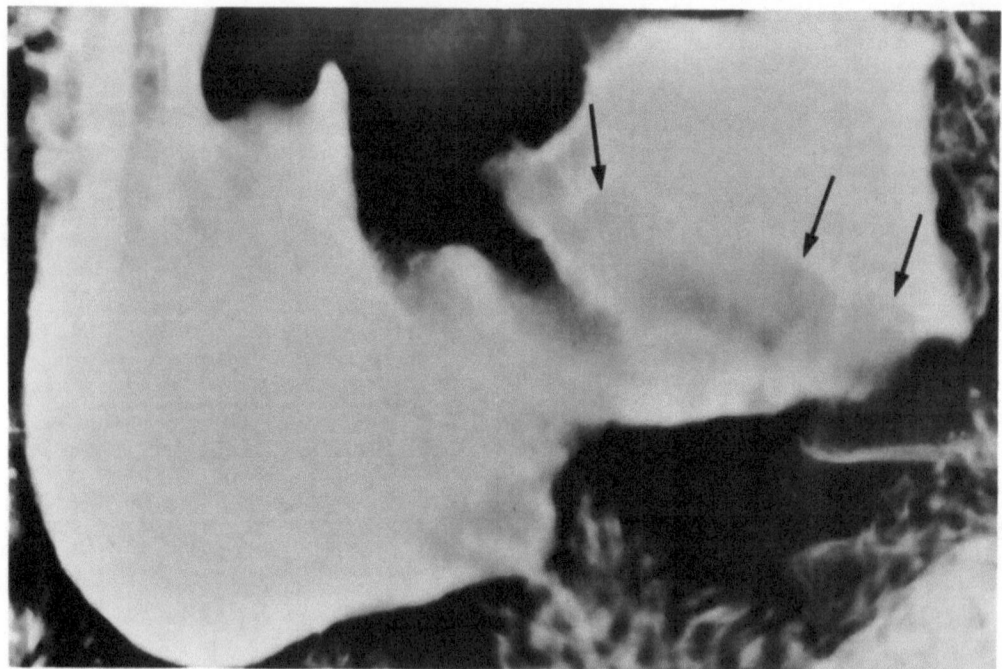

Fig. 101
PC study, prone position. Large lesion suggestive of a malignant tumor of the antrum with involvement of the duodenal bulb (arrows).

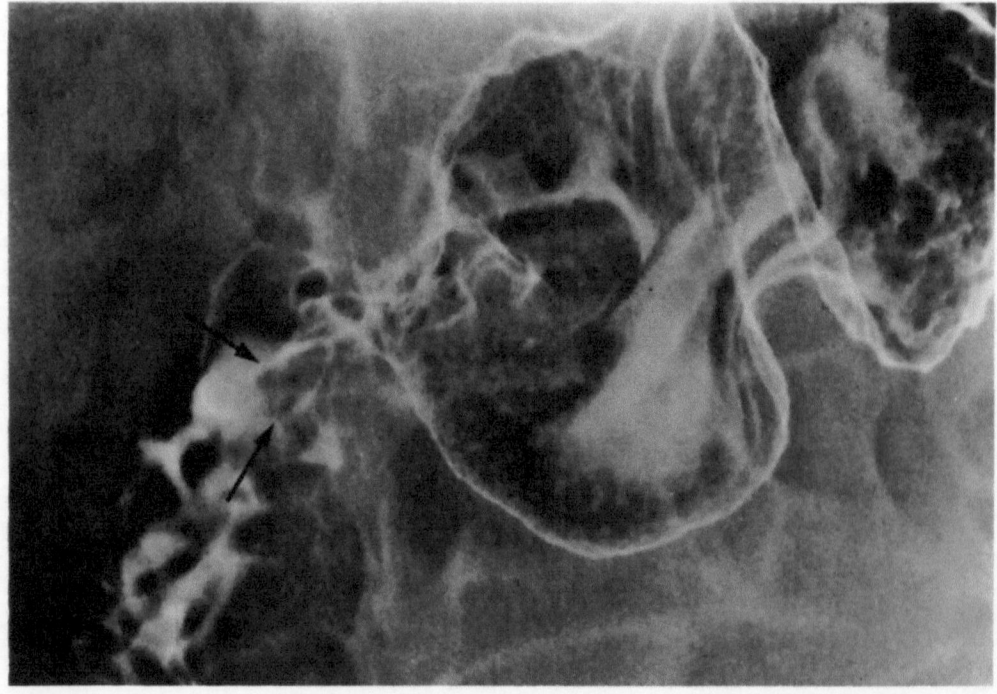

Fig. 102
DC study, supine position, LPO. Stricture of the prepyloric region suggesting a malignant lesion; probably involvement of the base of the duodenal bulb (arrows). Gastroscopy: malignant stenosis. Biopsies: adenocarcinoma. At operation the tumor was considered to be unresectable.

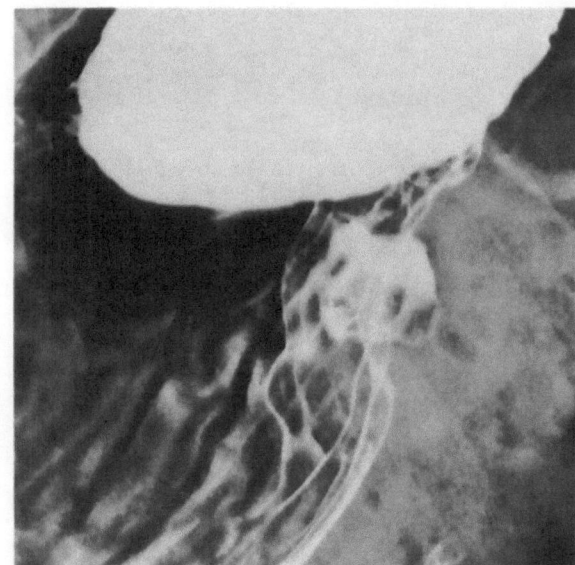

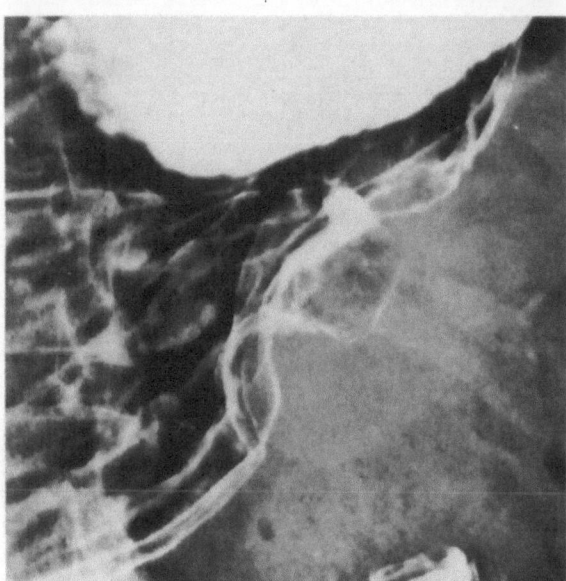

7.8. Metastatic tumors

Metastatic deposits in the stomach are rare. The primary tumors most likely to seed to the stomach are malignant melanoma, bronchogenic carcinoma and cancer of the breast (27, 81, 263). The diagnosis can also be made if multiple mass lesions with or without central dimpling (which may occur with or without ulceration) occur in the presence of a known primary tumor.

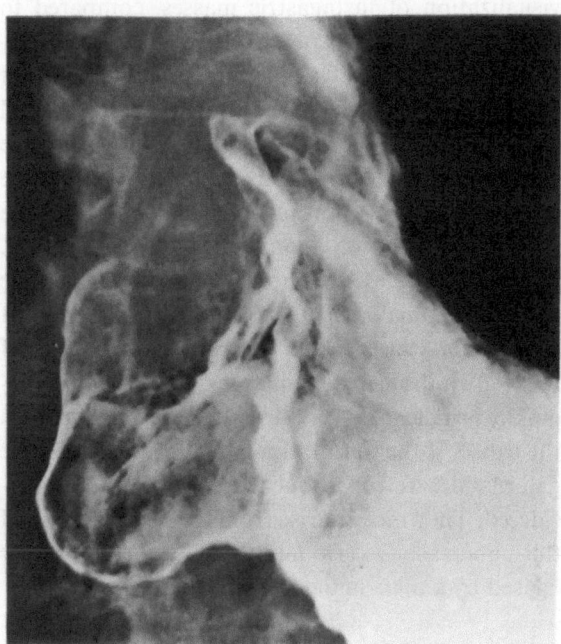

Fig. 103
a. DC study, supine position.
b. DC study, supine position, RPO. Protrusion with a diameter of more than 1 cm. with gently sloping edges on the greater curvature of the higher corpus. Central ulceration. Appearances suggest a tumor of submucosal origin, either a leiomyoma or a leiomyosarcoma. Histological examination of the resected specimen revealed a leiomyosarcoma.

Fig. 104
DC study, prone position. Filling defect in the fundus of a patient with multiple metastases of a malignant melanoma in the gastrointestinal tract. This mass lesion is also supposed to be a metastasis. (Courtesy of Department of Radiology, Leiden University Hospital, Leiden, The Netherlands.)

7.9. Indentations

An indentation of a hollow viscus which is caused by an extrinsic mass not fixed to that viscus, is inconstant under the forces of gravity, respiration or palpation. This fact is the basis of the differential diagnosis between an intramural mass and an indentation caused by extrinsic mass (128) (figs. 105, 106). An extrinsic mass fixed to the wall of a hollow viscus causes an indentation that is fairly constant. Such an indentation cannot be differentiated in a simple way from the configuration caused by an intramural mass (47). Diagnostic pneumoperitoneum (fig. 107) may assist.

Hypotonic DC gastrography greatly enhances the visualization of juxtagastric masses, compared to conventional radiography of the stomach. (The increased diagnostic yield may be compared to that of hypotonic DC duodenography versus conventional examination of the duodenum). Apart from the classical indentations, the hypotonic DC technique frequently reveals a normal dorsal indentation of the posterior wall in the region of the angulus (figs. 115, 116), produced by the duodenojejunal flexure. The gall-bladder may indent the lateral dorsal aspect of the antrum – the so-called "antral pad sign" (244). If this indentation is demonstrated, oral cholecystography is indicated to confirm that the gall-bladder is the cause. If the indentation is not produced by the gall-bladder, retroperitoneal masses have to be considered. They mostly arise from the head or body of the pancreas. Occasionally an antral pad sign is caused by a mass in the liver.

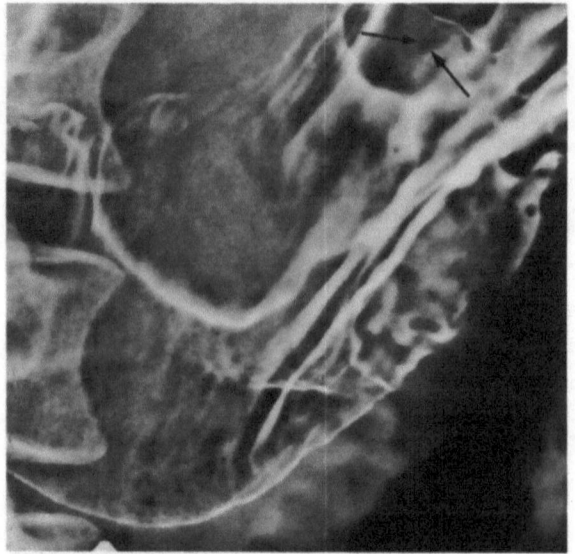

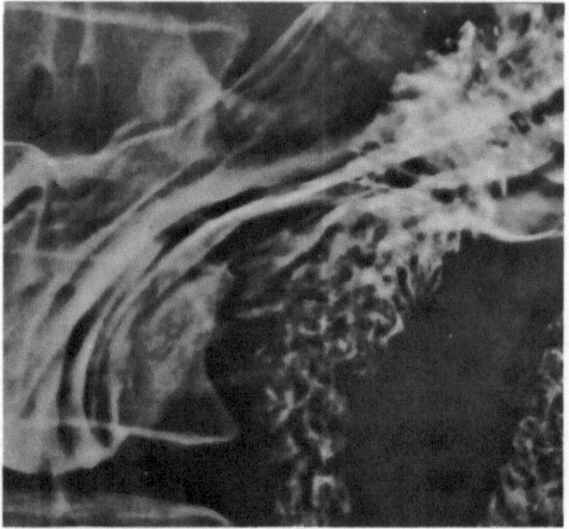

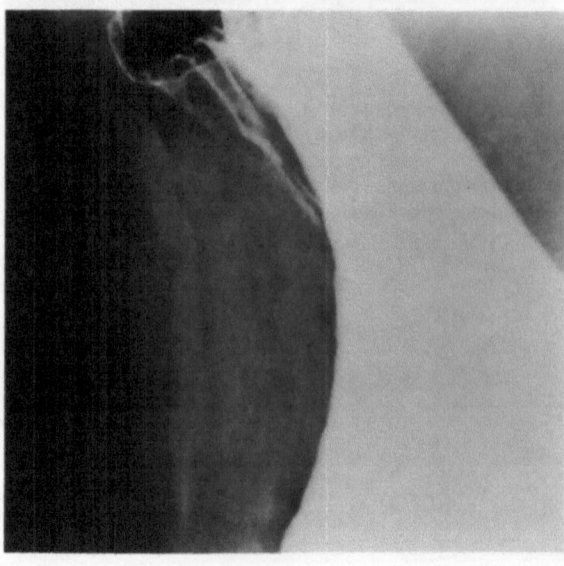

Fig. 105

a & b. DC studies, supine position. Filling defect in the region of the angulus. The filling defect changes during the respiration which indicates that we are dealing with an impression. In the region of the angulus a fold that can be located on the posterior wall which is seen to proceed in the region of the filling defect (arrows). This indicates that the indentation must be localised on the anterior wall (cf. Fig. 19).

c. PC study, lateral view, which confirms that the indentation is an anterior one. Operation: fibroma of the sheath of the rectus abdominis muscle.

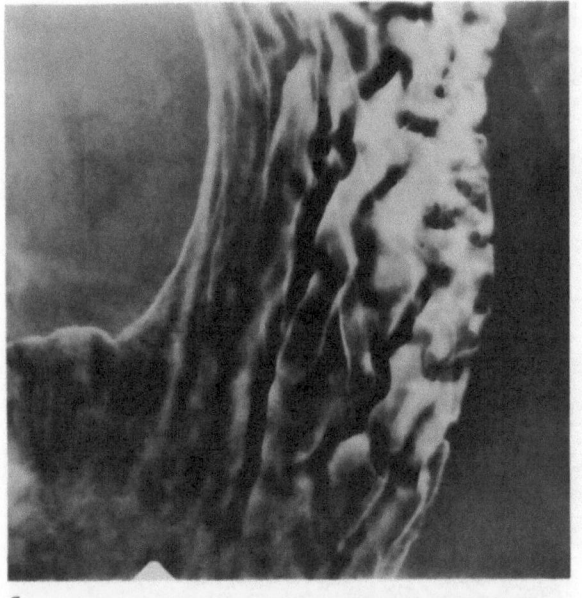

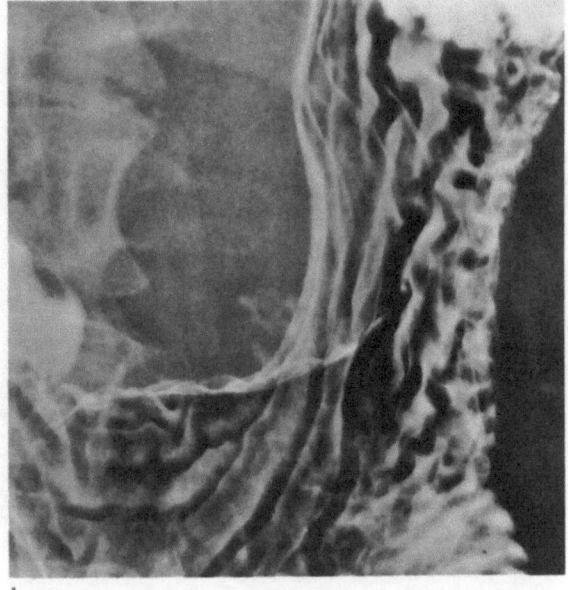

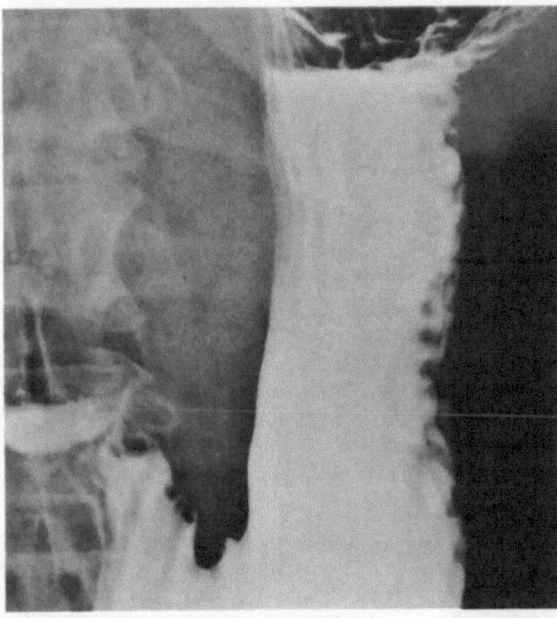

Fig. 106
a & *b*. DC studies, supine position.
c. PC study, erect position. Filling defect on the lesser curvature aspect just above the angulus. The filling defect is inconstant during changes of the forces of gravity. This is very characteristic of an indentation. At operation metastases of an adenocarcinoma of unknown origin were found in the liver.

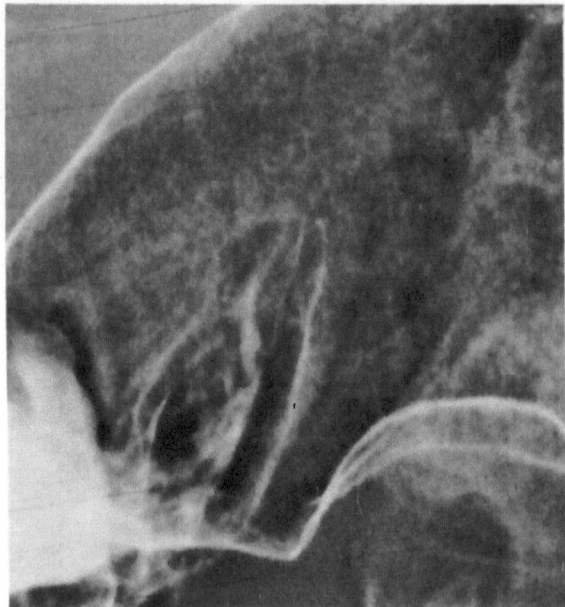

a

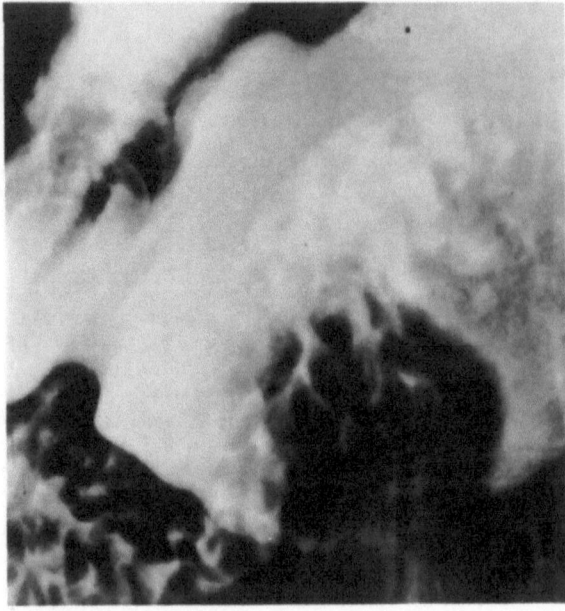

b

Fig. 107

a. DC study, supine position.

b. PC compression study, erect position. Filling defect on the greater curvature of the antrum that is constantly present. The form of the mass changes under the forces of gravity. It is impossible to differentiate between an intramural mass and an indentation caused by an extrinsic mass fixed to the gastric wall. The endoscopist observed uninterrupted peristaltic waves and considered an extrinsic mass.

c. Diagnostic pneumoperitoneum delineated an extragastric mass. Because no gas was seen between the mass (white arrows) and the gastric wall (black arrows), the mass was considered to be fixed to the wall. At operation an extragastric tumor connected to a stalk to the greater curvature was found. Histological examination revealed a leiomyoma.

c

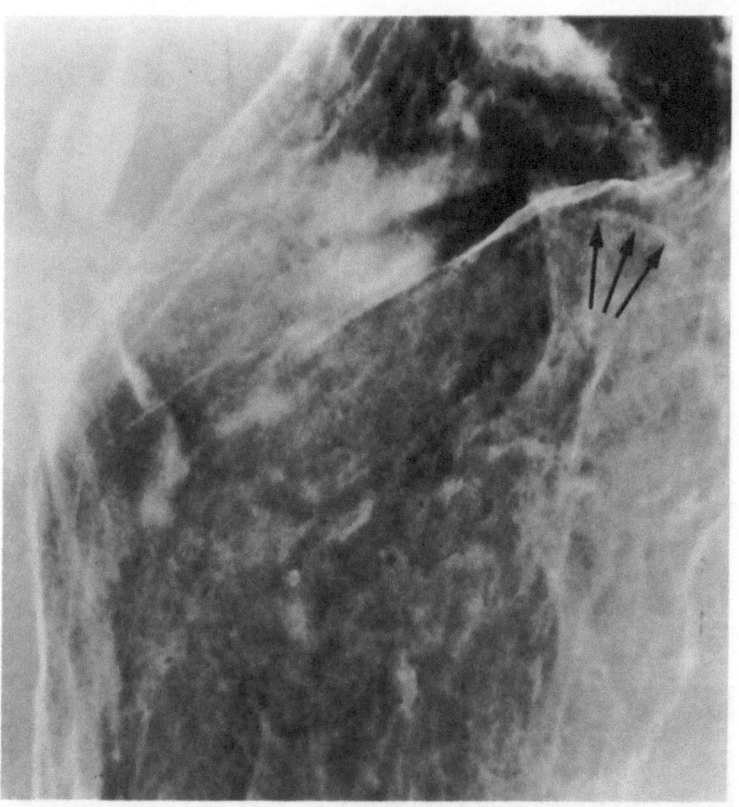

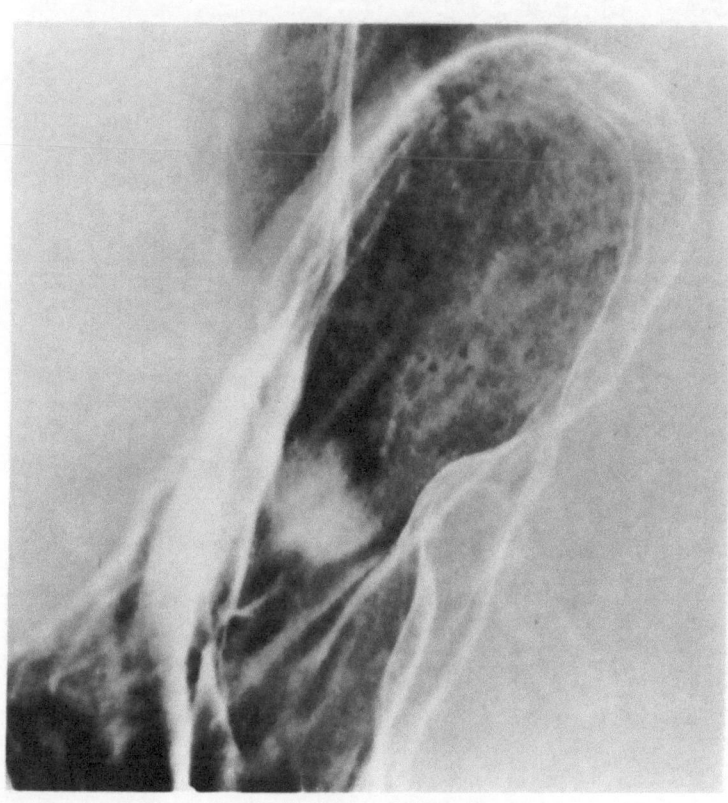

Fig. 108

a. DC study, supine position, RPO, table about 30° anti-Trendelenburg. Ridge-like impression on the posterior wall of the fundus. The orally convex calcification (arrows) strongly suggests an impression caused by the splenic artery.

b. DC study, lateral view, confirming that the indentation is caused by the splenic artery.

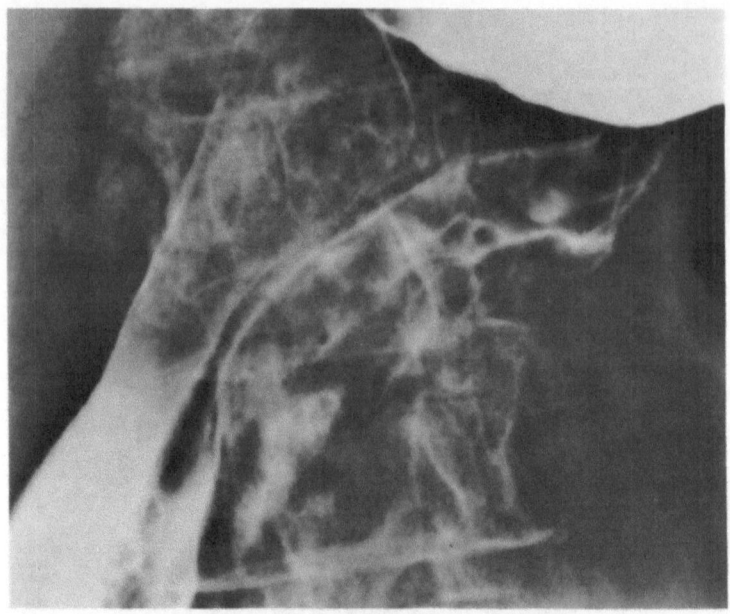

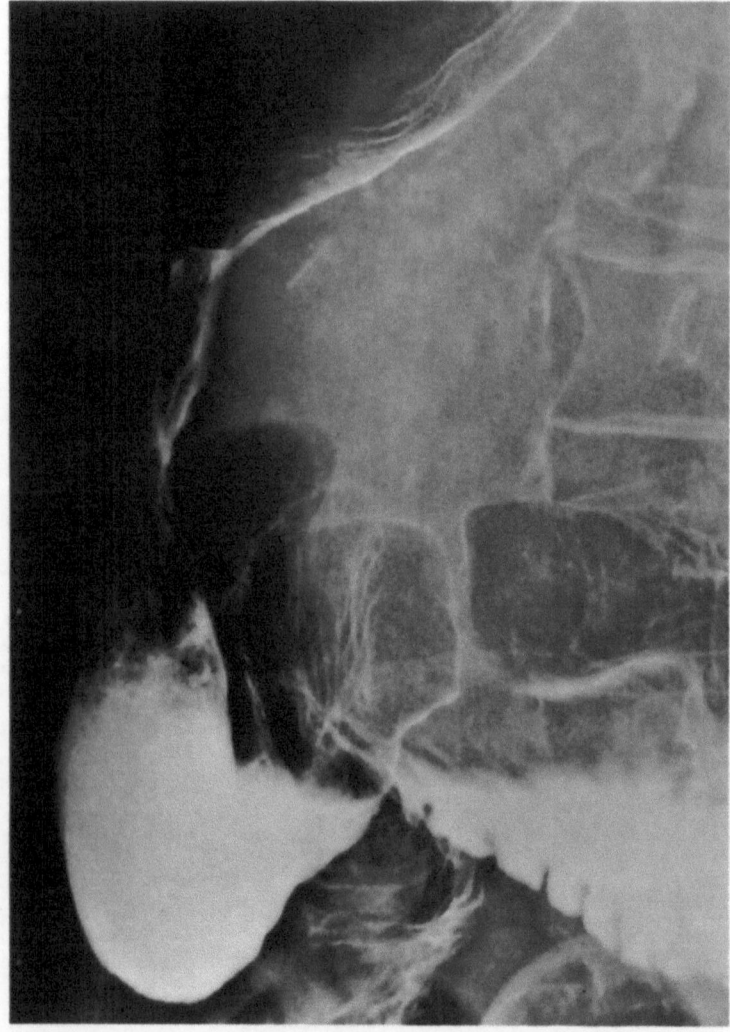

Fig. 109

a. DC study, supine position, table slightly
   anti-Trendelenburg. Filling defect on the
   greater curvature side of the higher corpus.
   The aspect of this filling defect was inconstant during the changing forces of gravity
   as observed fluoroscopically. This indicates
   that we are dealing with an impression.

b. Nearly erect position, RPO. This film demonstrates that the impression is caused by
   an aneurysm of the abdominal aorta.

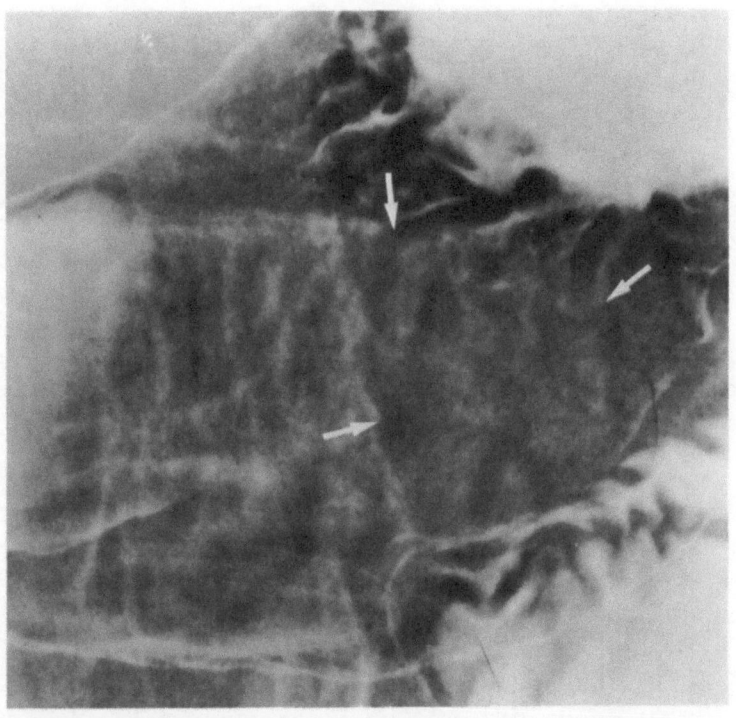

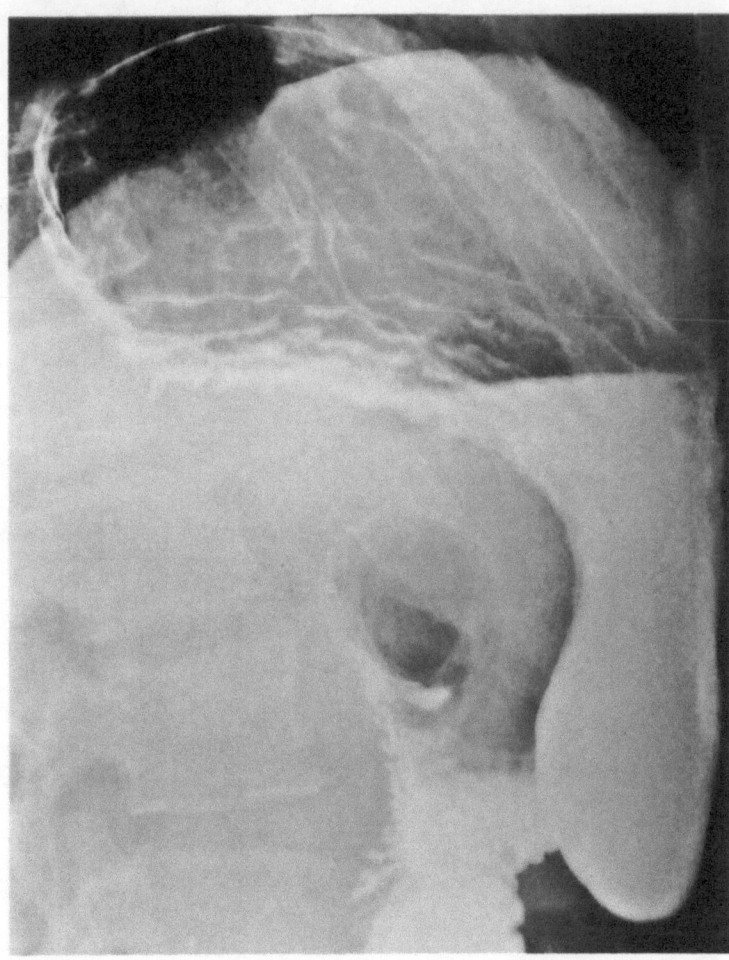

Fig. 110

a. DC study, supine position. The folds of the posterior wall near the gastric angulus are effaced (arrows). The picture is most suggestive of an impression.

b. Erect position, lateral view. The indentation is clearly demonstrated and is in all probability caused by a mass in the corpus of the pancreas. A further examination including pancreatic echography and a clinical follow-up, were highly in favour of the diagnosis chronic pancreatitis.

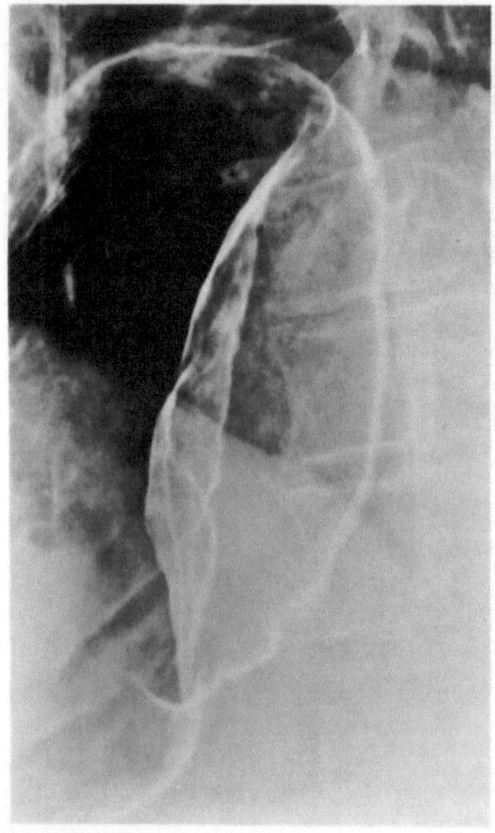

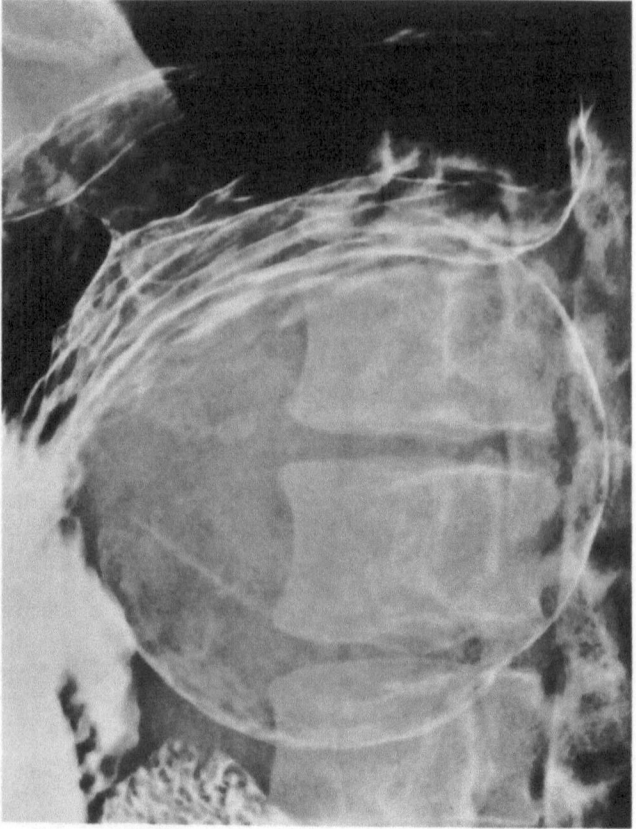

Fig. 111
DC study, nearly lateral view; table about 50° anti-Trendelenburg. Impression on the dorsal aspect of the fundus. Isotope studies and echography demonstrated a splenic cyst.

Fig. 112
DC study, patient nearly erect, RPO. Indentation of the dorsal aspect of the fundus and the corpus caused by a splenic cyst with a calcified wall. Histological examination after operation confirmed the diagnosis benign splenic cyst.

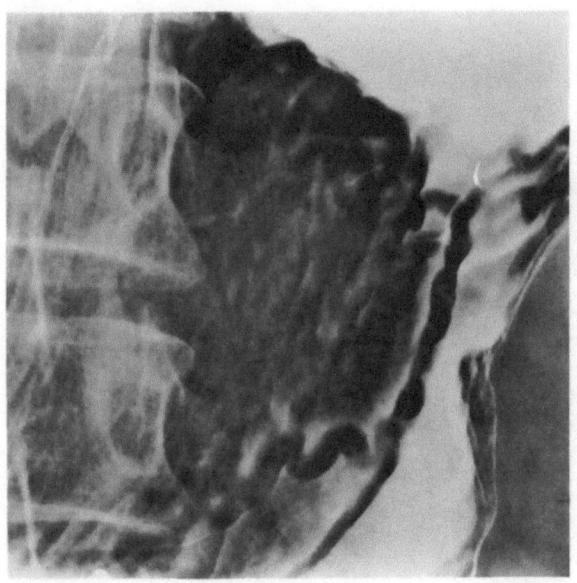 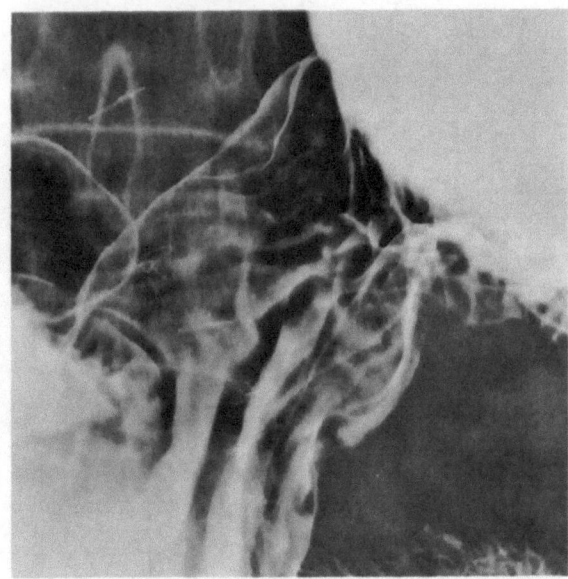

a   b

Fig. 113

a. DC study, supine position. The folds on the posterior aspect of
   the corpus are effaced.
b. A different view of the posterior wall of the corpus. There is less
   gaseous distension. This changing appearance favors the diagnosis: indentation of the posterior wall.
c. Supine position, horizontal beam projection. This film clearly
   demonstrates the indentation. At operation a carcinoma in the
   pancreatic corpus was found.

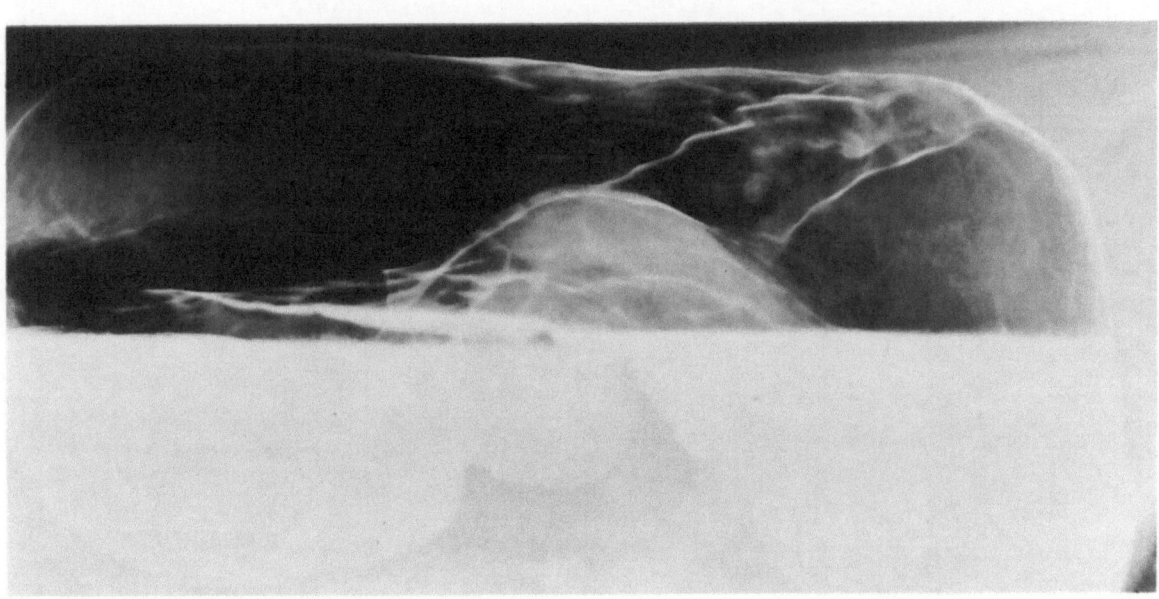

c

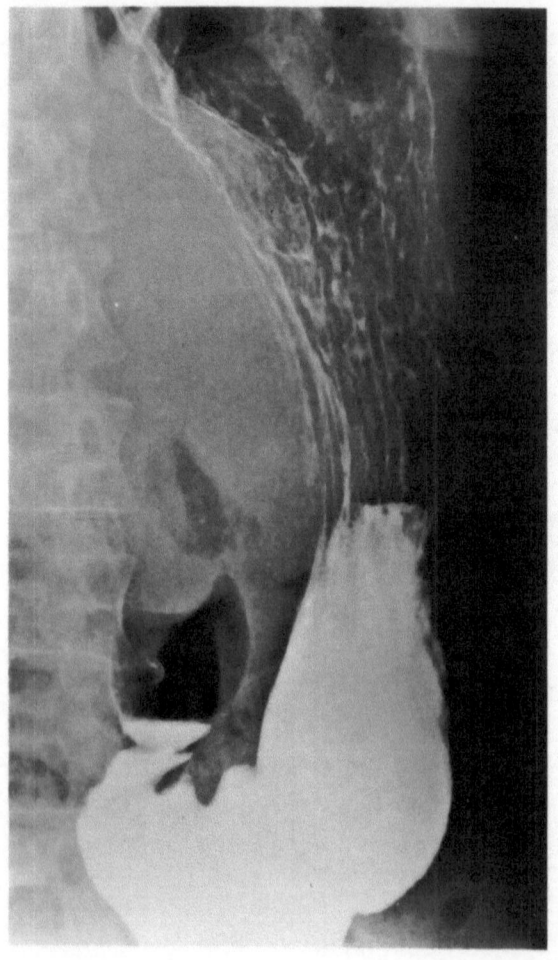

a

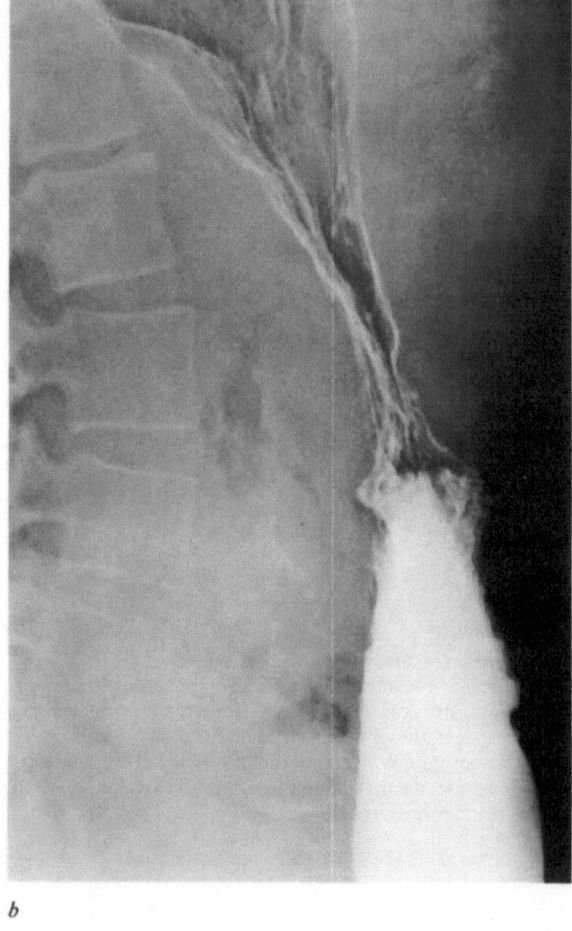

b

Fig. 114
a. Erect position, frontal view.

b. Erect position, lateral view.

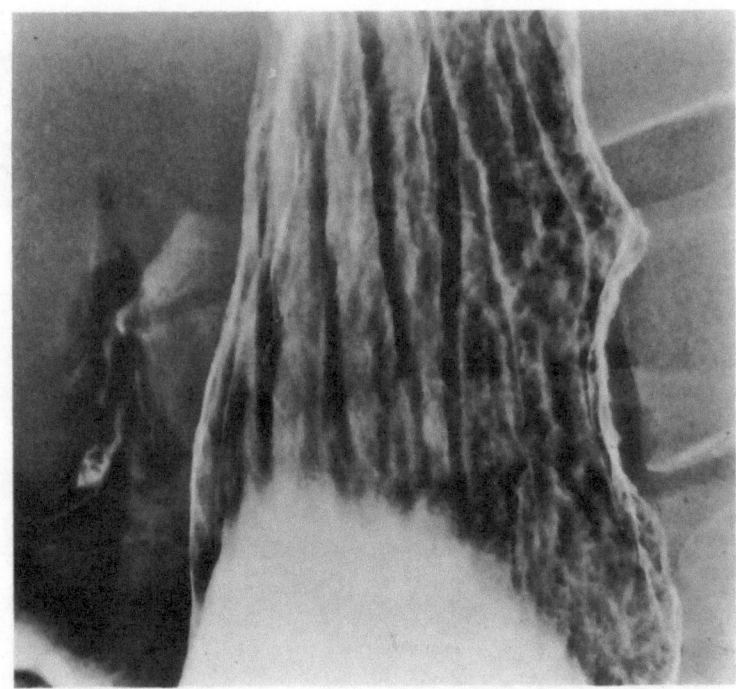

c. DC study, supine position, nearly lateral view.

d. Prone position, lateral view, horizontal beam projection. Indentations of the posterior and anterior wall of the stomach. Further examinations, including an IVP, isotope studies and an arteriography, demonstrated multiple cysts in the liver and kidneys.

c

d

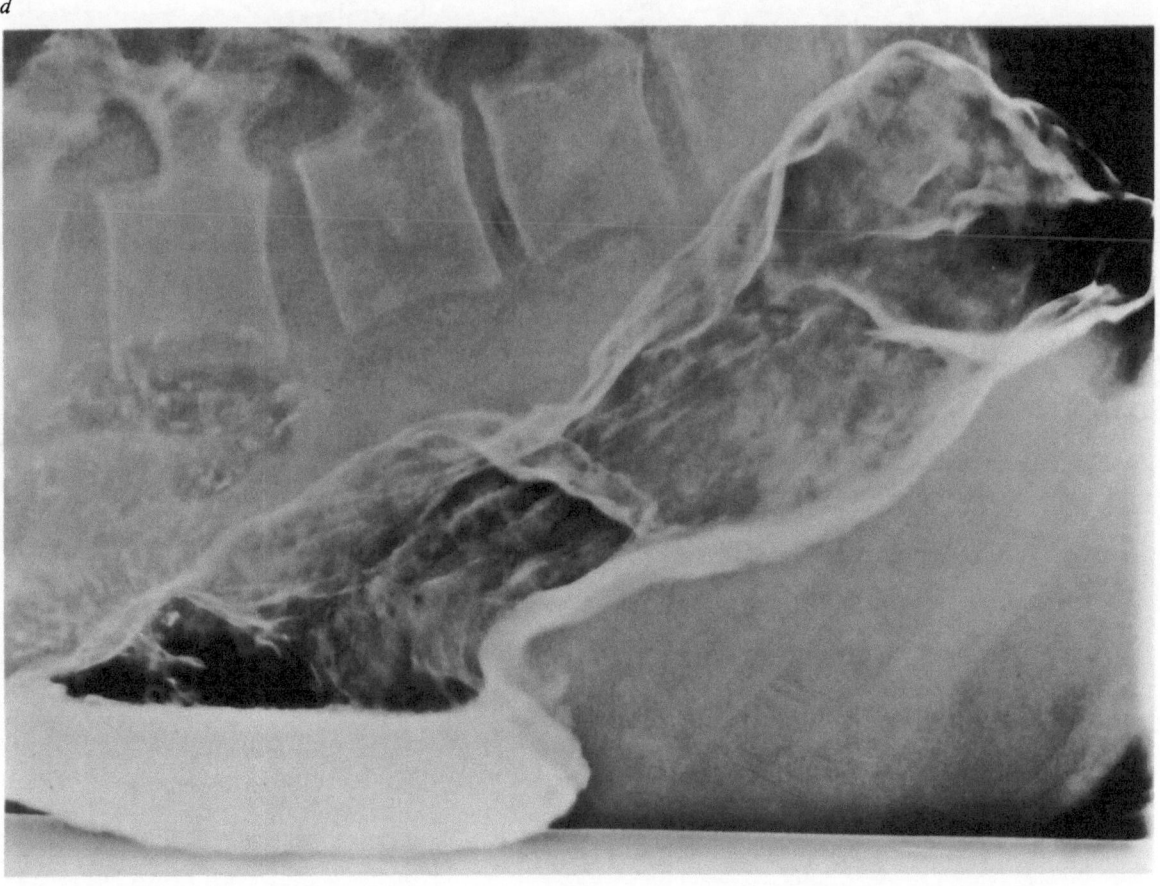

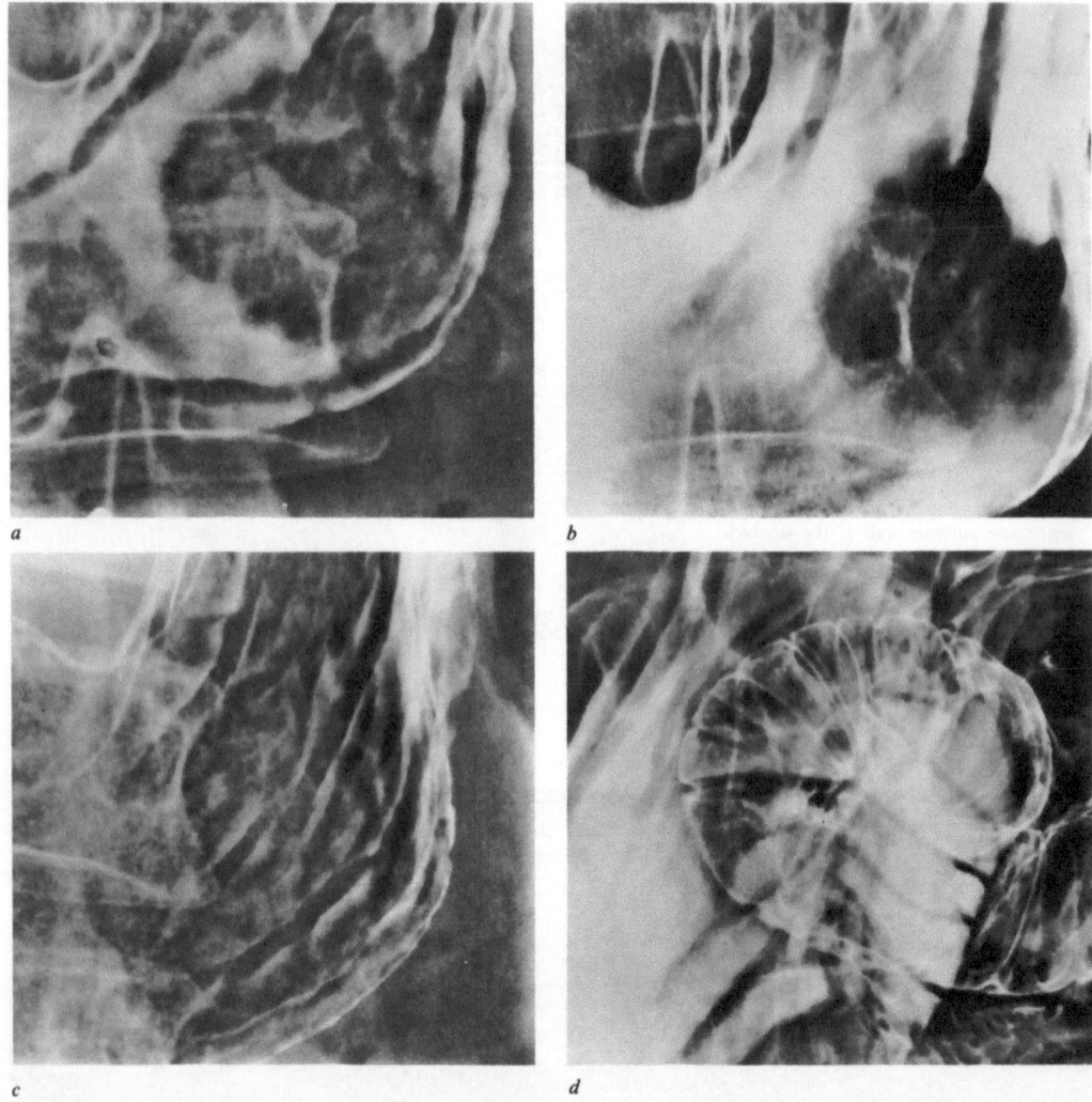

Fig. 115

a, b & c. DC studies, supine position, under changing conditions, including different gaseous distensions. Filling defect on the posterior wall with a changing aspect, which is characteristic of an indentation.

d. Filling of the small bowel demonstrates that the indentation is caused by the duodenojejunal flexure.

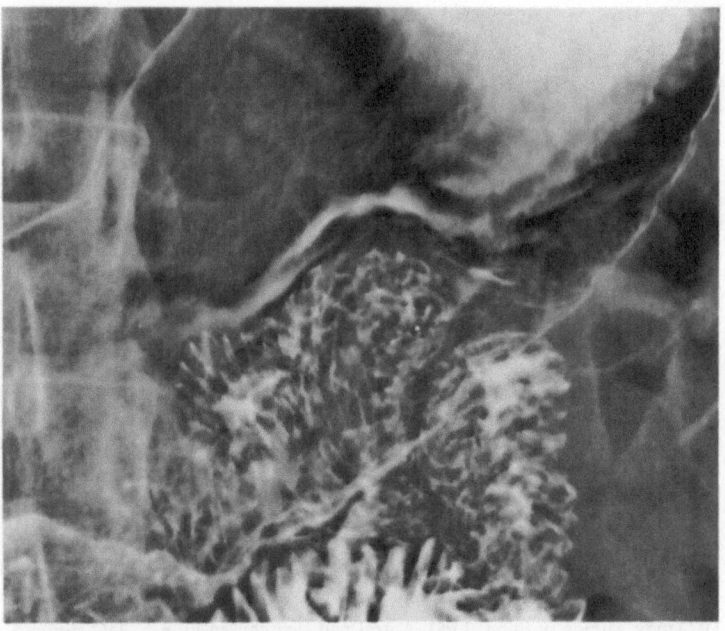

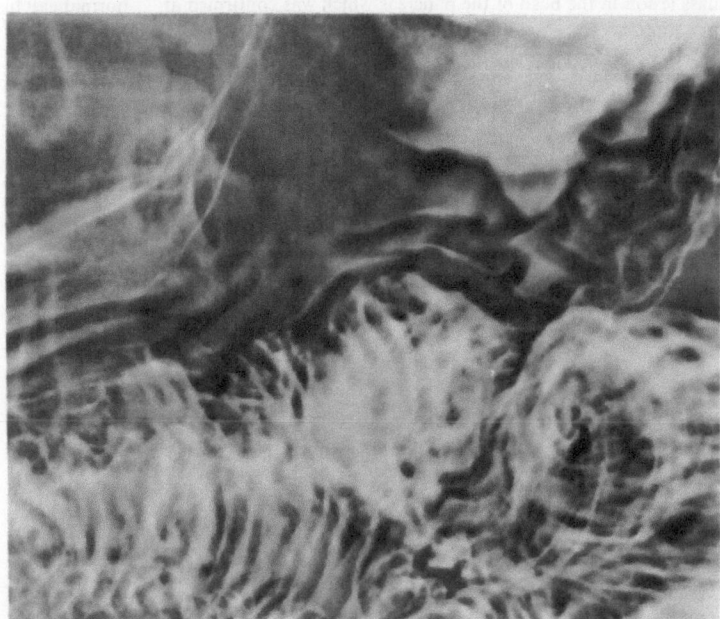

Fig. 116
a & *b*. DC studies, supine position, of 2 patients showing 2 more examples of normal
posterior wall indentations caused by the
duodenojejunal flexure.

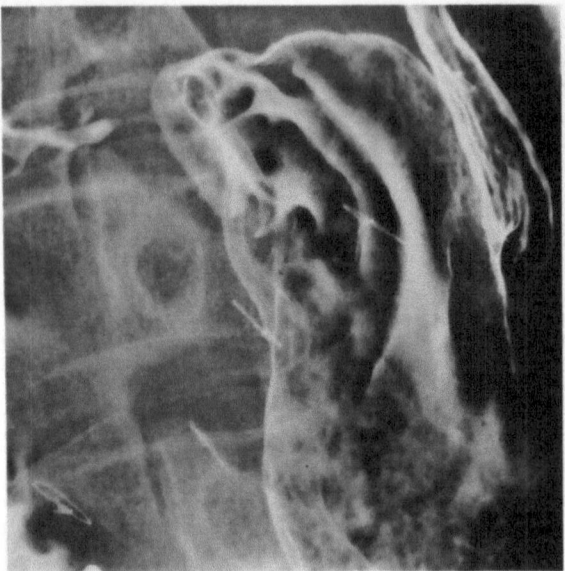

Fig. 117
DC study, supine position, LPO. Antral pad sign caused by a mass lesion in the head of the pancreas which was confirmed at operation.

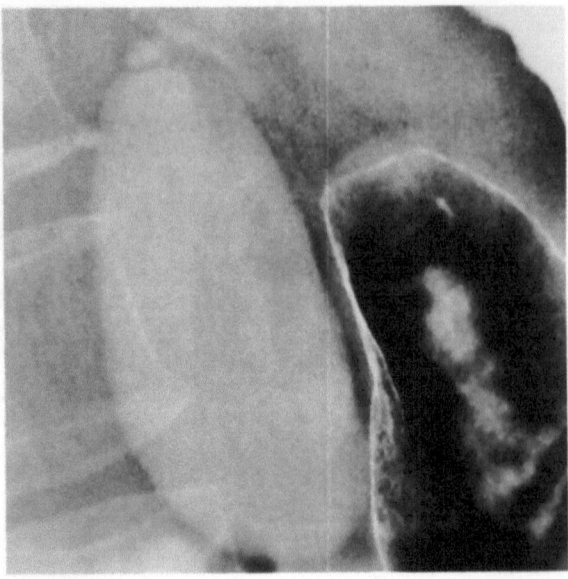

Fig. 118
DC study, supine position, LPO. Antral pad sign caused by a normal gall bladder.

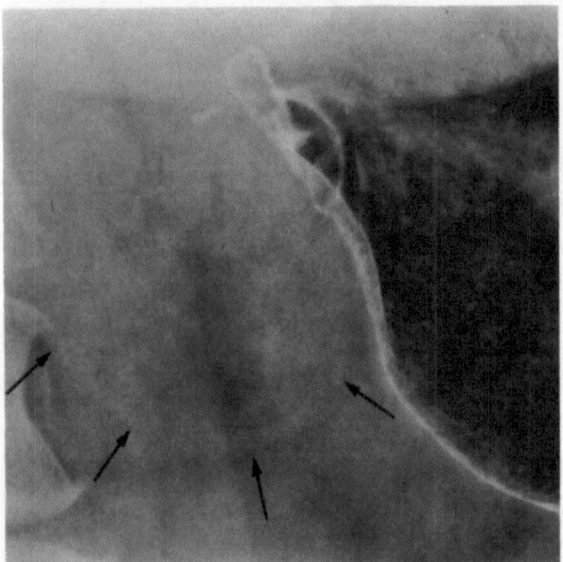

Fig. 119
DC study, supine position, LPO. Antral pad sign. The distended gall bladder is only faintly visualized (arrows).

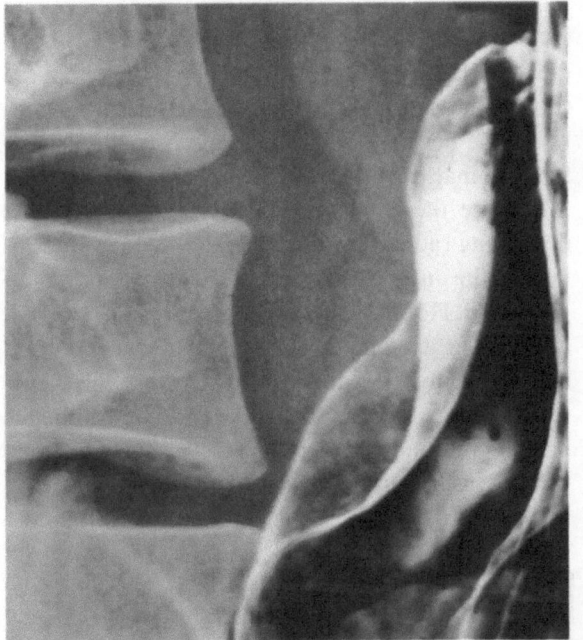
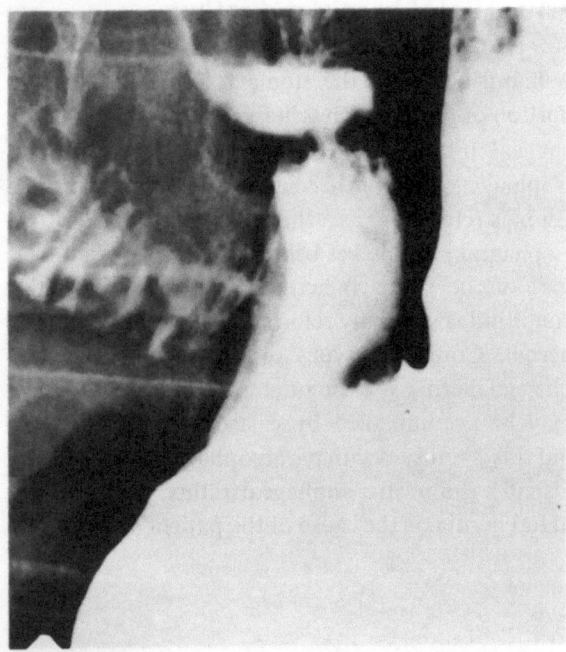

Fig. 120

a. DC study, supine position, LPO.

b. PC study, erect position, LPO. Antral pad sign. At operation a metastasis in the liver was found as the cause of this indentation.

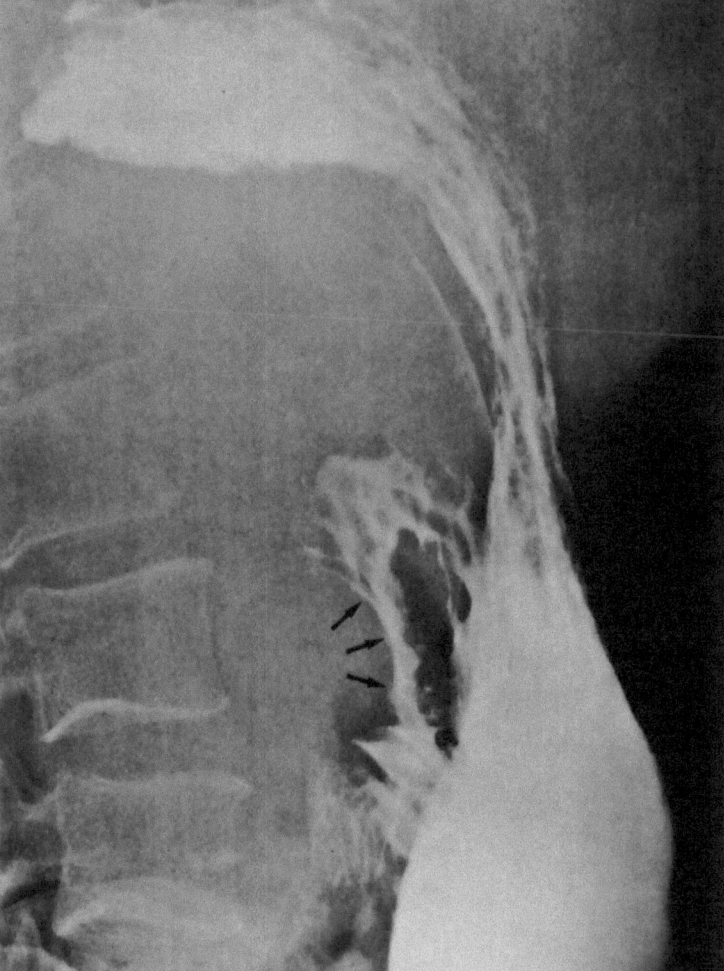

Fig. 121

Patient semi-erect, lateral view. An indentation of the dorsal wall of the gastric corpus and an indentation of the dorsal wall of the descending duodenum (arrows). This combination of a right and a left dorsal abdominal mass is highly suspicious of bilateral renal masses. Autopsy: polycystic renal disease.

7.10. Hiatal hernia and reflux

A hiatal hernia of the stomach is present when a portion of the stomach is herniated through the esophageal hiatus of the diaphragm. If the gastroesophageal junction herniates into the thorax, the lesion is referred to as a sliding hernia. If the gastroesophageal junction lies below the hiatus and another part of the stomach herniates into the chest, the condition is generally referred to as paraesophageal hernia. Combined types of sliding and paraesophageal hernia are encountered. A sliding hernia may be accompanied by gastroesophageal reflux, but this is unusual with paraesophageal hernia (242). Usually the gastroesophageal reflux, and not the hiatal hernia, is the cause of the patient's symptoms

(46). If a large part of the stomach is situated in the thorax, the radiological diagnosis of a hernia is easy, but if the hernia is small the diagnosis may be difficult to make.

Despite the extensive literature on this subject describing radiological signs of the various types of hernia, the author believes that they are not often of great help. However, if a supradiaphragmatic pouch is demonstrated and this pouch is shown to contract concentrically, then it can be stated that this structure is part of the esophagus because the esophagus has longitudinal and circular musculature. The gastric fundus has an oblique musculature and is therefor incapable of concentric contraction (45). Some-

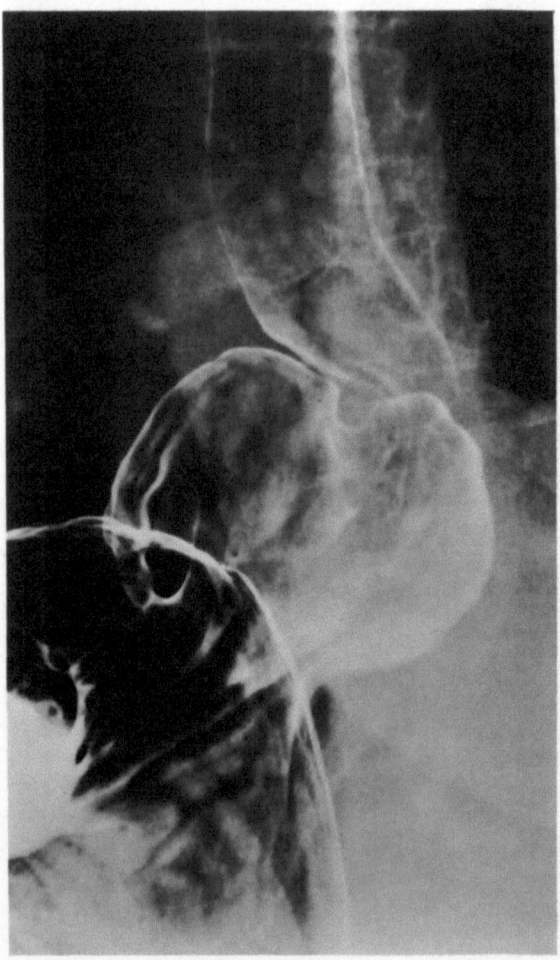

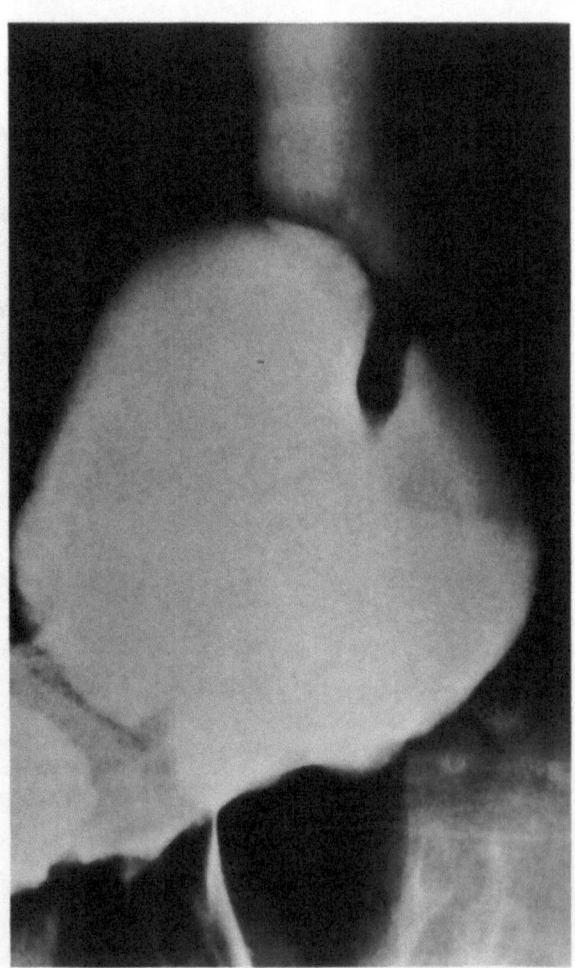

Fig. 122
a. DC study, supine position, LPO; table 40° anti-Trendelenburg. A portion of the stomach is herniated through the esophageal hiatus of the diaphragm, the gastroesophageal junction lies in the thorax: sliding hiatal hernia.
b. DC study, supine position, showing gastro-esophageal reflux.

times the number of folds in a supradiaphragmatic pouch – usually 4 or more – and their tortuosity can be used as proof of a hernia.

If the intra-abdominal pressure is raised by applying compression to the patient's abdominal wall, a small hernia or gastroesophageal reflux may be produced. During the act of vomiting, a rise in the intra-abdominal pressure is caused by descent and sudden spasm of the diaphragm with simultaneous contraction of muscles of the abdominal wall (219). The author has observed on several occasions, how a huge sliding hernia forms, at the moment that a patient starts to vomit during an examination (figs. 123, 124). While the Valsalva and Müller procedures may also be helpful, it may be argued that both provoke situations that exceed physiological conditions. The same holds true for the so-called water-siphonage test which is used by some radiologists to initiate gastroesophageal reflux (44).

It is uncertain if premedication with glucagon 0.5 mg influences the incidence of radiologically-demonstrable herniation or reflux.

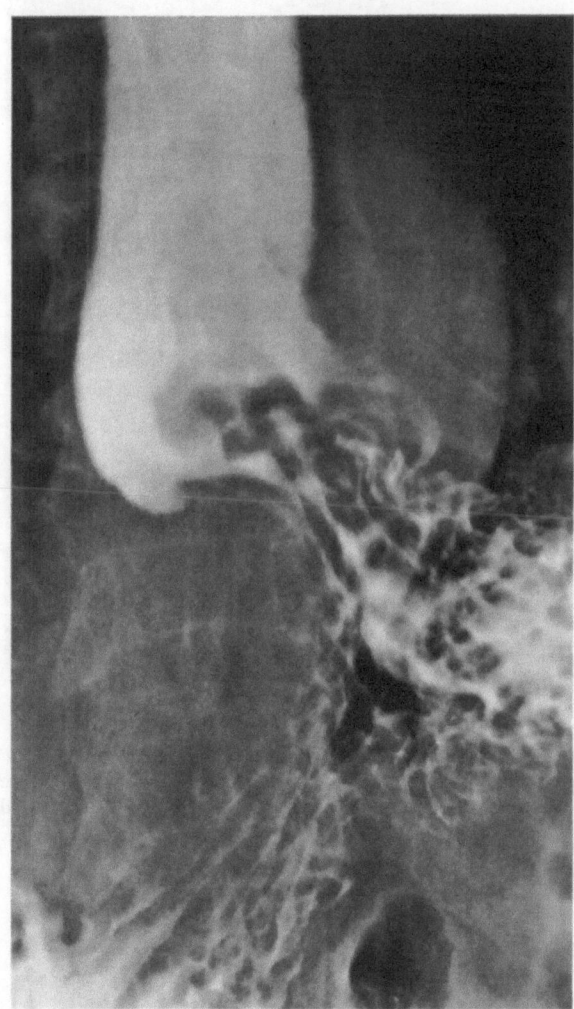

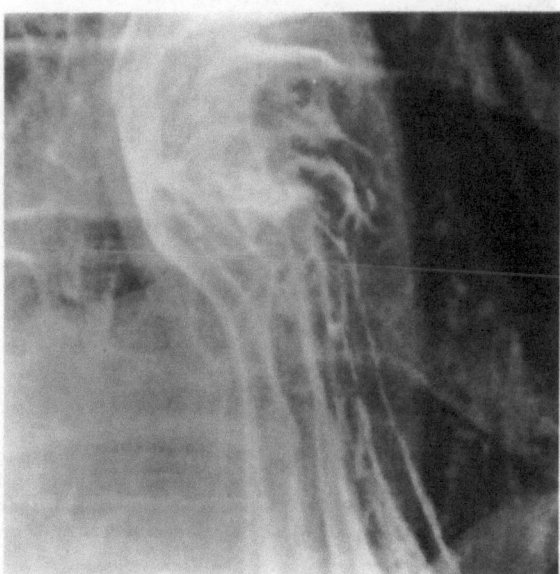

Fig. 124

Fig. 123

Figs. 123 & 124
DC studies of two patients who started to vomit during an examination. A huge sliding hernia is formed.

7.11. Gastric retention

It is generally believed that gastric retention renders the radiological examination valueless. However, personal experience has shown that a correct diagnosis can be made even if large quantaties of material are retained in the stomach. Gastric retention is nearly always caused by a lesion situated in the distal part of the stomach, the pylorus or the duodenal bulb. Pyloric or proximal duodenal lesions are only very rarely malignant. Concerning lesions of the gastric antrum, a DC examination will in many instances indicate whether the lesion is benign or malignant. In the presence of gastric retention, the patient requires additional amounts of contrast medium (barium suspension as well as gas). By rotating the patient frequently or, if this is impossible, after lying for a few minutes in the right lateral position, DC films of the antrum, pyloric region and duodenal bulb are obtained. For these the patient lies in the LPO position (figs. 125, 126).

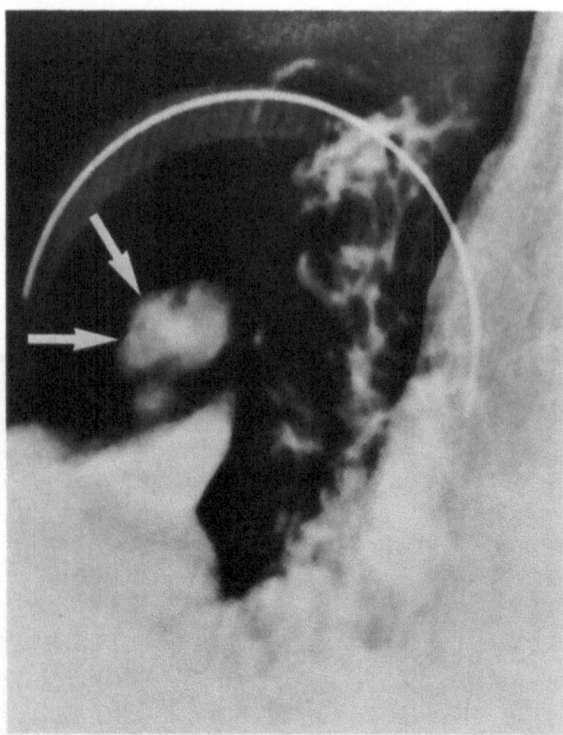 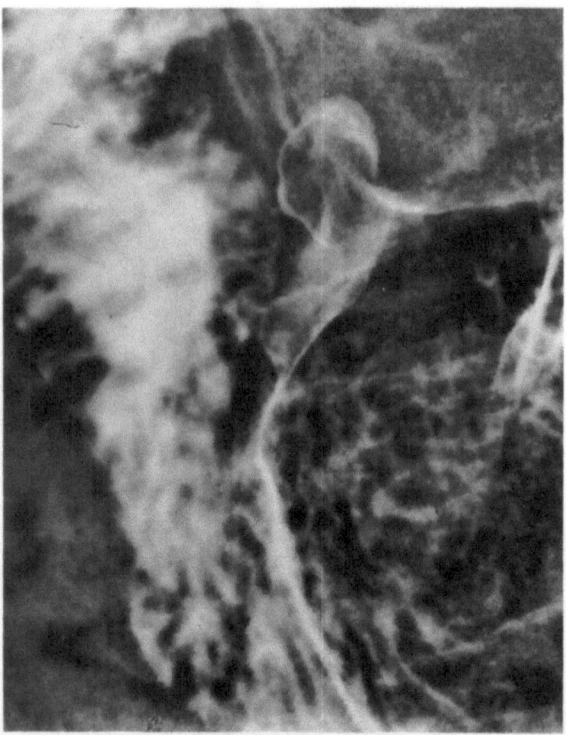

Fig. 125

a. PC study, erect position, RPO. An anteriorly-situated juxtapyloric ulcer niche is shown (arrows).

b. DC study, supine position, LPO. The juxtapyloric niche is shown as a ring shadow because of its situation on the anterior wall. Although this patient had considerable gastric retention, the distal part of the stomach could be well visualized using the technique described above. A juxtapyloric or pyloric niche nearly always proves to be benign, as in this case, which was proved by biopsy and follow-up studies.

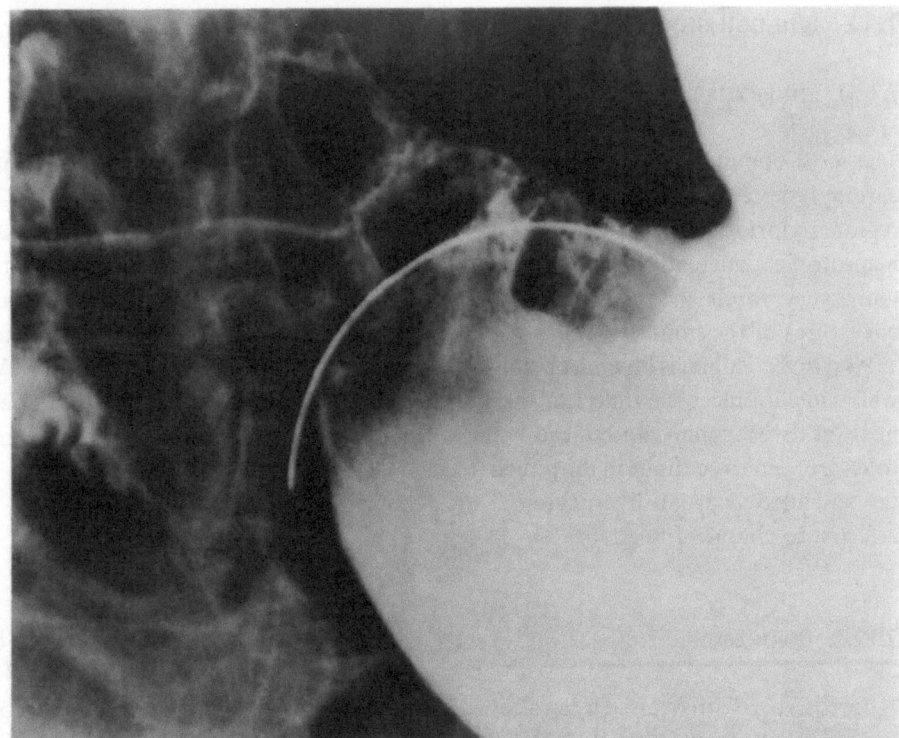

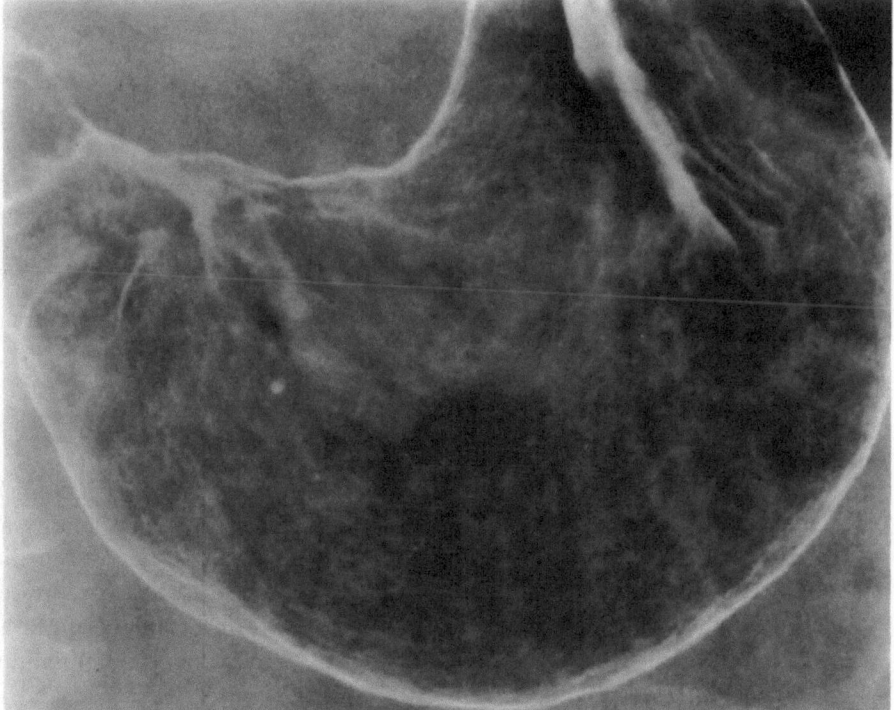

Fig. 126
a. PC compression study, erect position, LPO. This study visualizes only the retained food.
b. DC study, supine position, LPO. Good visualization of the antrum has been obtained. The deformity
   is virtually diagnostic of a malignant lesion. Gastroscopy: suspicious of a malignant lesion. Biopsy:
   highly suspicious of adenocarcinoma. In this patient there was also overwhelming clinical evidence in
   the form of hepatic metastases for the diagnosis of antral adenocarcinoma. This diagnosis could be
   made at the initial radiological examination, despite the retention of food in the stomach, by utilizing
   the described technique.

7.12. Miscellaneous

7.12.1. DIVERTICULUM

The most common site of gastric diverticula is the cardia; less frequently they are found in the pyloric region. Pyloric diverticula sometimes contain foci of heterotopic pancreatic tissue in their walls (227). Only very rarely are diverticula situated on the curvatures of the stomach (47).

As a diverticulum is an outpouching of the gastric wall while an ulcer is a defect of the wall, the diagnosis of diverticulum can be readily made if gastric folds are seen to continue in the pouch (fig. 127). For the so-called "partial diverticulum," the reader is referred to chapter 7, section 12.3.

7.12.2. CORROSION

A corrosive gastritis caused by swallowing an acid or lye can result in antral stricture. If a history of corrosive ingestion is lacking, it may be difficult to differentiate from other lesions of the antrum, e.g. carcinoma (83).

7.12.3. HETEROTOPIC PANCREATIC TISSUE

Heterotopic pancreatic tissue in the stomach presents itself mostly as a smooth mass on the greater curvature of the antrum or the prepyloric region (136). Often there is central umbilication. The pancreatic tissue is usually situated in the submucosa (173). The term "partial diverticulum" is sometimes used if the mucosa projects into the muscular coat of the stomach, resulting in a collar-stud accumulation of barium parallel to the longitudinal axis of the antrum. A small nest of pancreatic tissue often occurs in the wall (228, 259).

The site of the mass on the greater curvature, as well as its smooth surface, may enable the radiologist to make the correct diagnosis. In differentiating these lesions from other conditions with central umbilication such as leiomyoma, leiomyosarcoma, polyp or varioliform erosion, it should be remembered that the umbilication present in the latter group of conditions represents ulceration. Retrograde filling

of pancreatic ducts during endoscopy may be helpful in diagnosis.

7.12.4. PYLORIC HYPERTROPHY OF THE ADULT

Pyloric hypertrophy of the adult occurs with or without gastric ulceration: it is not clear if the ulcer is the primary event, or secondary to the pyloric hypertrophy (12, 28, 226). If an ulcer is present, it is often situated on the angulus. Variations in shape and caliber occur, which can be used to differentiate the lesion from antral carcinoma (9, 28, 226).

7.12.5. BEZOAR

A bezoar is an intragastric mass composed of accumulated ingested material. Differentiation from gastric tumors is usually easy, because bezoars are freely movable under the forces of palpation and gravity.

7.12.6. ANTRAL DIAPHRAGM

An antral mucosal diaphragm is a circumferential membrane of mucosa and submucosa. If present in the prepyloric region, it produces a confusing picture of the so-called "double duodenal cap" (fig. 136). The lesion is often asymptomatic but it can cause a gastric outlet syndrome (26, 78, 218). Hypotonic gastrography permits an easy radiological diagnosis.

7.12.7. CROHN'S DISEASE

Involvement of the stomach is rare in Crohn's disease. The early lesions are probably varioliform erosions or nodules in the antrum (64, 149, 216). As the disease progresses, the antrum becomes deformed, and the appearance has been described as a "ram's horn" configuration. Peristalsis over this segment is sluggish and infrequent (67, 141). An irregular network of thickened folds may be present (232), as well as fissured ulcerations (67). Demonstration of Crohn's disease affecting other parts of the bowel will point to the correct diagnosis (67, 95, 104, 155, 256).

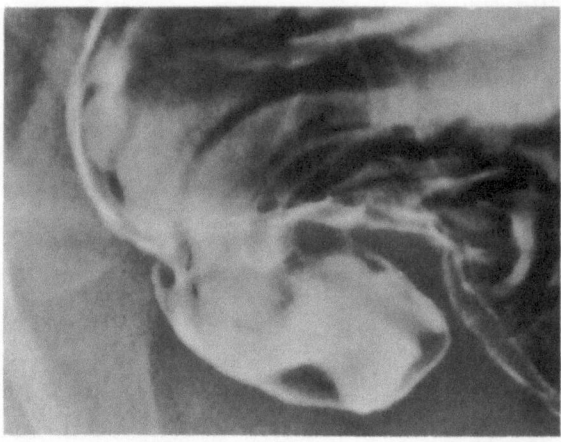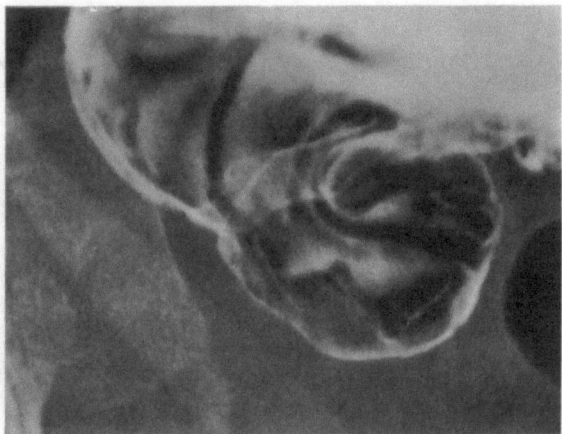

Fig. 127
a & b. DC studies, supine position, LPO: table 30° anti-Trendelenburg. Outpouching of the gastric wall near the cardia. The gastric folds are seen to continue in the pouch which proves a diverticulum and excludes an ulcer niche.

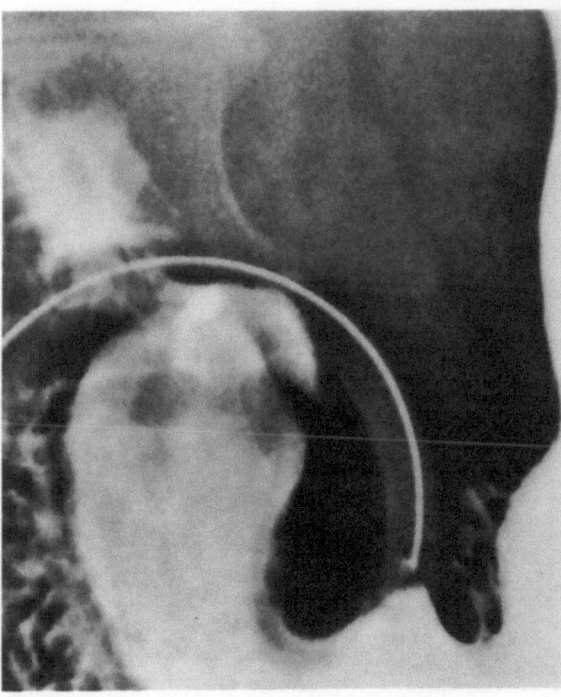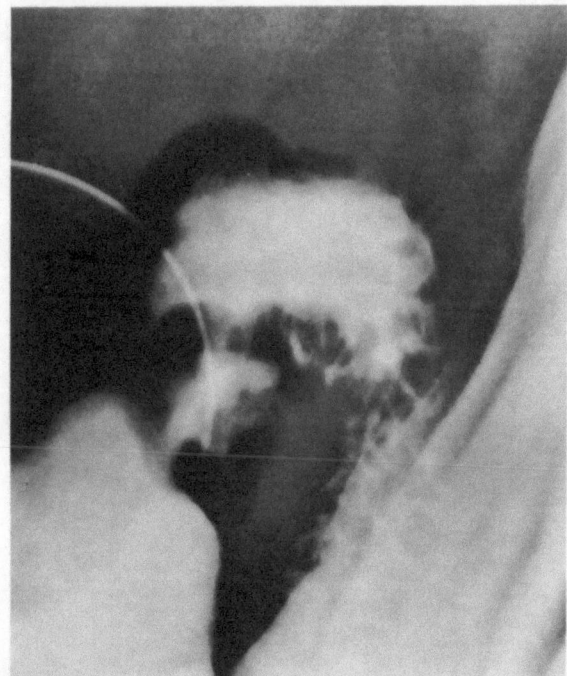

Fig. 128
a. PC study, erect position, LPO.
b. PC study, erect position, RPO. Filling defect on the dorsal side of the pylorus either caused by an ulcer niche or a diverticulum. The endoscopist made the diagnosis prepyloric diverticulum because he observed an outpouching with an intact mucosa.

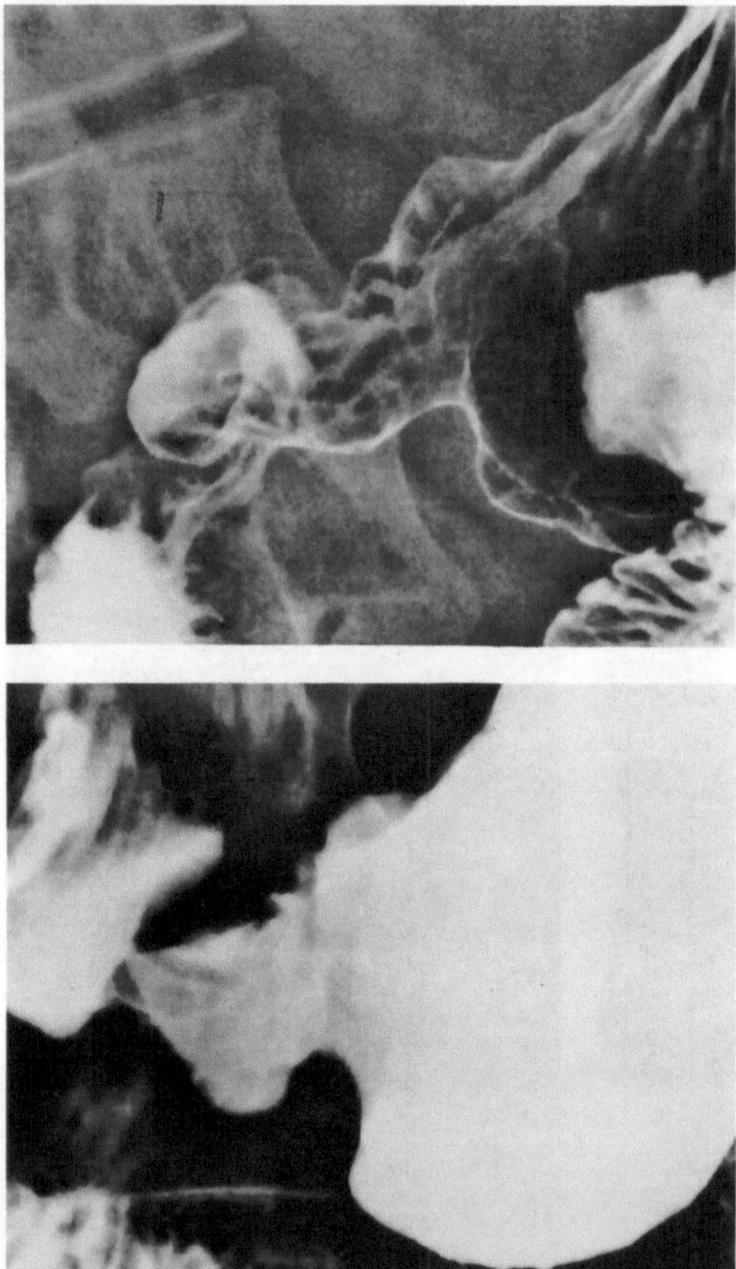

Fig. 129
a. DC study, supine position, LPO.
b. PC study, erect position, LPO. Antral stricture in a patient with a history of
   corrosive ingestion 3 weeks before.

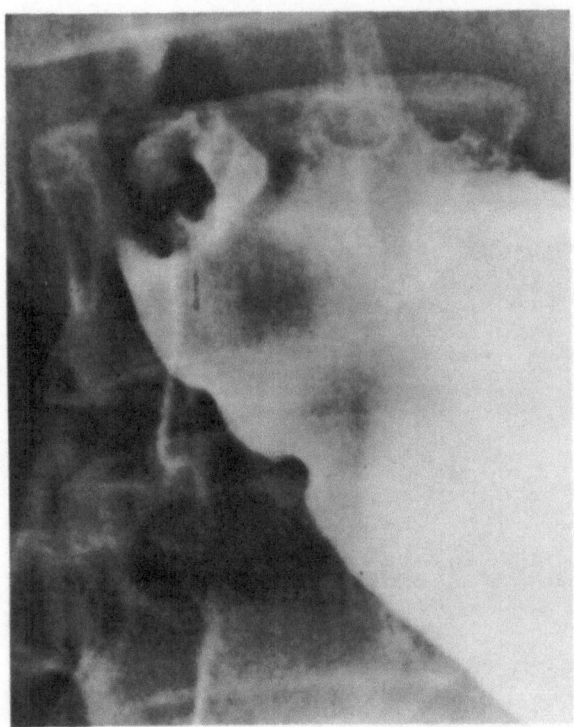 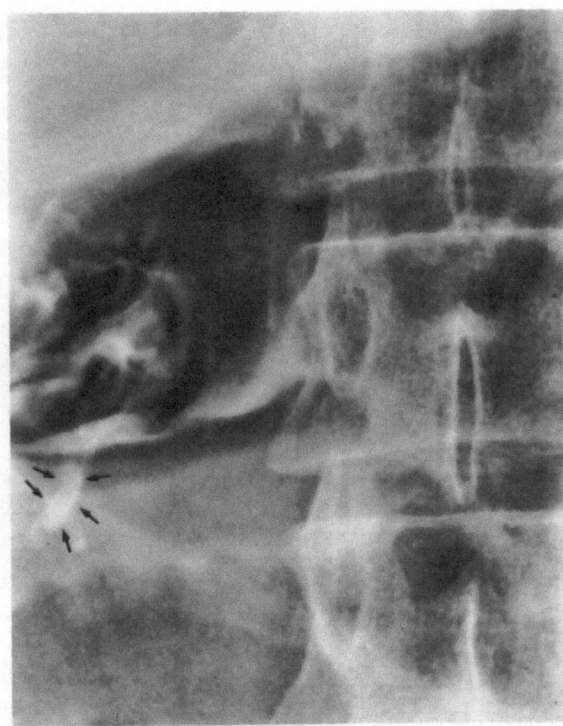

Fig. 130

a. Smooth mass with central umbilication on the greater curvature of the prepyloric region. The appearance is highly suggestive of heterotopic pancreatic tissue. The endoscopist observed a clear fluid flowing out of the central excavation.

b. Retrograde filling of a duct (arrows) during endoscopy which nearly confirms the diagnosis.

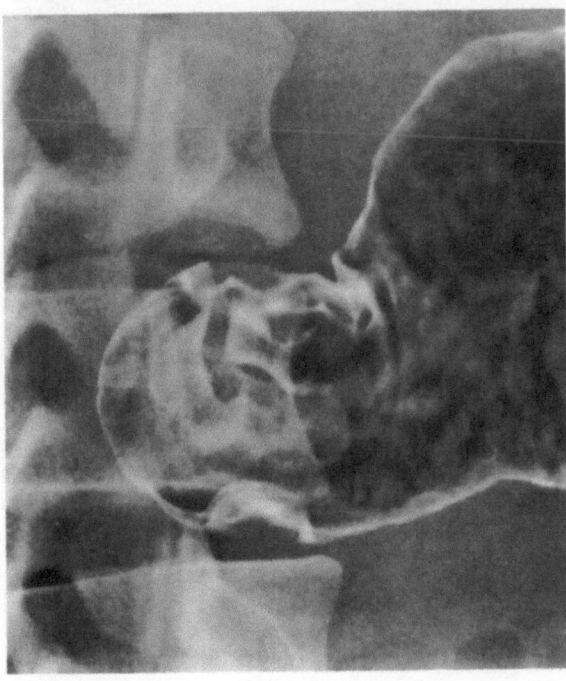 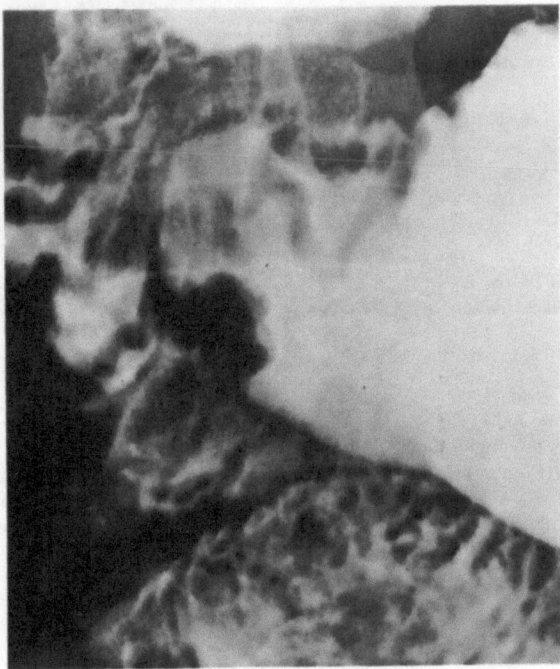

Fig. 131

a. DC study, supine position, LPO.

b. PC compression study, erect position, LPO. Smooth mass with central umbilication on the greater curvature of the prepyloric region. The appearance is highly suggestive of heterotopic pancreatic tissue. Endoscopy: a polypoid lesion (intact mucosa) and a central excavation.

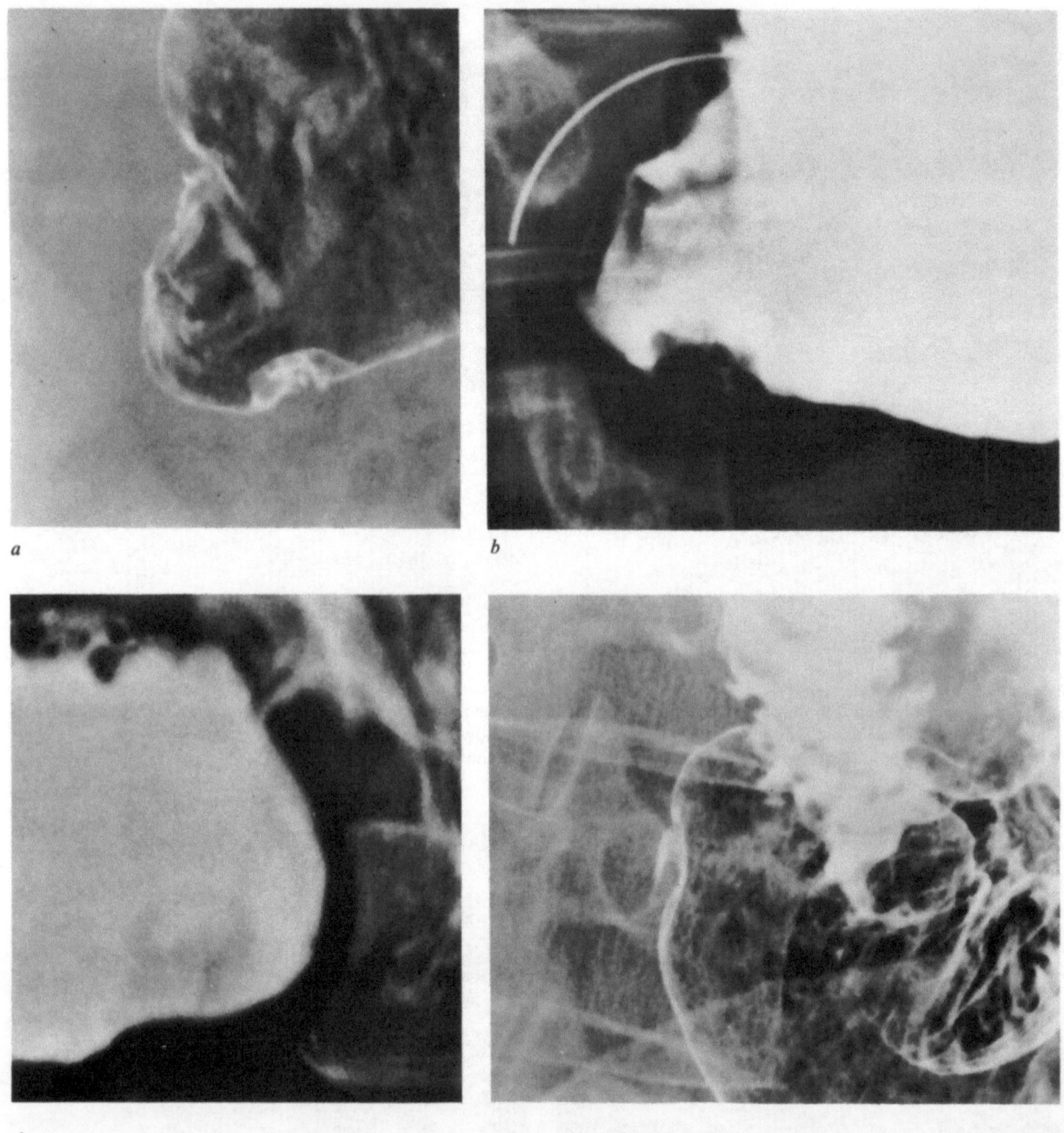

a

b

c

Fig. 132

a. DC study, supine position, LPO.

b. PC compression study, erect position, LPO.

c. PC study, prone position. Prepyloric mass on the greater curvature with the appearance of heterotopic pancreatic tissue.

Fig. 133

DC study, supine position, LPO. Collar-stud accumulation of barium parallel to the longitudinal axis of the antrum suggesting a partial diverticulum. Biopsies: no signs of malignancy. The lesion has been followed nonoperatively without change for 4 years.

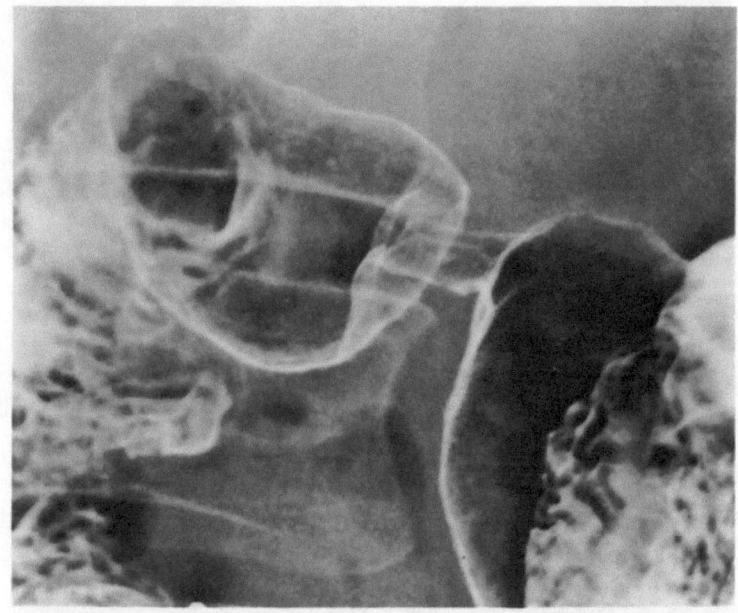

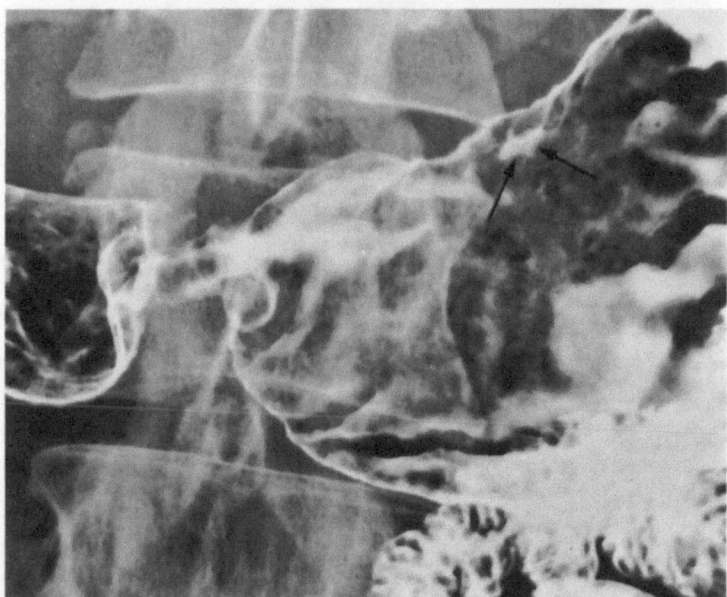

Fig. 134
a. DC study, supine position, LPO.
b. DC study, supine position. There is persistent elongation of the pyloric canal with
  an ulcer niche in the angulus (arrows). Several series of biopsies and a follow-up
  study proved benignancy. The findings were compatible with the diagnosis pyloric
  hypertrophy of the adult.

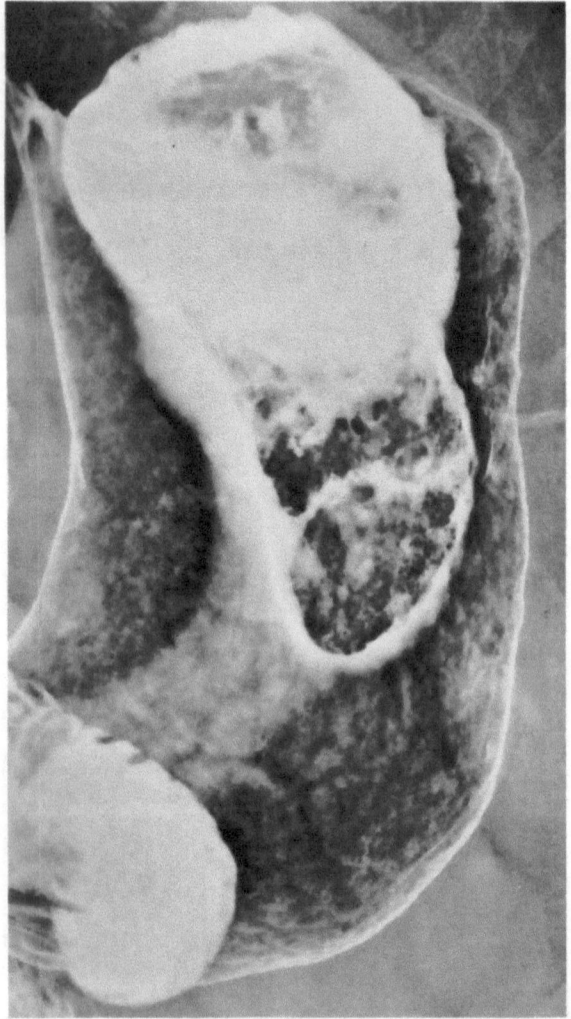

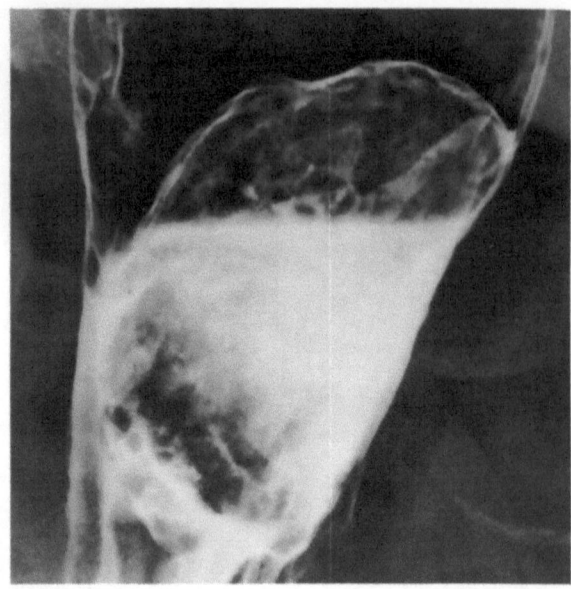

Fig. 135
a. DC study, supine position.
b. DC study, erect position. Intragastric mass which was freely
   movable under the forces of palpation and gravity: a bezoar.
   There is absence of rugae on the greater curvature. The endoscopist observed an atrophic mucosa. Biopsies: mucosal
   atrophy.

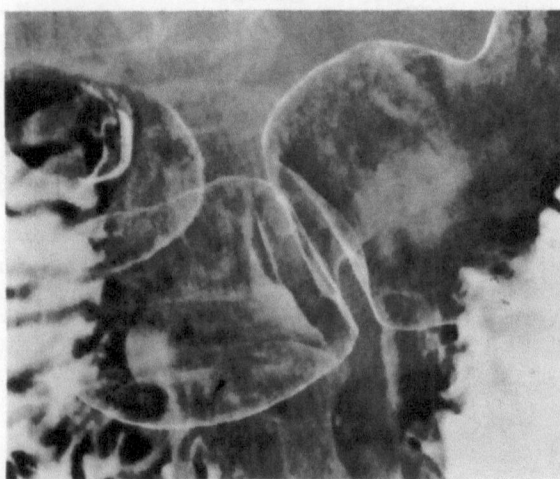

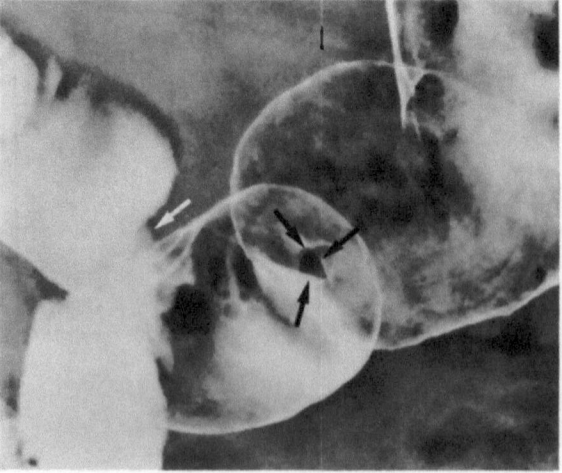

Fig. 136
a. DC study, supine position.
b. DC study, supine position, LPO. Antral mucosal diaphragm
   producing the confusing picture of the so-called "double duodenal cap." The black arrows point to the pseudo-pylorus; the
   white arrow points to the real pylorus.

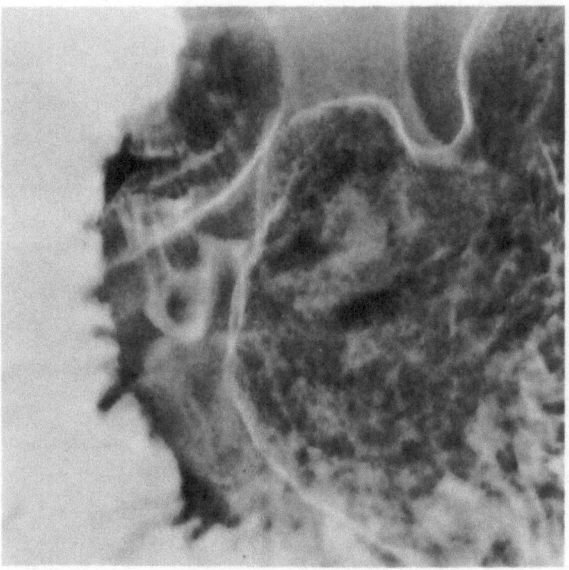 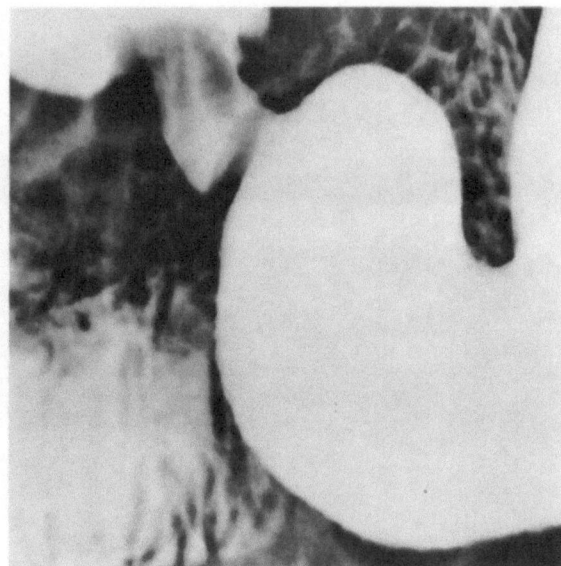

Fig. 137

a. DC study, supine position, LPO.

b. PC study, erect position, LPO. Another case of an antral mucosal diaphragm. The patient suffered from a gastric outlet syndrome.

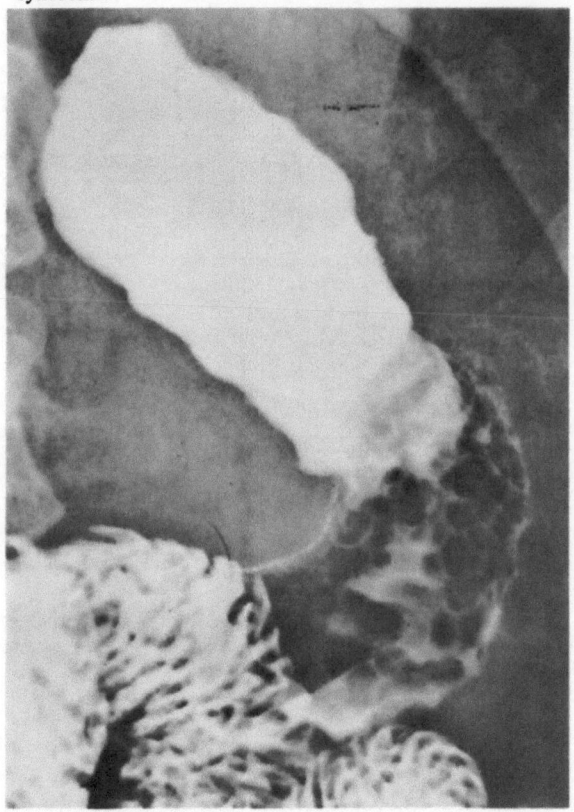 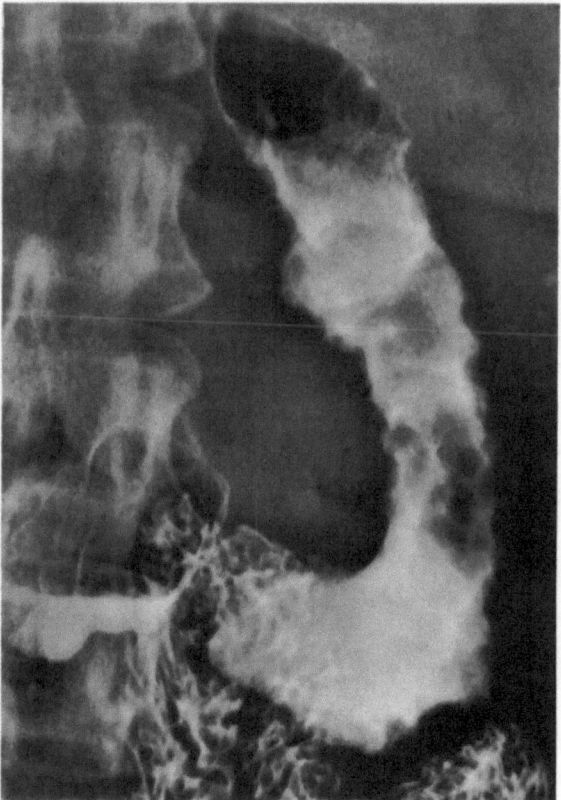

Fig. 138

a. DC study, supine position.

b. PC study, erect position. Shrinkage and nodularity of the corpus: Crohn's disease of the stomach (confirmed by Dr B.C. Morson, The Pathology Department of St. Mark's Hospital, London, England) (courtesy of Radiological Department of Hosital "St. Annadal," Maastricht, The Netherlands).

Chapter 8

DUODENUM

8.1. Normal and abnormal mucosal relief

8.1.1. NORMAL MUCOSAL RELIEF

The folds in the duodenal bulb are arranged in a longitudinal direction, although some irregularity may be present. The normal fold is approximately 2 mm. wide (204). Distension of the duodenal bulb effaces the folds. However, in the descending part of the duodenum, the transversely oriented folds of Kerkring remain visible even during complete distension.

The duodenal major papilla is a round or oval filling defect on the (posterior) medial wall of the descending part. The triad of promontory, straight segment and longitudinal fold (49) facilitates identification of the papilla (fig. 141). It can be visualized on both standard projections used in tubeless hypotonic duodenography, viz. supine LPO and prone. The major papilla is on average 8-10 mm. in length: 1.5 cm. is usually accepted as the upper limit of normal, although normal papillae of larger size have been reported (50).

The duodenal minor papilla bears a cephalo-ventral relation to the major papilla, the average distance between the two being 18-20 mm. Since the major papilla is a posteromedial structure in the descending duodenum, this means that the minor papilla lies on its anterior wall. It is a flat protrusion, several millimeters in diameter, with or without a central excavation. DC hypotonic duodenography in the prone position is the best method of visualizing it (196).

At the flexure between the bulb and the descending part of the duodenum, an appearance is frequently present which simulates an elevated lesion with central ulceration (figs. 143, 144). This configuration is a normal variant and may be related to several factors including distortion produced by flexion, sphincter function and extrinsic compression (22).

8.1.2. ABNORMAL MUCOSAL RELIEF

Fold thickening may occur in a variety of disorders including peptic ulcer disease, duodenitis, Zollinger-Ellison's syndrome, pancreatitis, renal failure, Crohn's disease, adenocarcinoma, malignant lymphoma and parasitic infections (giardiasis, strongyloides stercoralis). Vascular disorders such as duodenal varices, mesenteric arterial collateral vessels, and intramural hemorrhage may produce confusing but similar pictures (29, 51).

"Atrophy" of folds is often caused by destruction of the mucosal surface as a result of an inflammatory process or an abnormal circulation (230).

Nodularity with thickened folds may occur in malignant lymphoma and Crohn's disease (52, 235).

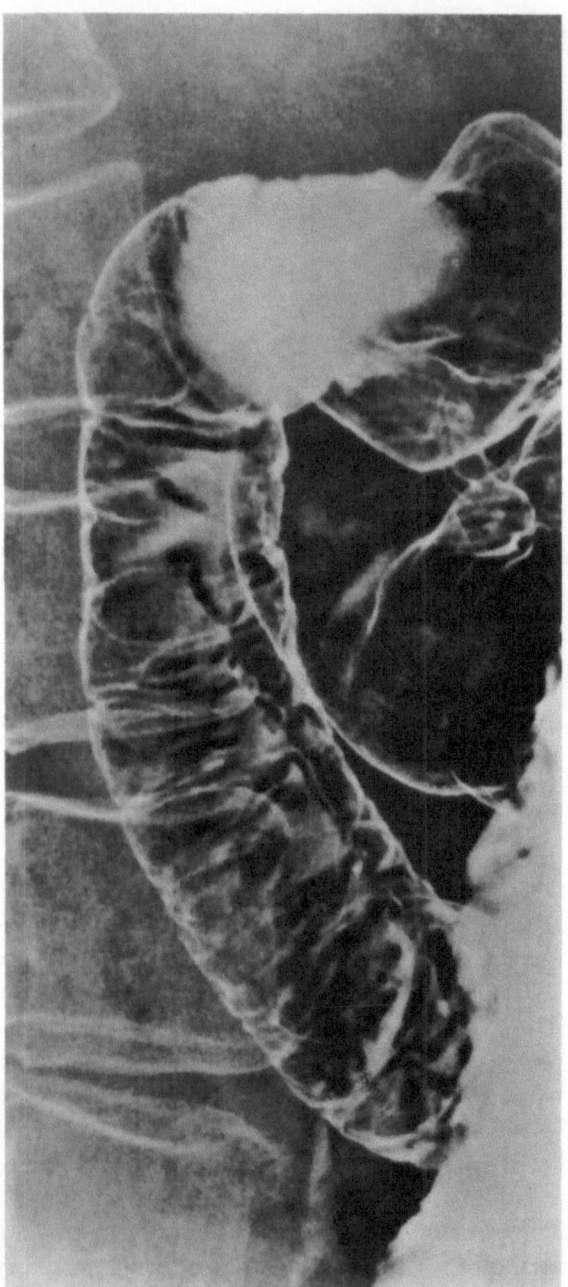 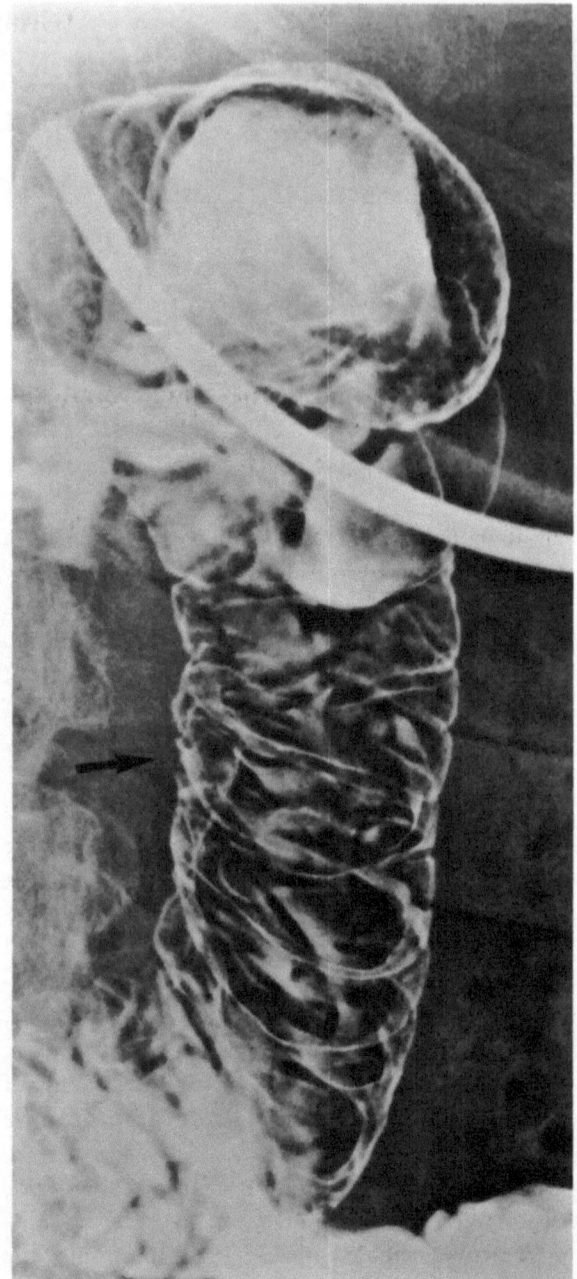

Fig. 139

a. DC hypotonic duodenography, supine position, LPO.

b. DC hypotonic duodenography, prone position. The transversely oriented folds of Kerkring remain visible even during
complete distension. The arrow points to the duodenal major
papilla. In the region where the minor papilla could be expect-
ed, there is troublesome superimposition of barium contrast in
the gastric antrum.

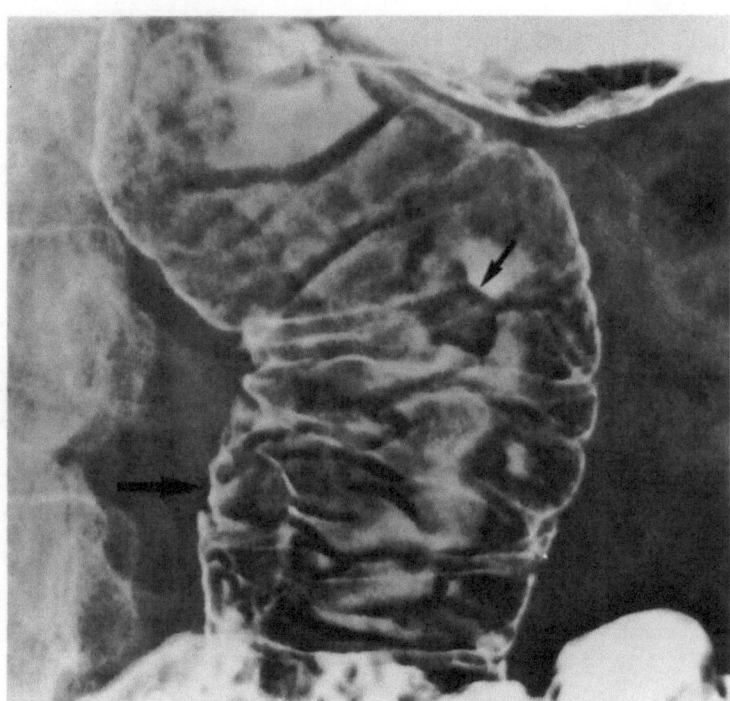

c. Same examination, prone position. Careful compression with a paddle between the patient and the table, eliminated the superimposition of the barium filled antrum and the DC filled duodenal loop. Visualization of both the major (large arrow) and the minor (small arrow) papillae. (Reproduced by permission of Fortschritte Röntgenstrahlen.)

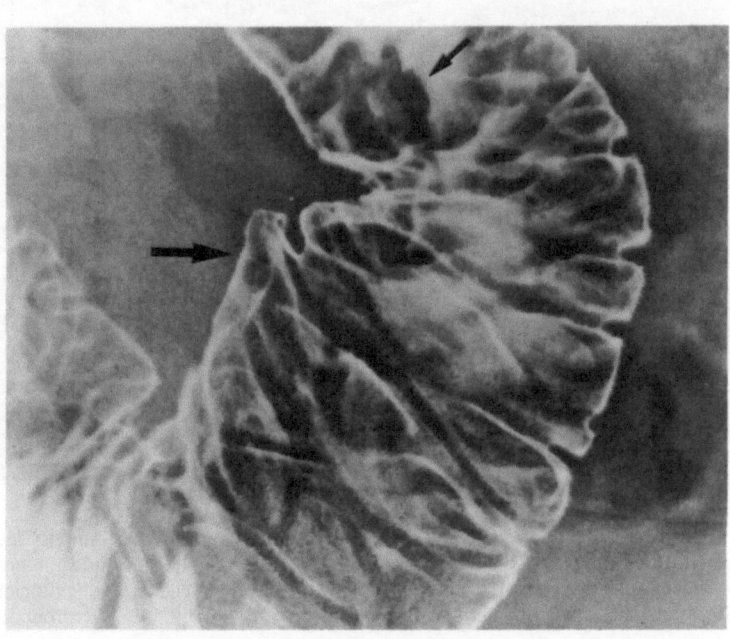

Fig. 140
DC hypotonic duodenography, prone position. Visualization of the major papilla (large arrow) and the minor papilla (small arrow). (Reproduced by permission of Fortschritte Röntgenstrahlen.)

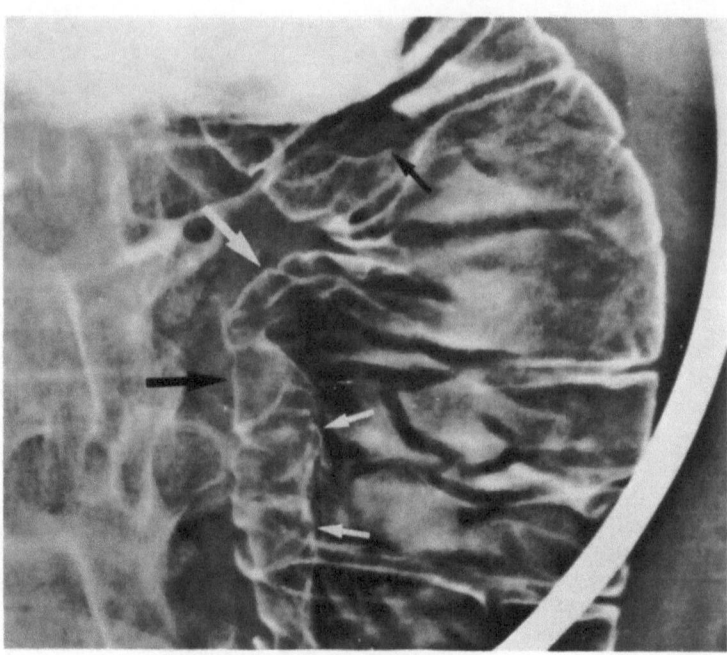

Fig. 141
DC hypotonic duodenography, prone position. The large black arrow points to the major
papilla; the small black arrow points to the
minor papilla. Visualization of the promontory (large white arrow) and the longitudinal
fold (small white arrows).

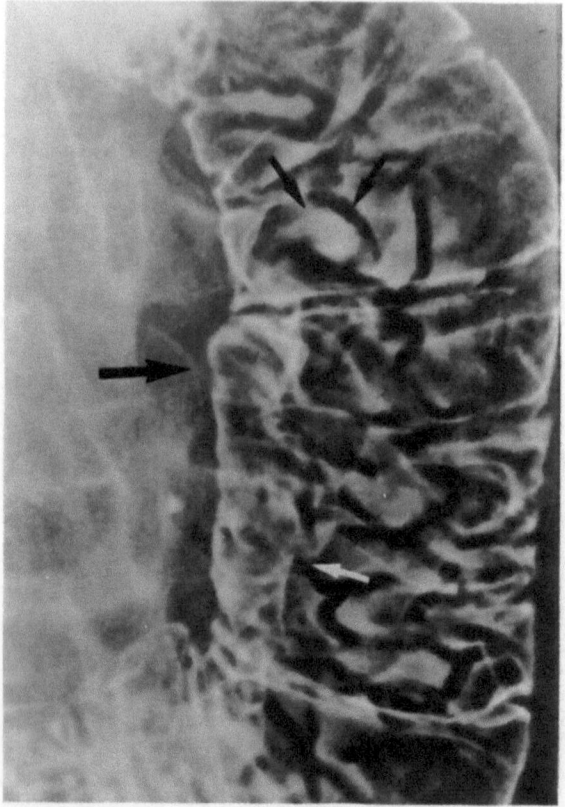

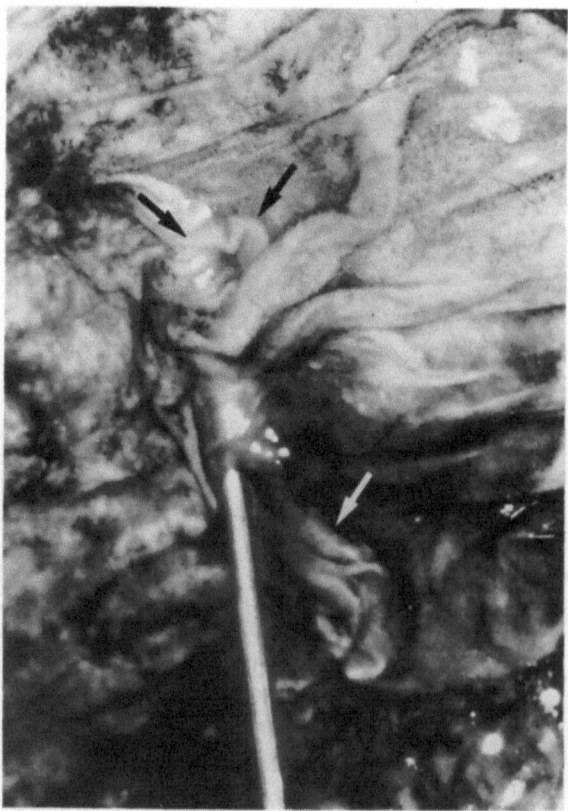

Fig. 142

a. DC hypotonic duodenography, prone position. The large arrow points to the probable localization of the major papilla.
The small white arrow points to the longitudinal fold. The
small black arrows point to the minor papilla.

b. Autopsy specimen of this patient. A probe has been introduced
into the major papilla. The small white arrow points to the
longitudinal fold; the small black arrows to the minor papilla.
(Reproduced by permission of Fortschritte Röntgenstrahlen.)

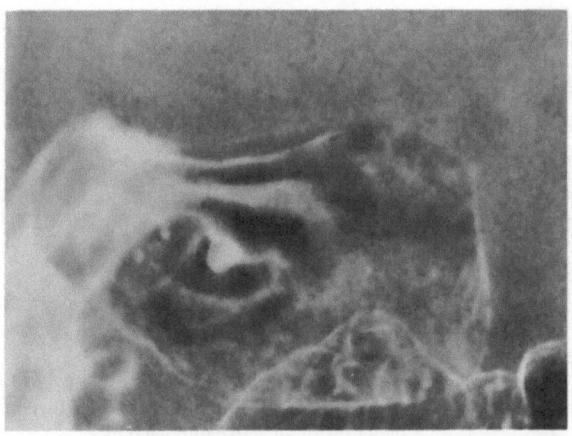

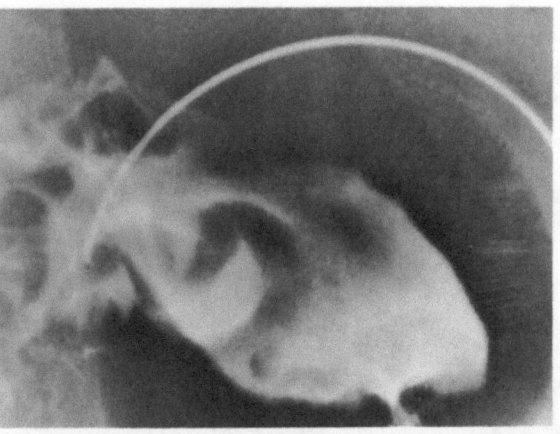

Fig. 143
DC study, supine position, LPO. Near the flexure between the bulb and the descending part of the duodenum an appearance which simulates an elevated lesion with central ulceration. This configuration is a normal variant.

Fig. 144
PC compression study, erect position, LPO. Same type of variant as shown in fig. 143. Endoscopy revealed an appearance that was compatible with this picture. The duodenal mucosa was considered to be normal; biopsies: no abnormality.

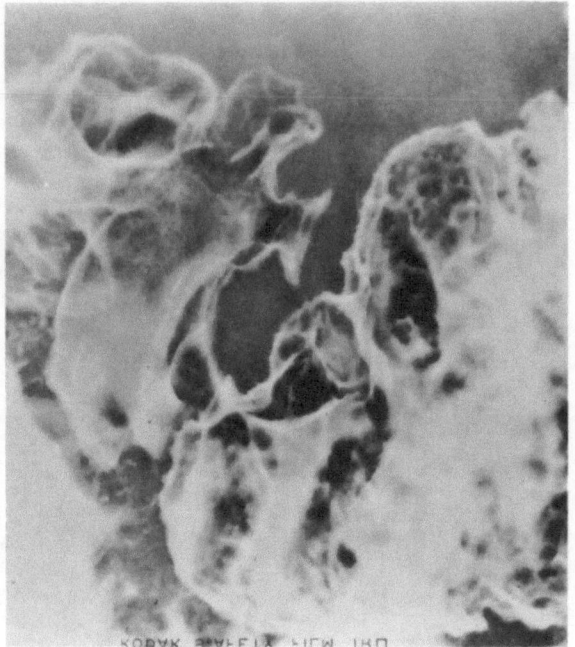

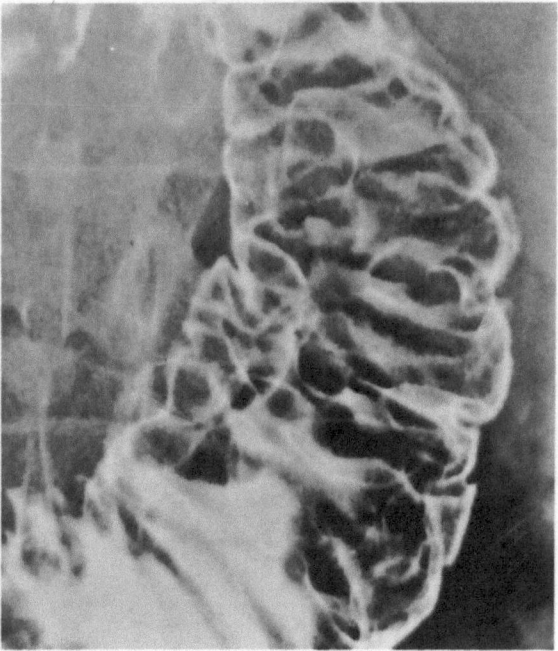

Fig. 145
a. DC study, supine position, LPO.
b. DC hypotonic duodenography, prone position. Coarse folds

with nodularity in the duodenal bulb and in the descending duodenum of a patient with malignant lymphoma of the gastrointestinal tract. See also figs. 37 and 98 of this patient.

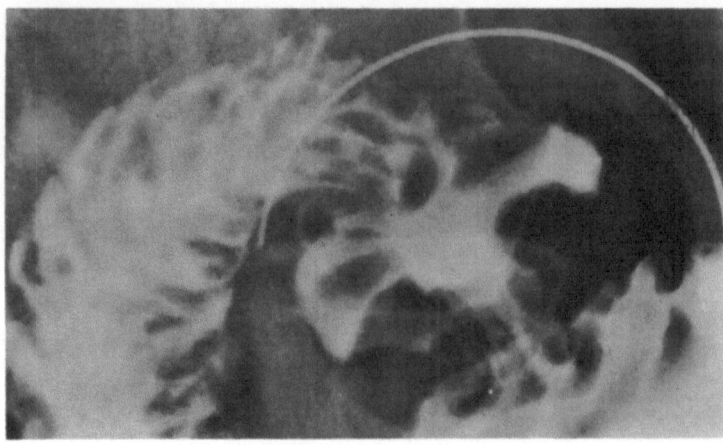

Fig. 146
PC compression study, erect position, LPO.
Thickened folds in the duodenal bulb of a
patient with an active duodenal ulcer.

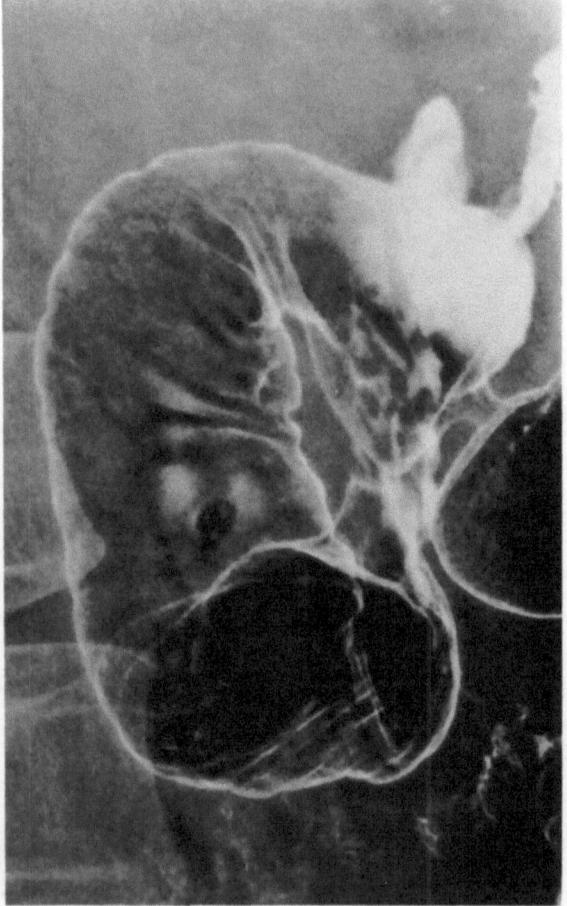 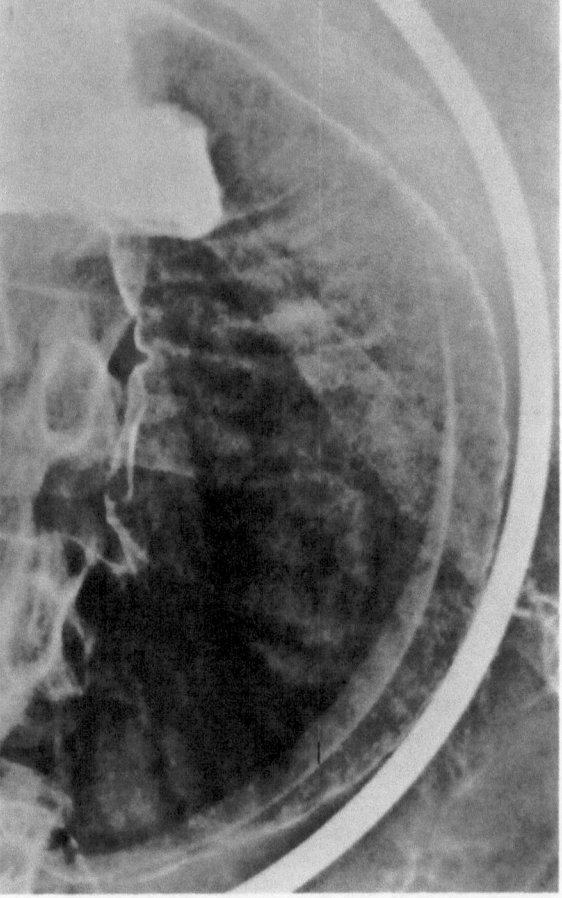

Fig. 147
a. DC hypotonic duodenography, supine position, LPO.
b. DC hypotonic duodenography, prone position, "Atrophy" of
folds. This patient suffered from an enterocolitis. Endoscopy
revealed heavily inflammatory changes with a destruction of
the duodenal mucosa. Biopsies: non-specific inflammatory
reaction.

8.2. Ulcers

Most duodenal ulcers occur in the duodenal bulb. Healing of a bulbar ulcer can occur without deformity; more often, however, scar formation results. Ultimately this may lead to shrinking and extreme deformity.

As in the diagnosis of a gastric ulcer, the radiological diagnosis of a duodenal ulcer depends on the demonstration of an ulcer niche. If the patient's physique permits adequate compression, PC studies in the erect LPO position are highly effective for demonstrating ulcer niches in the duodenal bulb. For localizing ulcers either on the anterior or the posterior wall, studies in the erect RPO position or DC pictures made in the supine LPO position are required. When adequate compression is impossible, the DC films made in this position may be adequate to reveal even small niches in the posterior wall and deep, abruptly marginated excavations on the anterior wall (figs. 15, 150, 151). It is vitally important for the radiologist to remember that a DC picture of the duodenal bulb which is perfectly normal, may hide an anterior-wall ulcer niche with gently sloping edges (fig. 149). If there is extreme scarring and deformity of the bulb, it may be impossible either to demonstrate or to exclude an active ulcer in the bulb. In such patients, endoscopy is mandatory.

Post-bulbar ulcers are relatively rare. They occur mostly on the proximal and medial aspect of the descending part of the duodenum (59) and are often associated with strictures (214). When scarring occurs, a ring-stricture results (14), which cannot be differentiated easily from the deformity, produced by an annular pancreas. Personal experience has shown that hypotonic duodenography greatly increases the percentage of cases in which a post-bulbar ulcer can be identified and diagnosed correctly.

The differential diagnosis between an ulcer niche in the descending part of the duodenum and a diverticulum is easy, provided it is remembered that an ulcer niche is a mucosal defect without folds passing in it, while a diverticulum is an outpouching of the duodenal wall with folds entering the lesion.

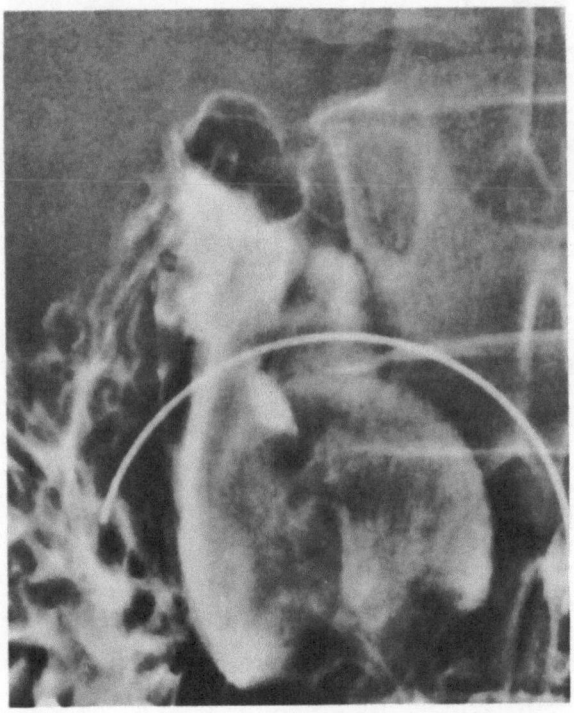

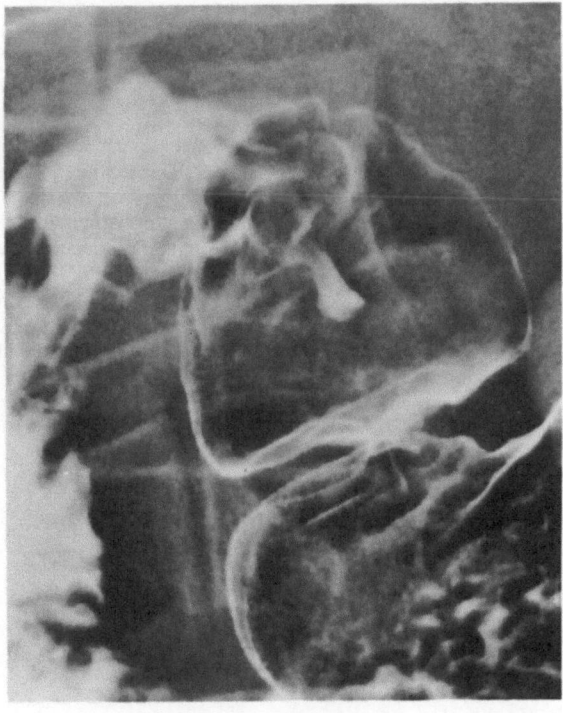

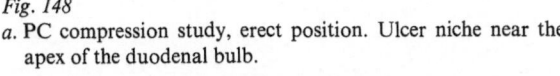

Fig. 148
a. PC compression study, erect position. Ulcer niche near the apex of the duodenal bulb.

b. DC study, supine position, LPO. Since the collection of barium remains visible in the supine position, the ulcer niche must be localized in the posterior wall of the duodenal bulb.

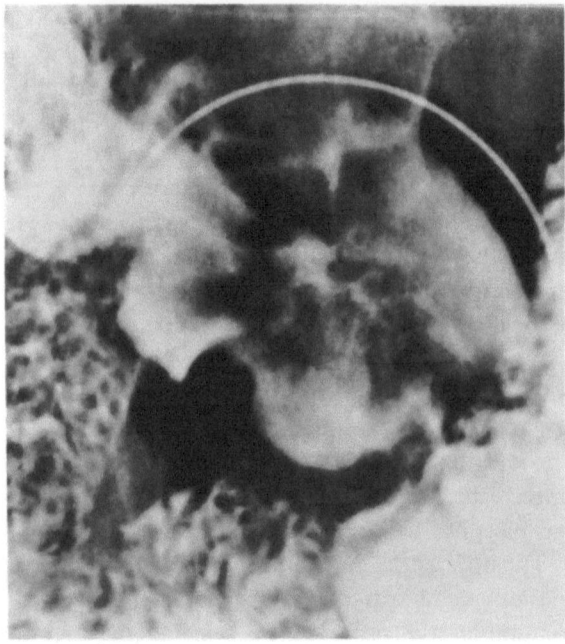

a

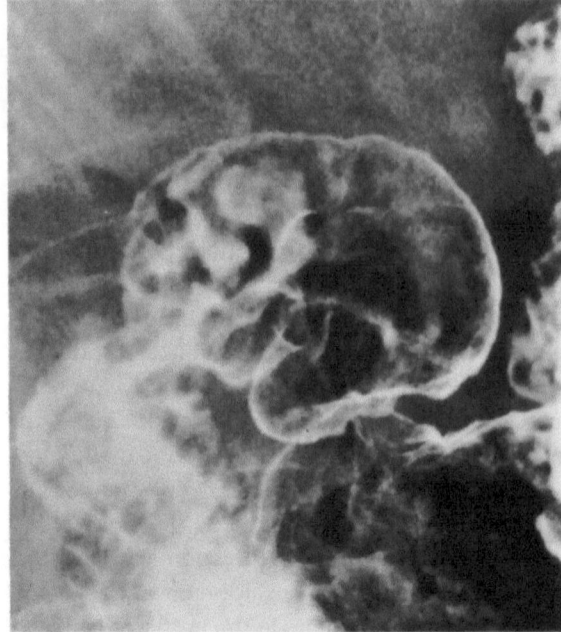

b

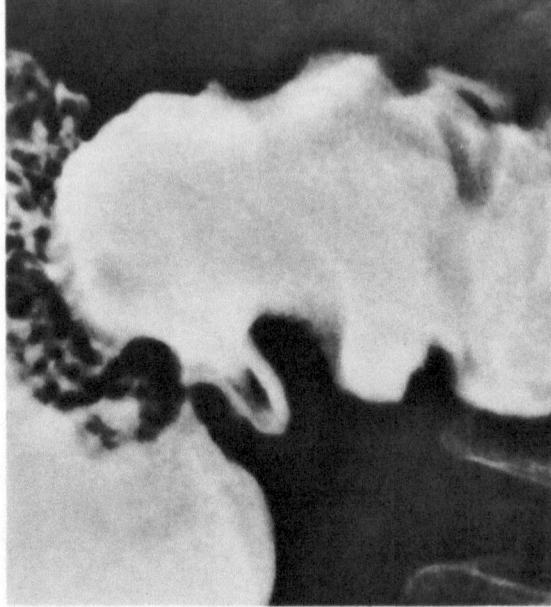

c

Fig. 149

a. PC compression study, erect position, LPO. Ulcer niche in the centre of the bulb.

b. DC study, supine position, LPO. Manipulating barium suspension along the posterior wall, no niche in the posterior could be demonstrated. As there is neither a ring shadow indicating an abruptly marginated ulcer in the anterior wall, nor a collection of barium on the posterior wall, it can be concluded that we are dealing with an ulcer niche, which has gently sloping edges, that lies in the anterior wall (cf. fig. 17).

c. PC study, prone position. Due to inadequate compression the ulcer niche is not visualized.

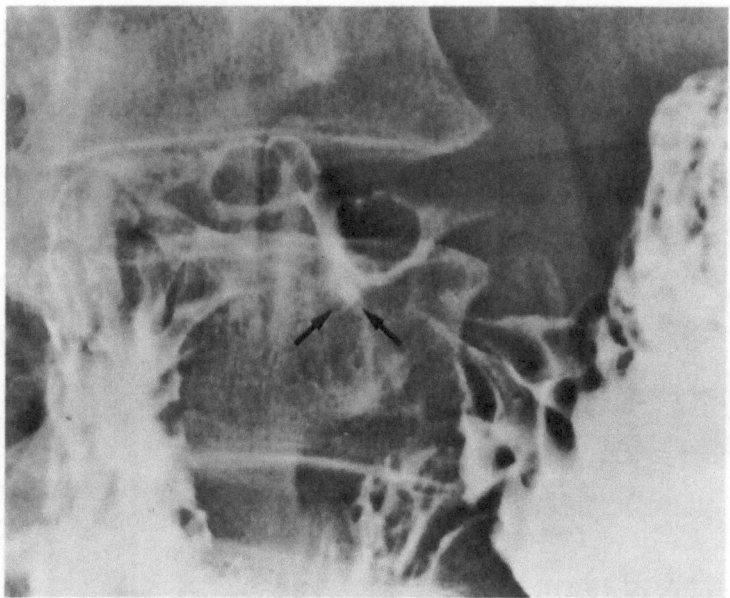

a

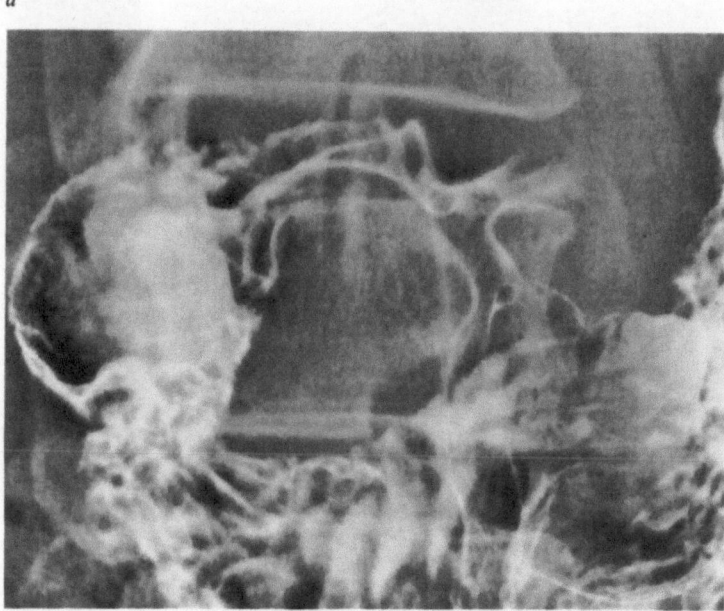

b

Fig. 150

a. PC compression study, erect position, LPO. The arrows point to an ulcer niche.

b. DC study, supine position, LPO. Ring shadow in the deformed duodenal cap. No barium suspension could be caught in the ring shadow by altering the patient's position or by tilting the table. This proves that the lesion is an abruptly marginated ulcer in the anterior wall (cf. fig. 15).

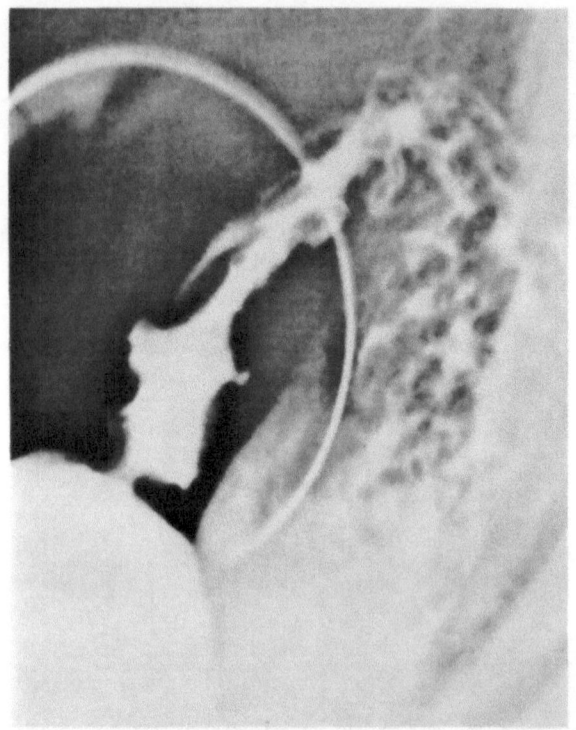

a

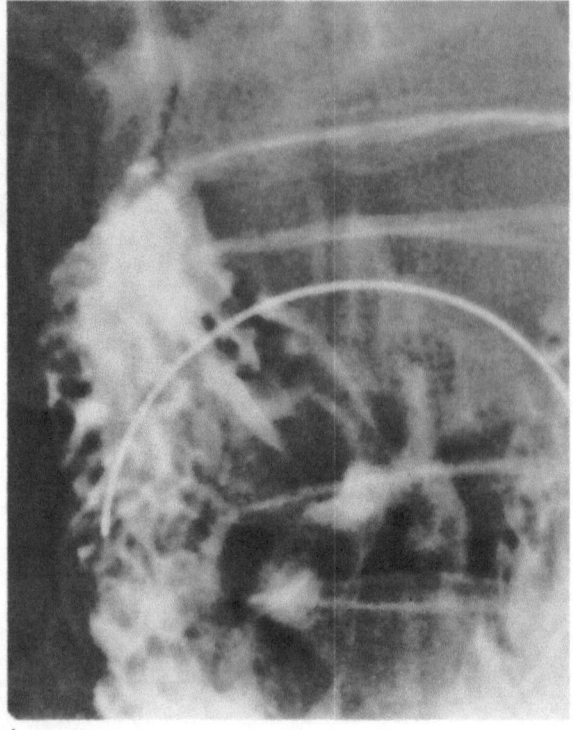

b

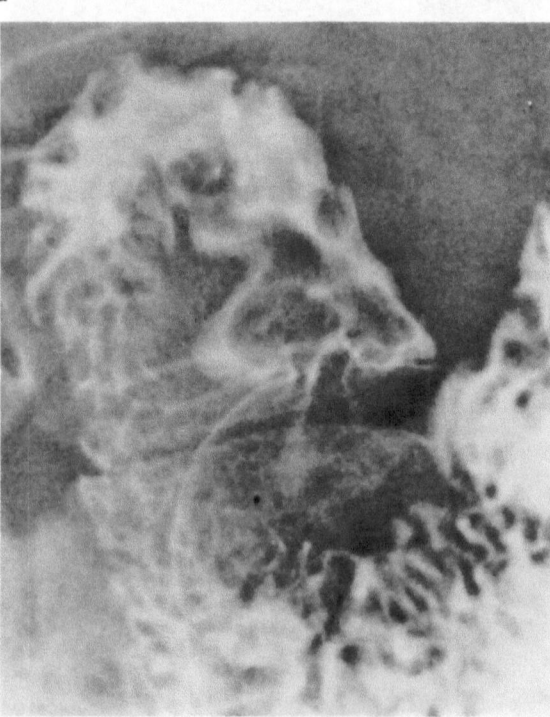

c

Fig. 151

a. PC compression study, erect position, RPO. Kissing ulcers; the rather large ulcer lies in the anterior wall, the smaller one in the posterior wall.

b. PC compression study, erect position, LPO, showing super-imposition of the two ulcer niches.

c. DC study, supine position, LPO. In this position only the small ulcer niche in the posterior wall is demonstrated.

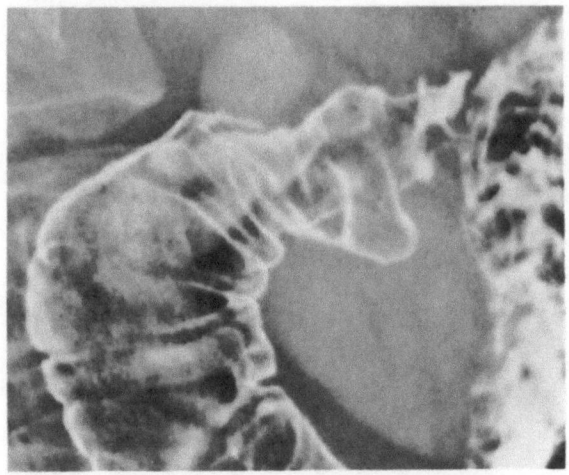

Fig. 152
DC hypotonic duodenography, supine position, LPO. There is
scarring and deformity of the bulb. It was impossible to demonstrate or to exclude a small active ulcer.

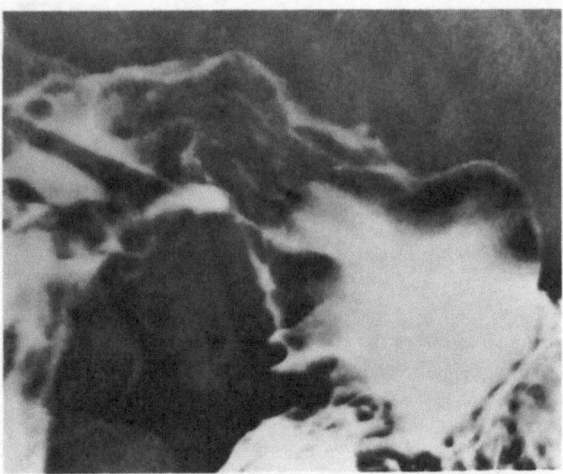

Fig. 153
DC study, supine position, LPO. Ulcer niche at the flexure between the bulb and the descending part of the duodenum.

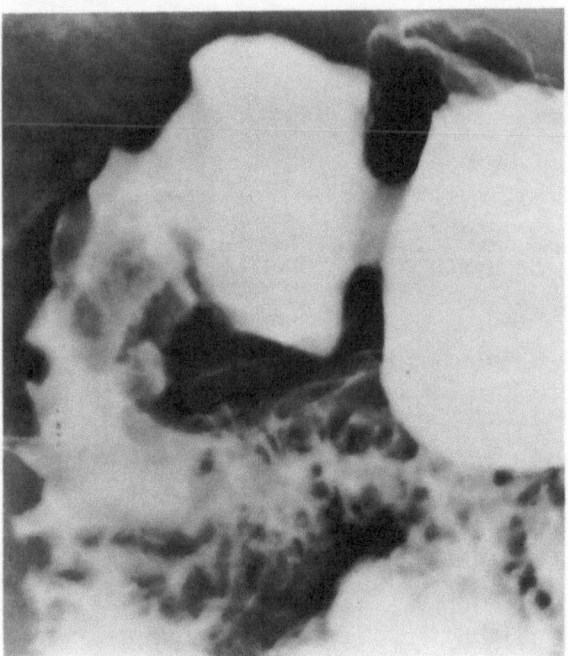

Fig. 154

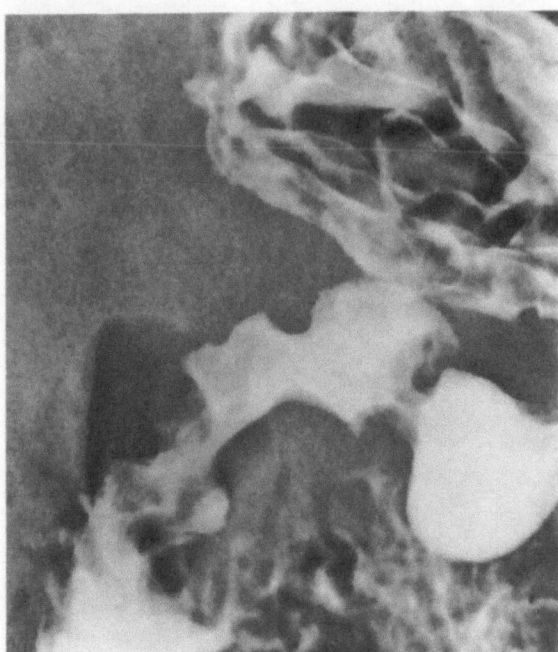

Fig. 155

Figs. 154 & 155
2 cases of endoscopically confirmed post-bulbar ulcers on the proximal and medial aspect of the descending part of the duodenum.
In fig. 155 there is a notch-like indentation on the lateral aspect of the descending duodenum.

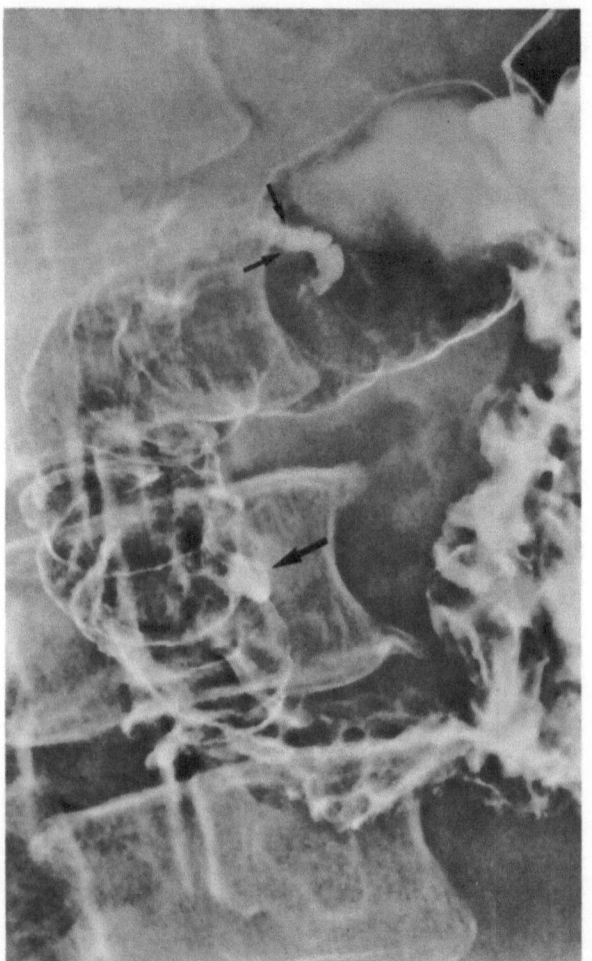 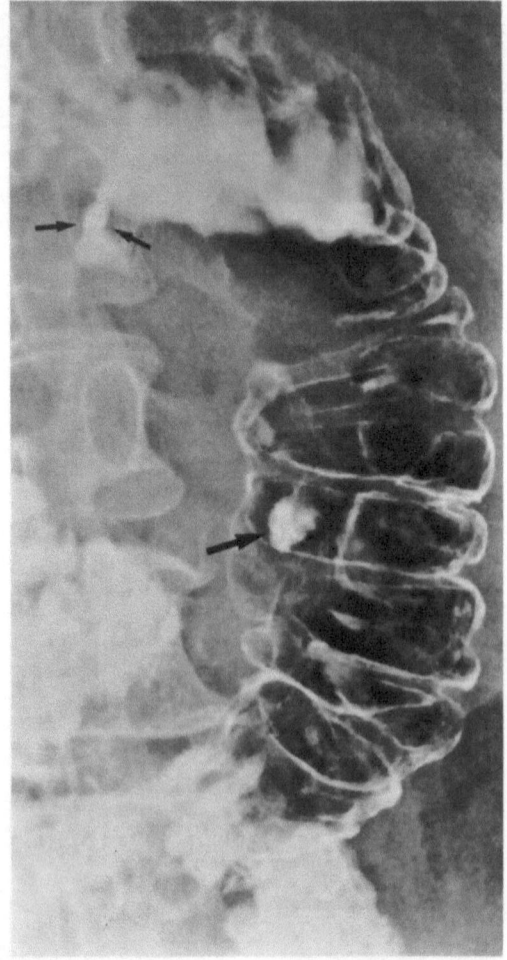

Fig. 156

a. DC hypotonic duodenography, supine position, LPO, of a
patient suffering from chronic pancreatitis.

b. DC hypotonic duodenography, prone position. Thickened
duodenal folds. The large arrow points to a post-bulbar ulcer
niche that was verified endoscopically. Retrograde filling of the
common bile duct (small arrows) which could be explained by a
previous choledocho-duodenostomy.

8.3. Benign tumors

(Including tumor-like lesions such as hyperplasia of Brunner's glands, benign lymphoid hyperplasia, heterotopic gastric epithelium, heterotopic pancreatic tissue.)

Tumors of the duodenum are rare. The benign tumors most frequently seen are adenomas (adenomatous polyps and villous adenomas), leiomyomas and lipomas (68, 249). Adenomatous polyps are usually small; they may be pedunculated or sessile (274). Villous adenomas of the duodenum have a characteristic cauliflower appearance; as in the colon, there is a high incidence of malignant degeneration (113, 209). Leiomyomas usually have a typical intramural configuration but intra- and extraluminal growth may distort the picture (58, 274). There is often central ulceration.

From the radiological point of view, lesions such as hyperplasia of Brunner's glands, benign lymphoid hyperplasia and islets of heterotopic gastric epithelium must be considered in this chapter. They often present as multiple, shallow filling defects in the duodenal bulb (80, 96). Heterotopic pancreatic tissue of the duodenum usually occurs as a single submucosal nodule; as in the stomach, the diagnosis may be suggested if barium fills duct-like structures (56). In most of these conditions, the radiological appearances do not permit definite diagnosis. Endoscopy and biopsy are frequently indicated.

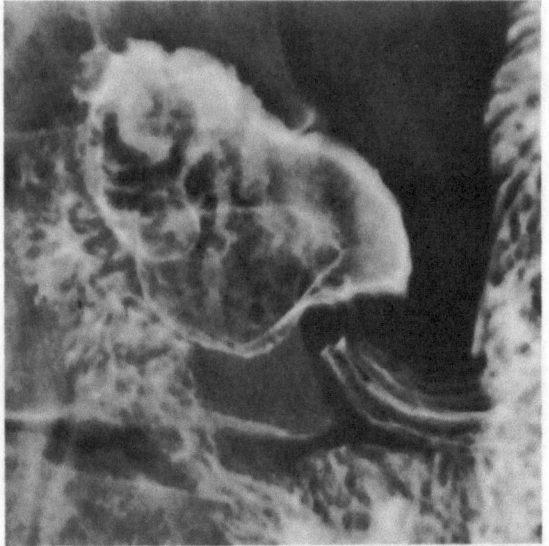

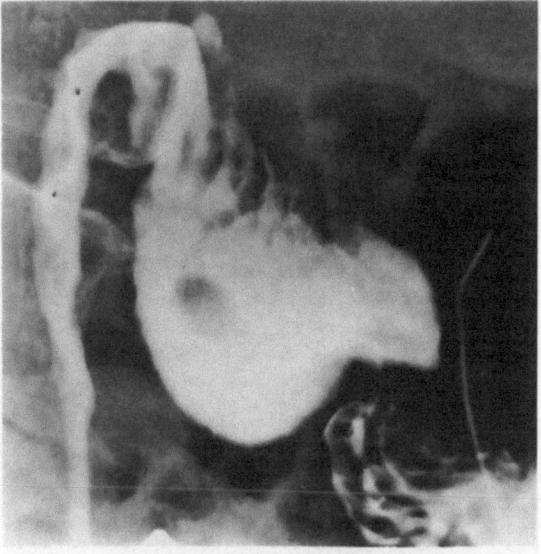

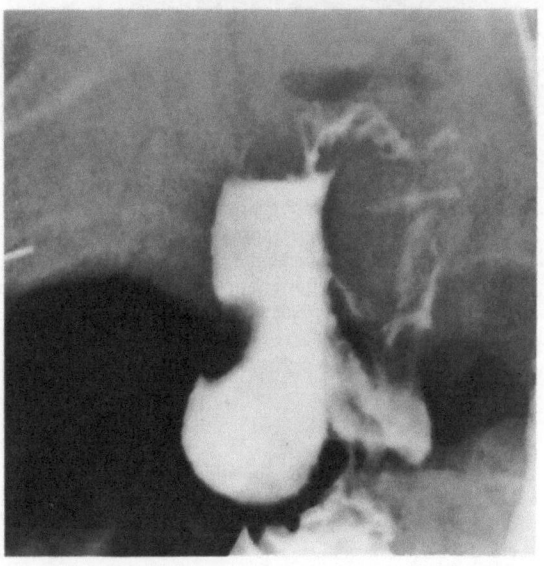

Fig. 157

a. DC study, supine position, LPO. Multiple small polypoid lesions on the posterior wall of the duodenum. Superimposed on the relief of the posterior wall a ring shadow caused by an abruptly marginated polypoid lesion that must be localized on the anterior wall.

b. PC compression study, LPO.

c. PC compression study, RPO, confirming that the large polypoid lesion is localized on the anterior wall. Biopsies from the large polyp: no definite diagnosis, no malignancy.

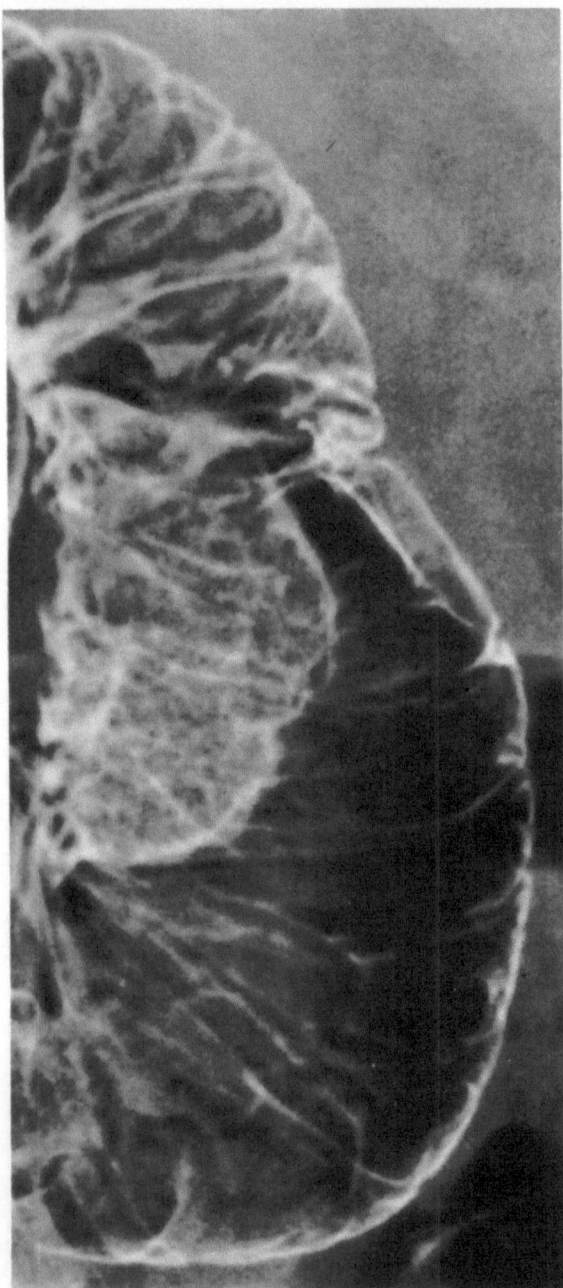

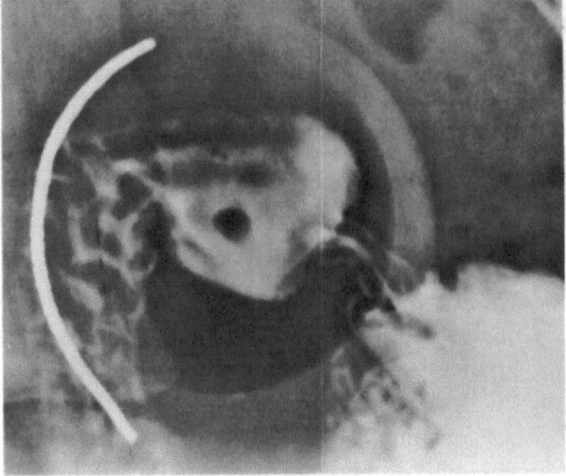

Fig. 159
PC compression study, erect position, LPO. Endoscopic confirmation. Biopsies: lipoma.

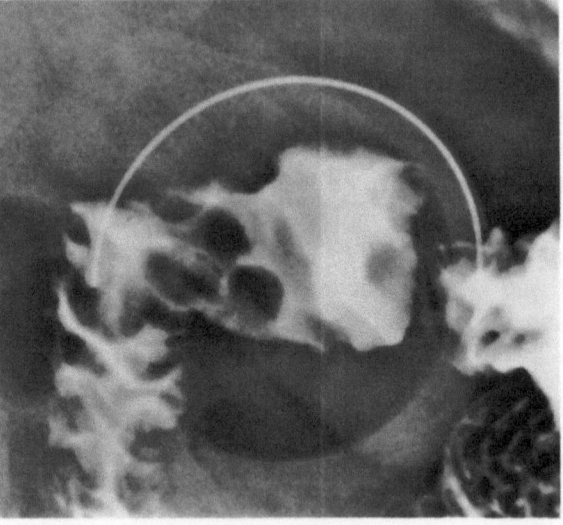

a

Fig. 158
DC hypotonic duodenography, prone position. Large filling defect with a cauliflower appearance on the medial aspect of the descending part of the duodenum. Endoscopy revealed a polypoid tumor with a cauliflower appearance. Histological examination of the resected specimen: villous adenoma.

Fig. 160   →
a. PC compression study, erect position, LPO.
b. DC study, supine position, LPO. Several filling defects in the duodenal bulb. Biopsies showed hyperplasia of Brunner's glands.

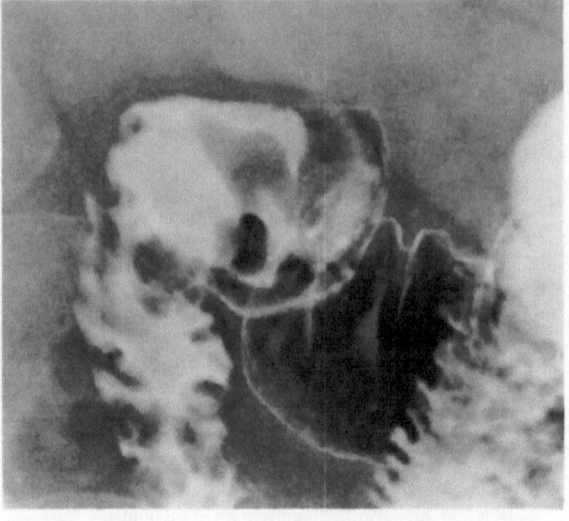

b

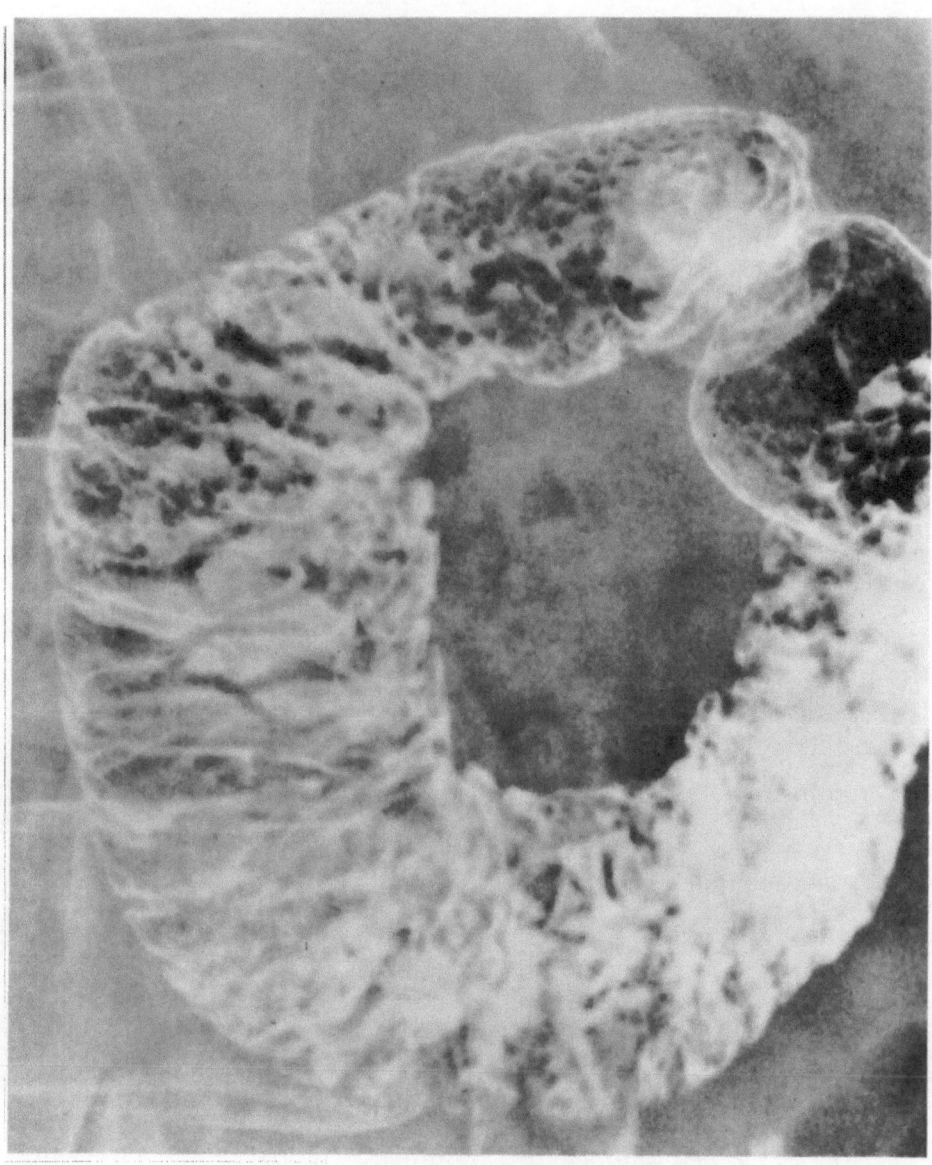

Fig. 161
DC hypotonic duodenography, LPO. Multiple tiny nodules in the duodenal bulb and the proximal part of the descending duodenum. Endoscopic confirmation. Biopsies revealed benign lymphoid hyperplasia.

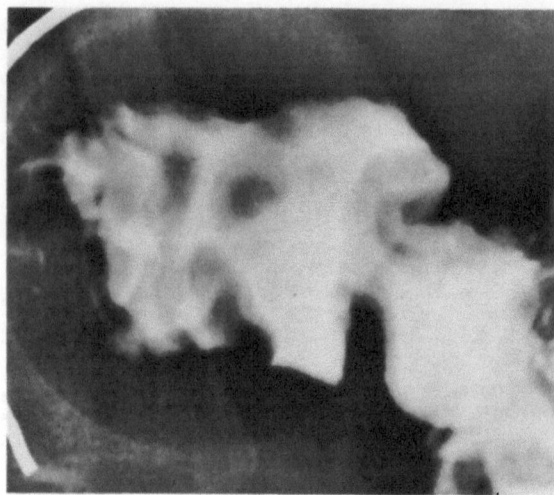

Fig. 162
PC study, erect position, LPO. Several filling defects in the duodenal bulb. Biopsies showed heterotopic gastric epithelium.

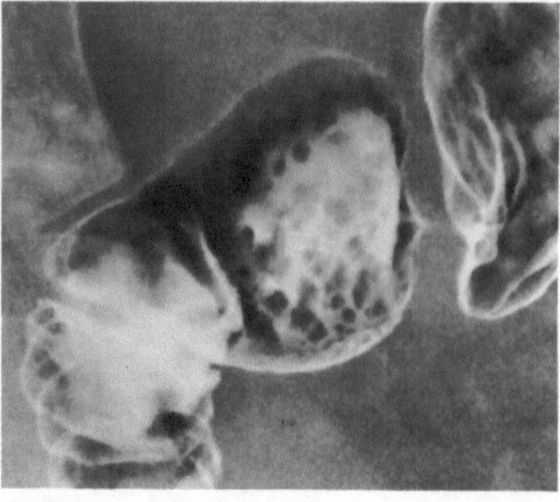

Fig. 163
DC study, supine position, LPO. Multiple filling defects on the posterior wall of the duodenal bulb. Biopsy specimens demonstrated heterotopic gastric epithelium.

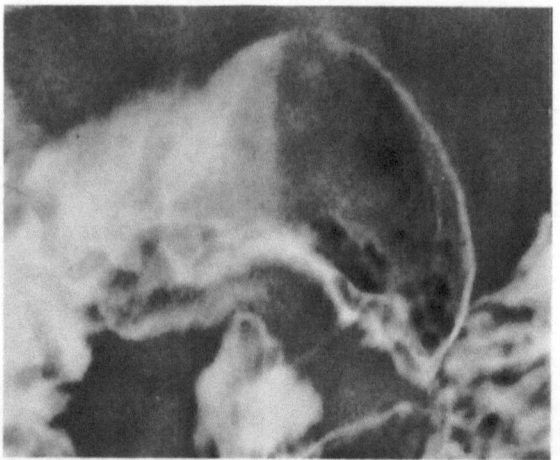

a

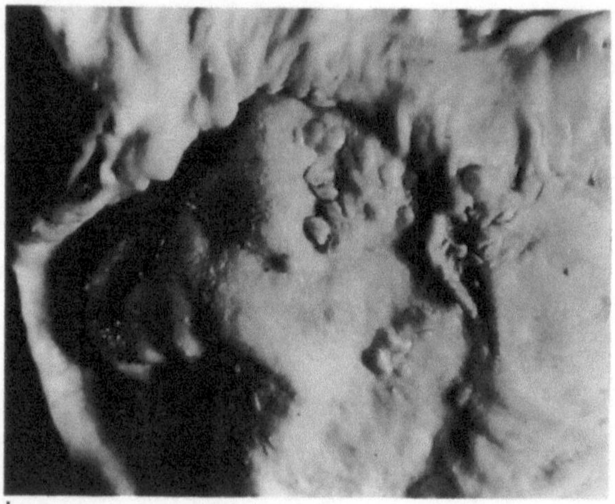

b

Fig. 164
a. DC study, supine position, LPO. Filling defects in the base of the duodenal bulb.
b. Autopsy specimen. Histological examination proved that the polypoid lesions were caused by islets of heterotopic gastric epithelium.

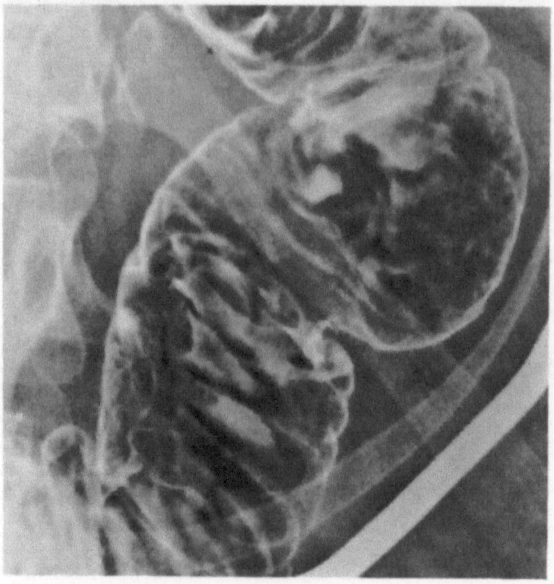

Fig. 165
DC hypotonic duodenography, prone position. Elevated lesion with a central excavation on the anterior wall of the descending duodenum. Endoscopy showed an elevated lesion with a central dimple. Biopsies did not show abnormalities. Heterotopic pancreatic tissue, leiomyoma and a large minor papilla have to be considered.

8.4. Malignant tumors

The incidence of primary small bowel malignancy is low, but absolute involvement of the duodenum is high (16, 42, 99).

The commonest malignant duodenal tumor is the adenocarcinoma, and the second commonest is leiomyosarcoma (16). Malignant lymphoma, which is probably the most common malignant growth in the small intestine (233), is encountered relatively frequently in the duodenum (7). Villous adenomas and carcinoids are tumors with a variable malignant potential, and the latter appears to have a predilection for the duodenal bulb (249). Whenever a mass lesion is visualized in the duodenum, the possibility of an alien cancer must be considered (265). An alien cancer can be a metastasis or a contiguous cancer (see 8.6. Indentations), originating from an adjacent organ such as the pancreas, biliary tract or gall bladder, stomach, colon or kidney. Although several of the above-mentioned conditions may show characteristic growth patters, e.g. malignant lymphoma (7, 161, 234), in most cases biopsy is necessary for definite diagnosis.

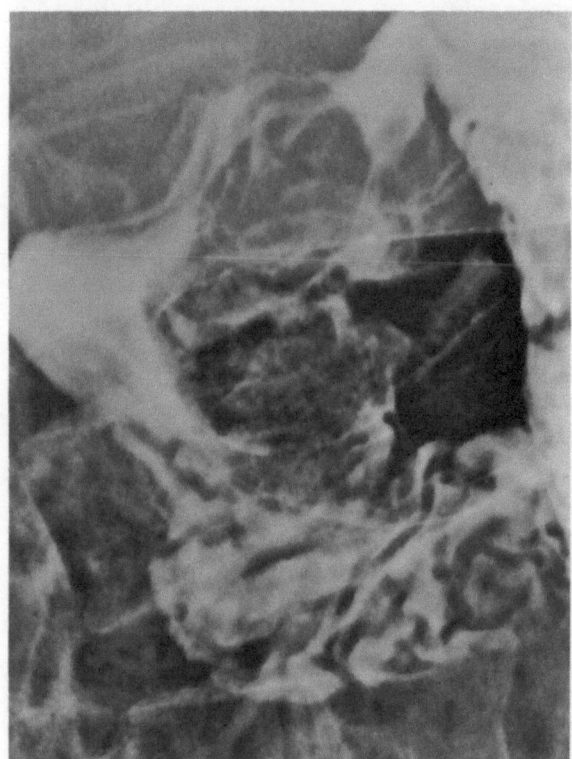 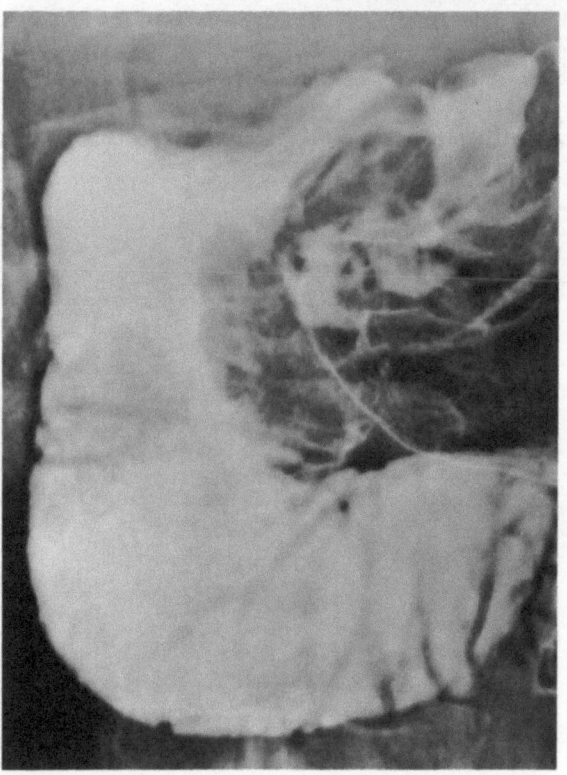

Fig. 166
a & *b*. Hypotonic duodenography, supine position, LPO. Filling defect on the medial aspect of the descending duodenum. It is difficult to differentiate between a lesion of the duodenum and an indentation caused by a mass lesion in the head of the pancreas. No endoscopy. At operation a polypoid tumor of the duodenum was found. Histological examination of the resected specimen demonstrated adenocarcinoma.

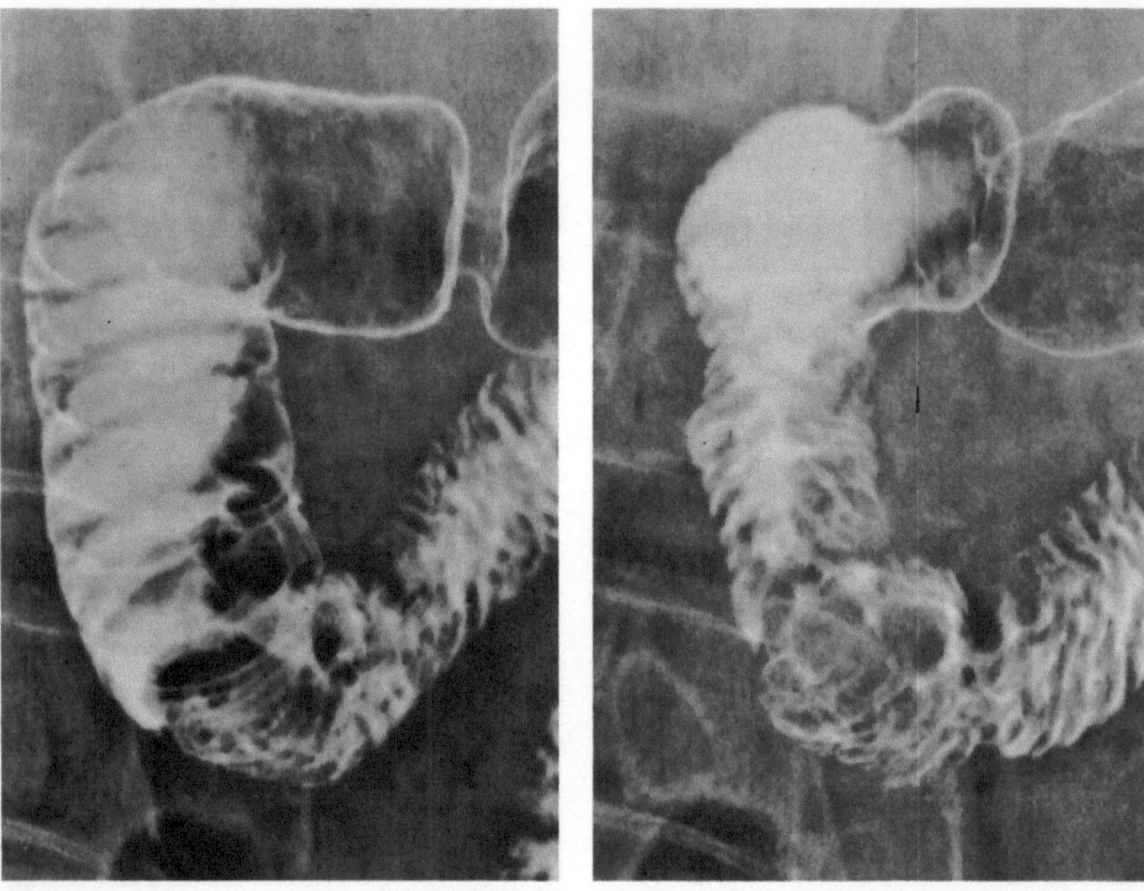

Fig. 167
a & b. DC hypotonic duodenography, supine position, LPO. Lobulated filling defect in the distal part of the descending duodenum.
    Autopsy: adenocarcinoma.

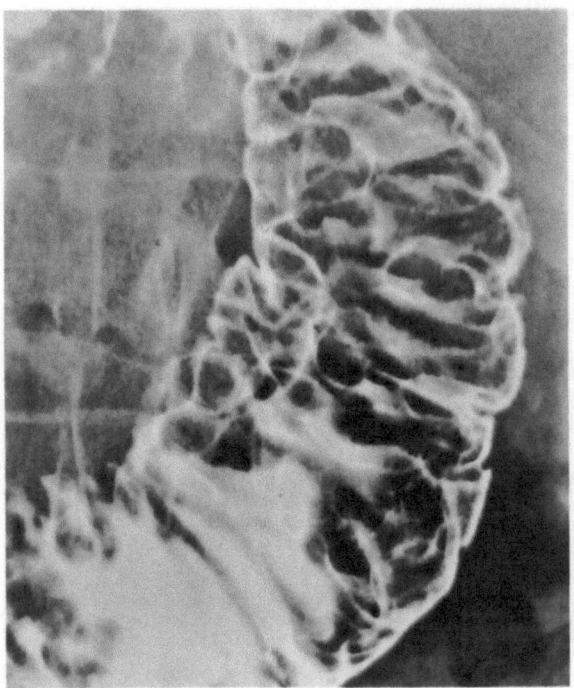

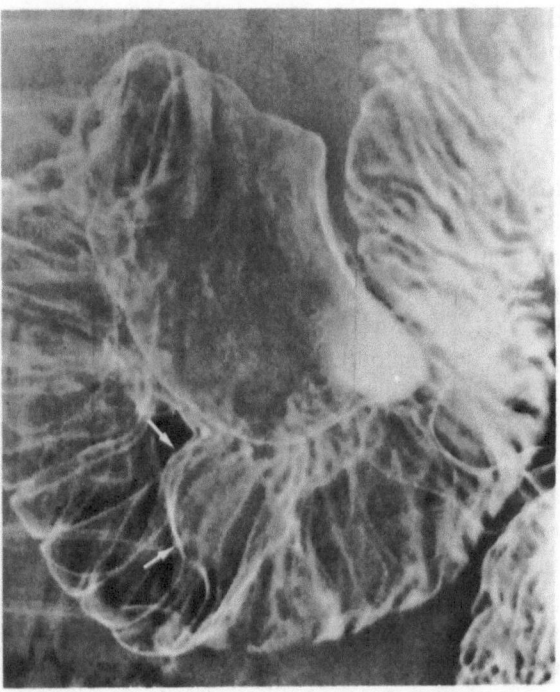

Fig. 168
DC hypotonic duodenography, prone position. Coarse folds with nodularity in the descending duodenum of a patient with malignant lymphoma of the gastrointestinal tract. See also figs. 37, 98 and 145 of this patient.

Fig. 169
DC hypotonic duodenography, supine position, LPO. Filling defect caused by a probably submucosal mass in the third part of the duodenum (arrows). At autopsy multiple metastases of a bronchogenic carcinoma were found.

8.5. Enlargement of the major duodenal papilla

Although a normal major duodenal papilla may be as long as 3 cm. it is usually considered abnormal if longer than 1.5 cm. (17, 53, 69, 120). Papillary enlargement may be the result of edema or neoplastic infiltration. Edema can be caused by pancreatitis, peptic ulcer or stone in the distal common bile duct (17, 54, 120). In the case of edema, the enlarged papilla has a smooth surface.

A periampullary adenocarcinoma, arising from the papilla or the ampulla of Vater, the head of the pancreas or the duodenal mucosa, usually produces an irregular filling defect. However, a carcinoma of the ampulla, may have a smooth surface (55). Benign tumors of the ampulla of Vater are very rare (121), giving an appearance that cannot be differentiated from edematous papillary swelling. In order to exclude an impacted stone – presumably the commonest cause of smooth-surfaced enlargment of the major duodenal papilla – the next logical step is cholangiography.

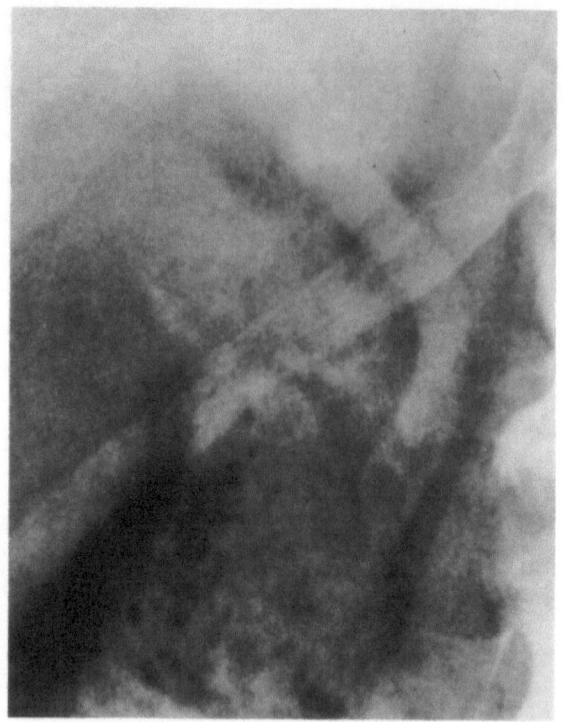

b

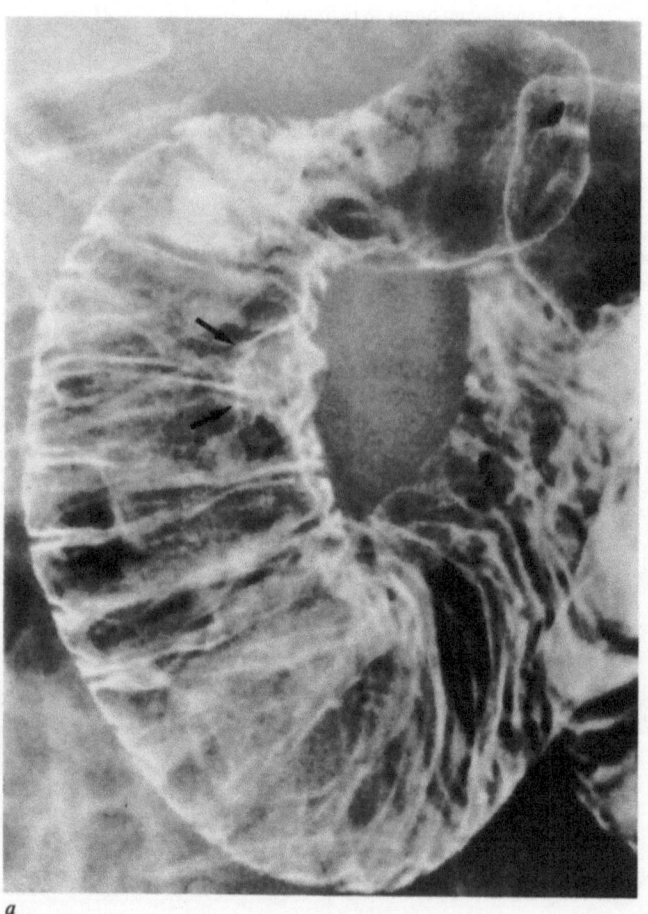

a

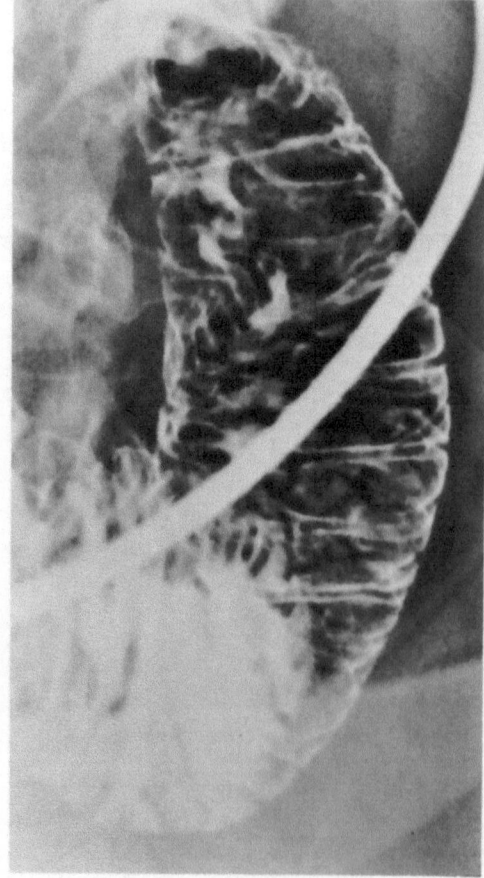

c

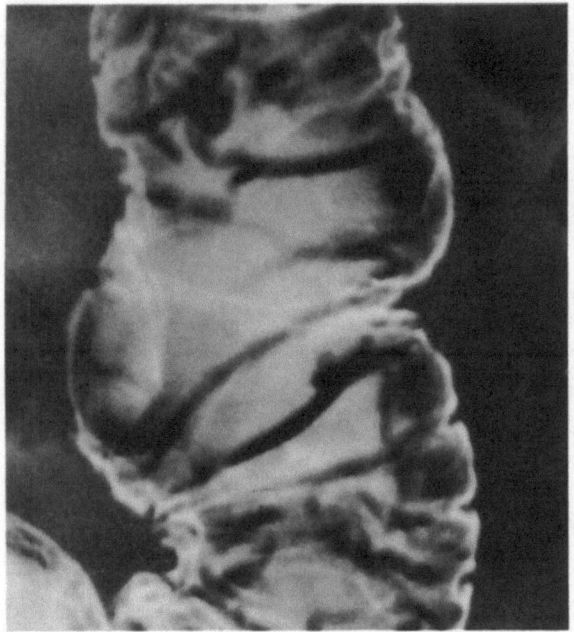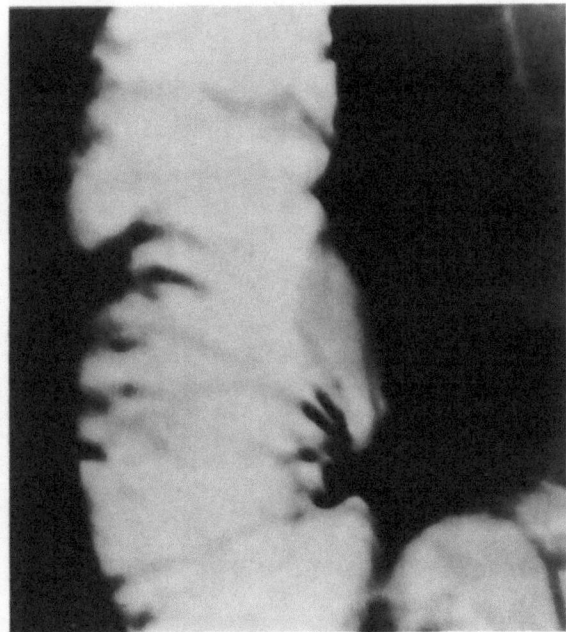

Fig. 171

a. DC hypotonic duodenography, prone position. A patient with obstructive jaundice.

b. PC hypotonic duodenography, supine position. Filling defect on the medial side of the descending duodenum. Endoscopy revealed an edematous major papilla. Endoscopic retrograde pancreatico-cholangiography demonstrated some stones in the distal common bile duct which were supposed to have caused edema of the major papilla.

8.6. Indentations

During the hypotonic examination the duodenum can be viewed as a mold formed by adjacent organs. Mass lesions of these organs can be diagnosed by deformity of this mold.

The lateral aspect of the flexure between the duodenal bulb and the descending part of the duodenum is often indented by the gall-bladder, either normal or pathological (figs. 172, 173, 174). In cases of pericholecystitic abcess, this impression may be irregular. A dilated common bile duct may indent the posterior aspect of the apex of the duodenal bulb (57) (fig. 175). The lateral aspect of the descending part lies in close relation to the right kidney, and often results in a normal impression (88). Mass lesions of the right kidney or an abnormally horizontal

longitudinal axis of the right kidney produces a larger impression (figs. 176, 177). Mass lesions in the liver may impress several sites on the lateral aspect (fig. 178). Contiguity of the hepatic flexure of the colon to the descending part of the duodenum facilitates the spread of a neoplasm (165).

Indentations on the medial aspect of the duodenum are in most instances caused by mass lesions in the head of the pancreas. Personal experience and that of others (122, 221) has shown that hypotonic duodenography fails to differentiate between a mass in the head of the pancreas caused by a carcinoma and one caused by chronic pancreatitis. Sometimes it is difficult even to differentiate a lesion of the duodenum from a mass lesion in the head of the pancreas (figs. 166, 179).

←

Fig. 170

a. DC hypotonic duodenography, LPO. The folds in the duodenal bulb are effaced by gaseous distension. In the descending duodenum the transversely oriented folds of Kerkring remain visible. Filling defect on the postero-medial side of the descending duodenum (arrows).

c. DC hypotonic duodenography, prone position, confirming the defect. This appearance is compatible with a large duodenal major papilla.

b. Cholangiography revealed a stone in the distal common bile duct. The filling defect demonstrated in a and b probably represents edema of the duodenal major papilla.

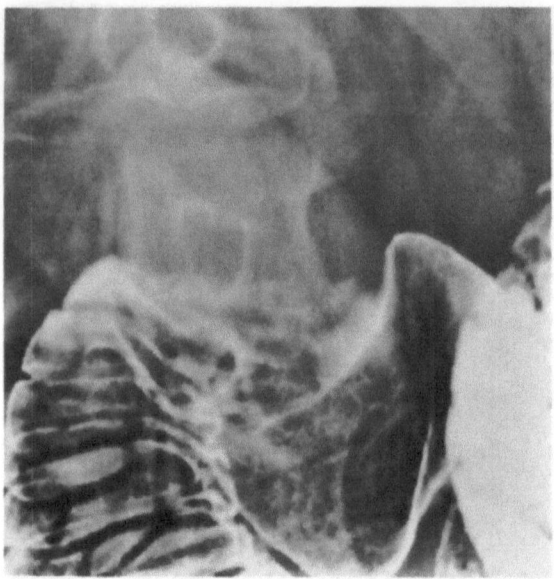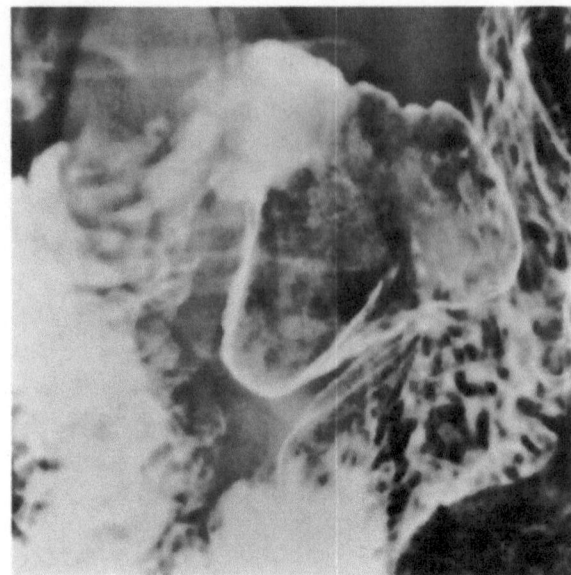

Fig. 172

a &b. DC hypotonic duodenography, supine position, LPO. Filling defect on the lateral aspect of the flexure between the deodenal bulb and the descending part of the duodenum. The filling defect is inconstant during changes of forces of gravity: indentation caused by a normal gall bladder which is faintly opacified.

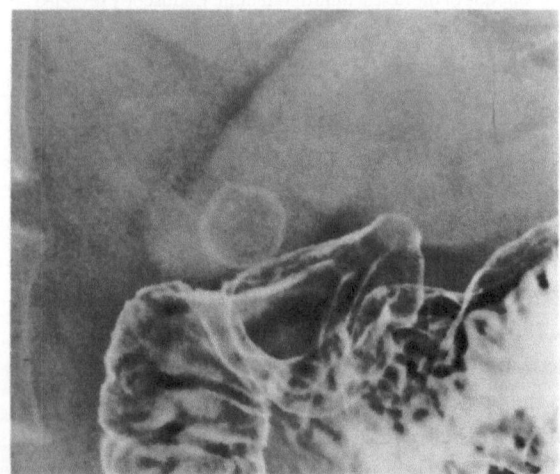

←
Fig. 173

DC hypotonic duodenography, supine position, LPO. The duodenal bulb is indented by the gall bladder which contains a stone.

Fig. 174

a & b. DC hypotonic duodenography, supine position, LPO. Irregular indentation in a patient with the clinical features of a cholecystitis. Operation revealed a pericholecystitic abcess.

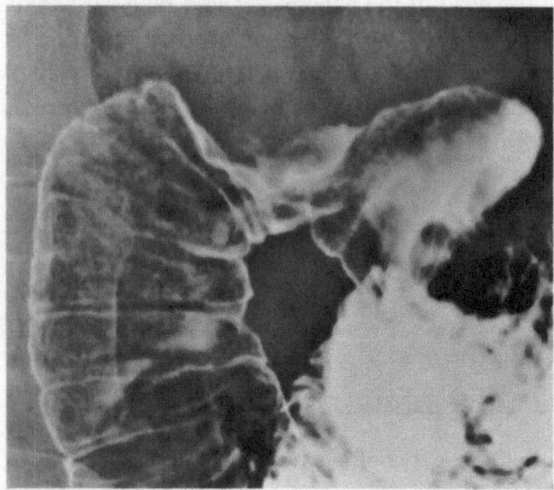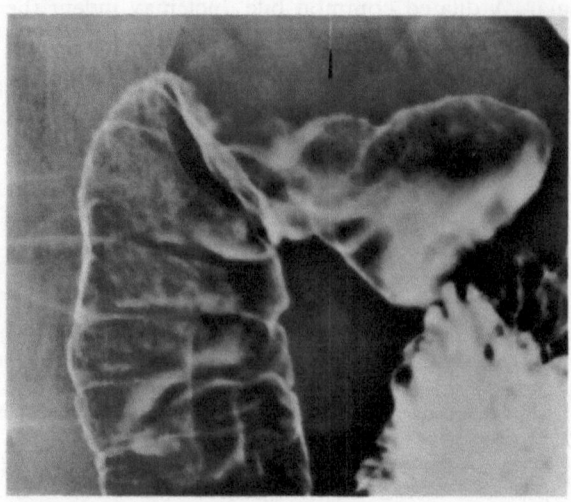

a   *b*

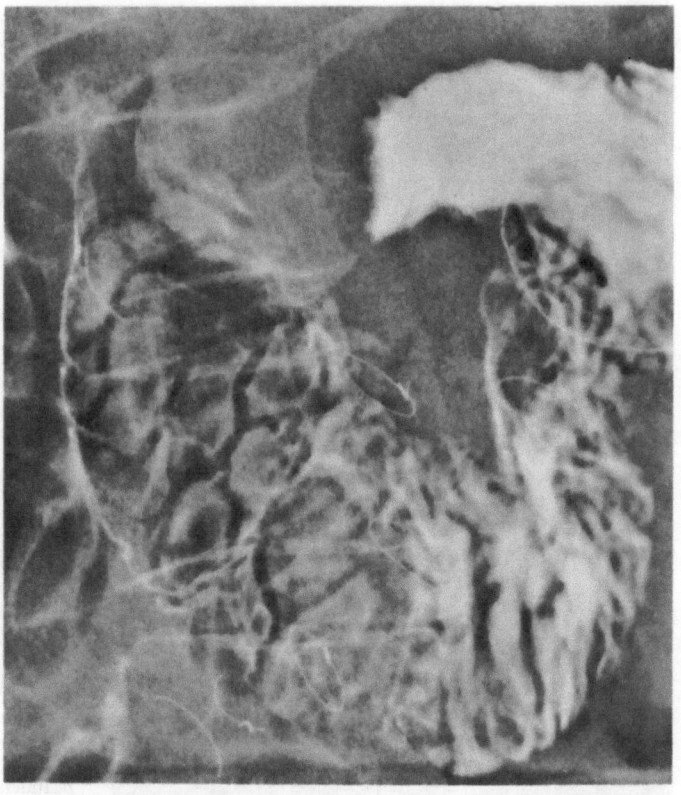

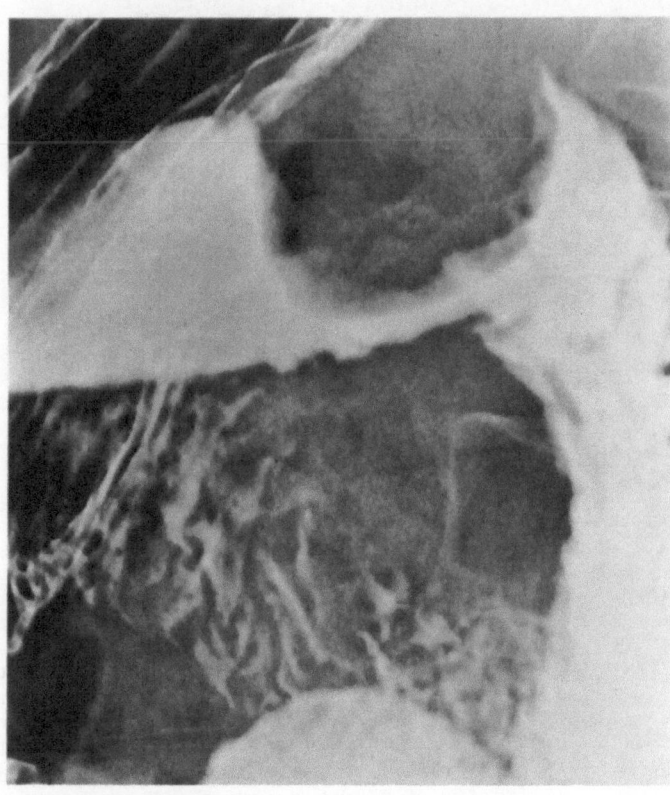

Fig. 175

a. DC hypotonic duodenography, supine position,
   LPO.

b. PC hypotonic duodenography, right procubitus
   position. The patient had previously been operated
   upon because of congenital anomalies of the biliary
   tract. Autopsy demonstrated an impression caused
   by a bile containing cavity which was probably an
   extremely dilated choledochal duct.

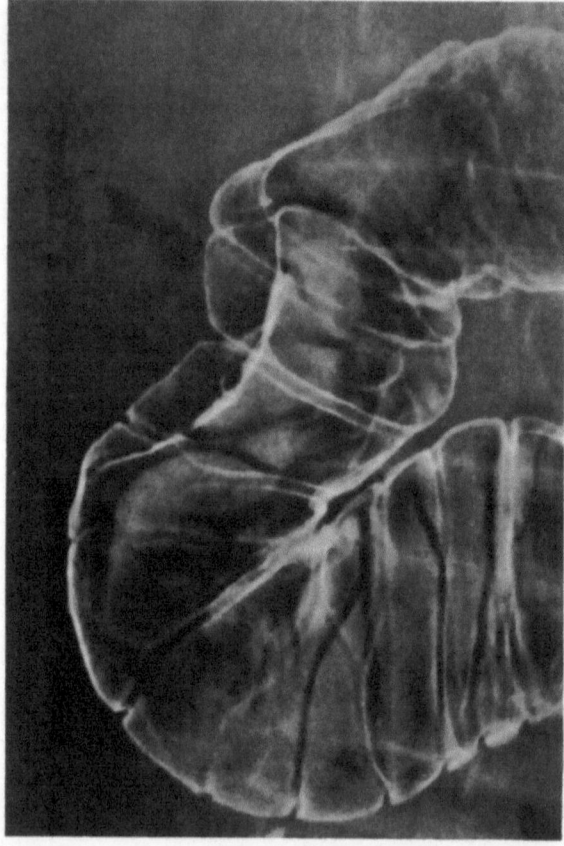

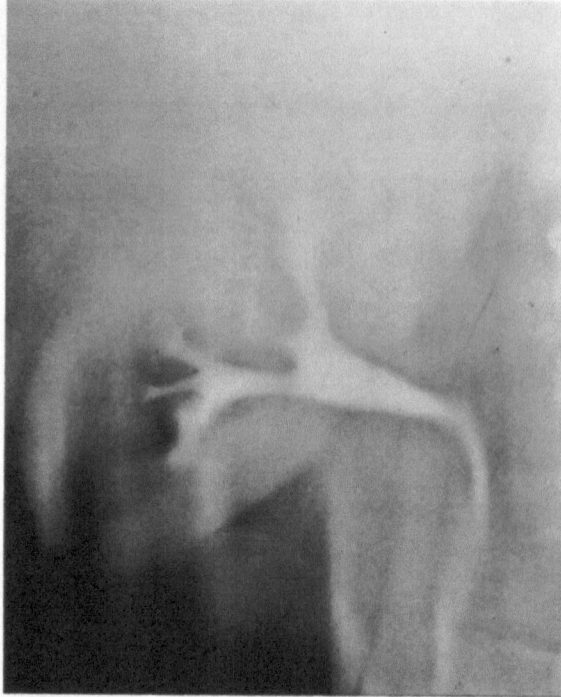

a

Fig. 176

a. DC hypotonic duodenography, supine position, LPO.

b. Indentation on the lateral aspect of the descending duodenum caused by an abnormally longitudinal axis of the right kidney as was confirmed by an IVP.

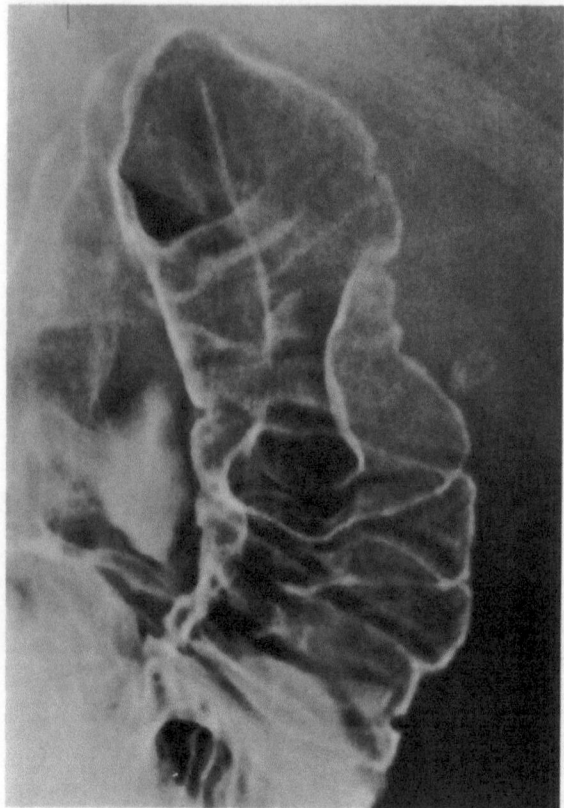

Fig. 177

DC hypotonic duodenography, prone position. Indentation of the lateral aspect of the descending part of the duodenum. This patient was suffering from polycystic renal disease. Autopsy confirmed that the indentation was caused by a renal cyst. Same patient as shown in fig. 121.

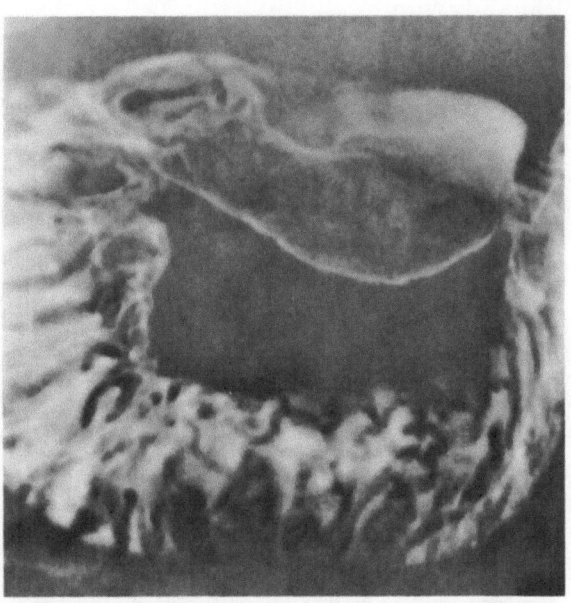

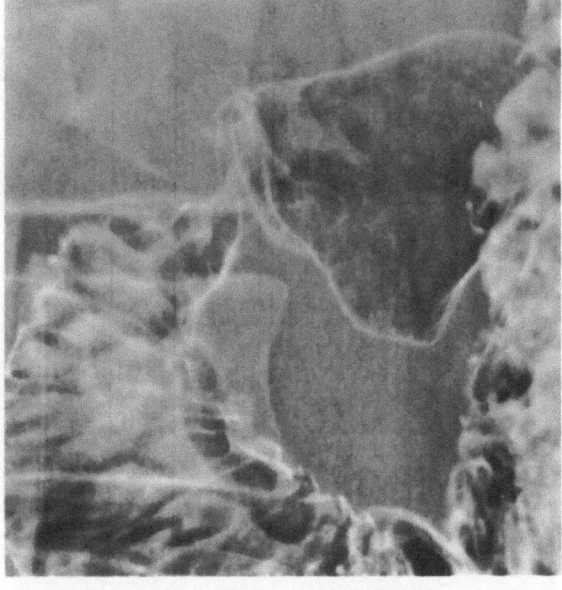

Fig. 178
DC study of the duodenal bulb, supine position, LPO. Indentation of the lesser curvature of the duodenal bulb. Autopsy demonstrated that the indentation was caused by a metastasis in the liver.

Fig. 180
DC hypotonic duodenography, supine position, LPO. Stricture of the proximal part of the descending duodenum. At operation a mass in the head of the pancreas was found. Biopsies revealed a chronic pancreatitis. A follow-up study confirmed the diagnosis.

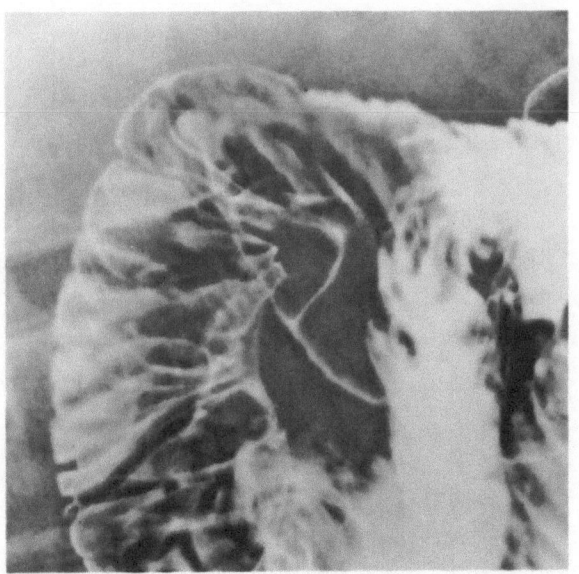

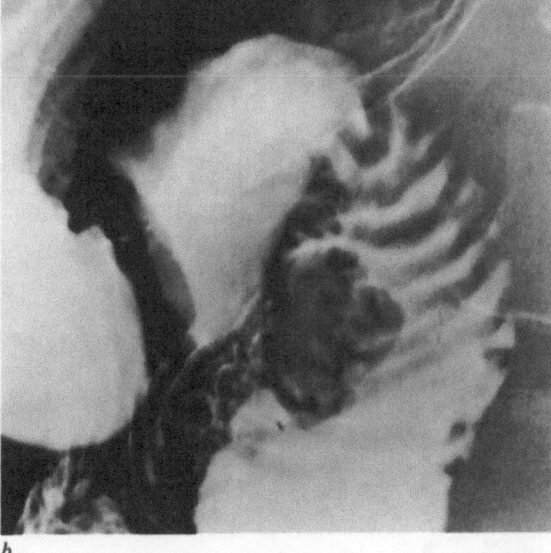

Fig. 179
a. DC hypotonic duodenography, supine position, LPO.
b. PC hypotonic duodenography, right procubitus position. Mass lesion on the medial aspect of the proximal part of the descending duodenum. It was difficult to differentiate between a lesion of the duodenum and a mass lesion in the head of the pancreas. Endoscopy showed an intact duodenal mucosa. Further examinations and a follow-up study were compatible with the diagnosis chronic pancreatitis.

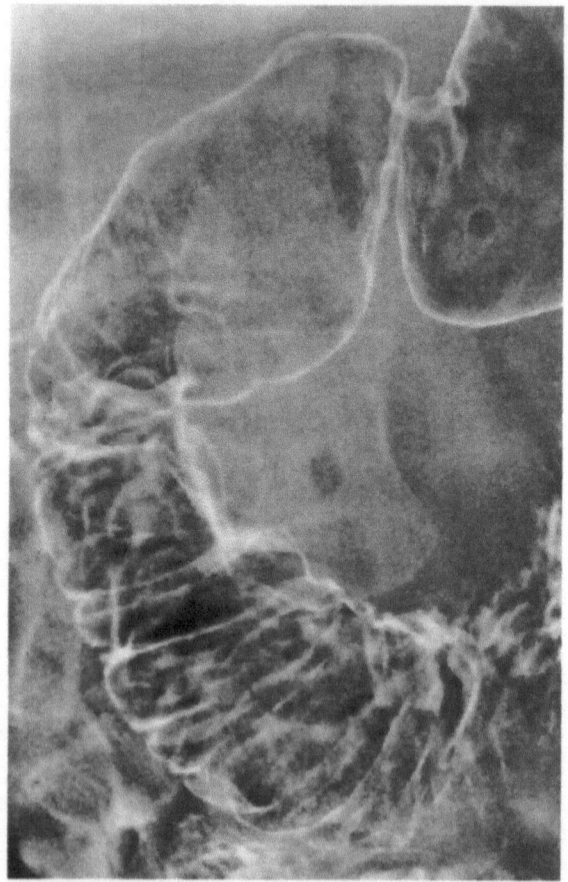

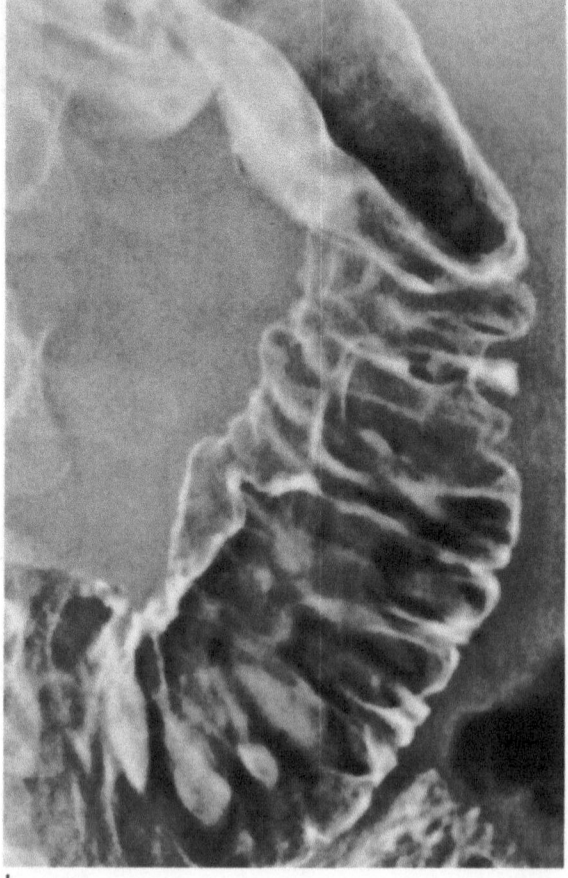

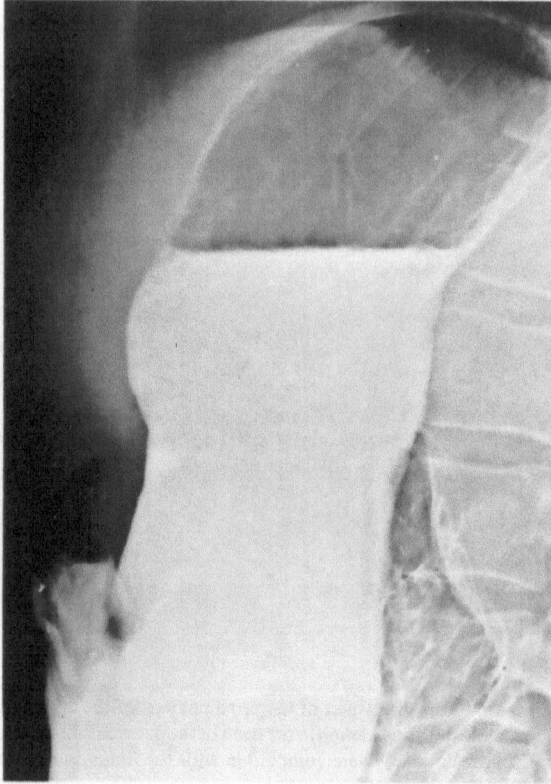

Fig. 181

a. DC hypotonic duodenography, supine position, LPO.

b. DC hypotonic duodenography, prone position. Indentation of the medial aspect of the duodenal bulb and the descending duodenum.

c. DC hypotonic duodenography, erect right lateral position, showing a dorsal indentation of the descending duodenum. At operation a mass in the head of the pancreas was found. Biopsies: chronic pancreatitis. Diagnosis confirmed by a follow-up study.

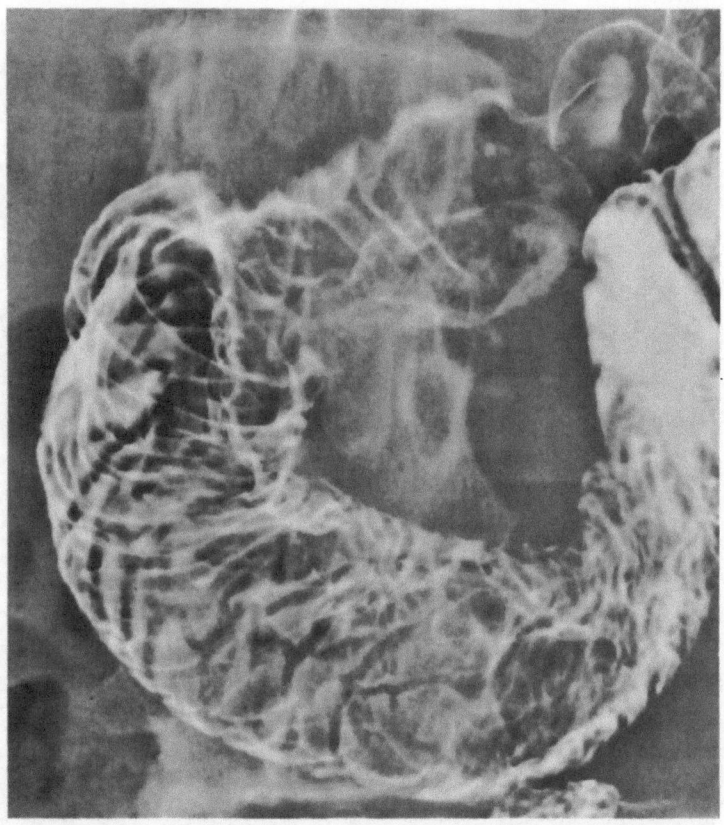

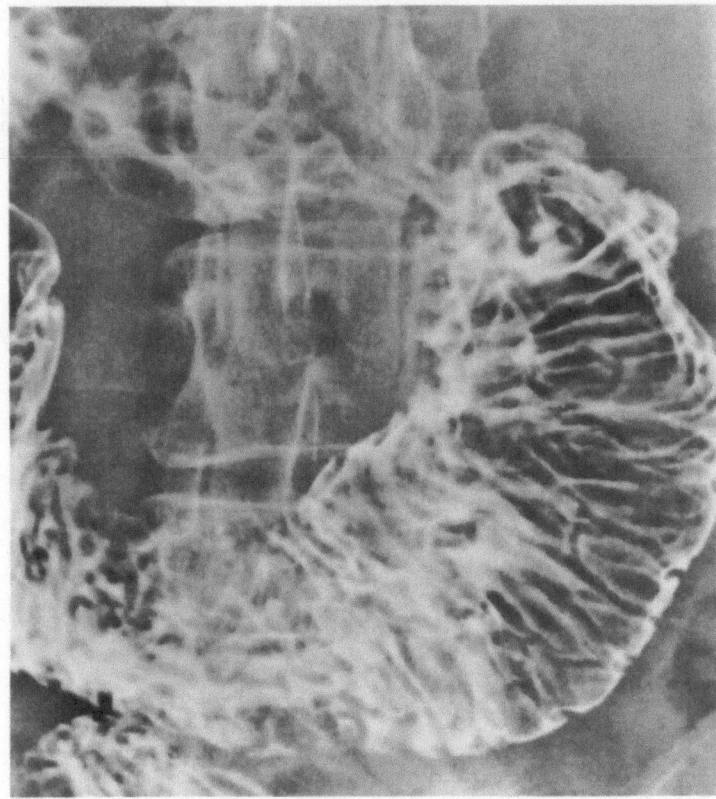

Fig. 182

a. DC hypotonic duodenography, supine position.

b. DC hypotonic duodenography, prone position. Irregular indentation of the medial aspect of the duodenal bulb and the descending duodenum. Autopsy demonstrated a carcinoma in the head of the pancreas.

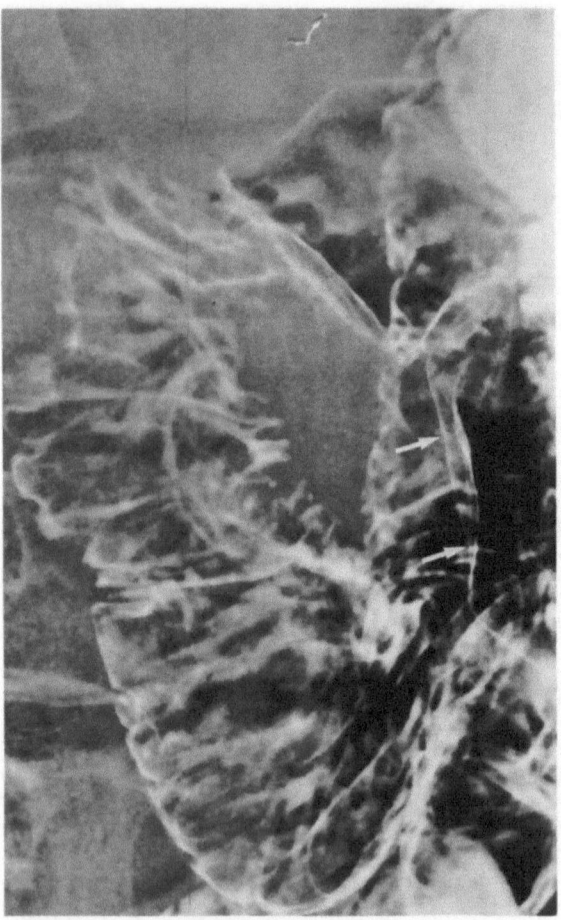 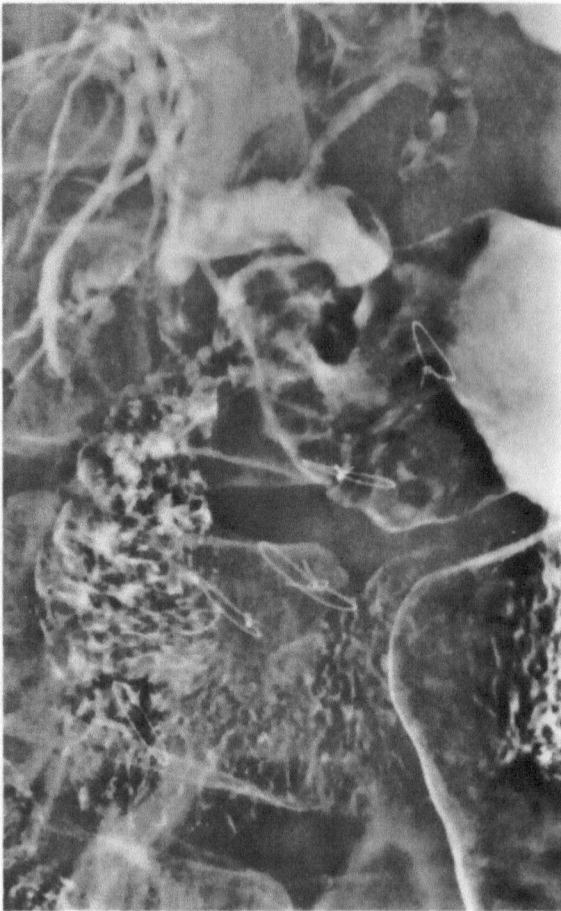

Fig. 183

a. DC hypotonic duodenography, supine position, LPO. Irregular indentation of the medial aspect of the descending duodenum. Smooth indentation of the duodenal bulb and the postero-lateral aspect of the gastric antrum: antral pad sign (arrows). At operation a carcinoma in the head of the pancreas was found; the gall bladder was extremely dilated. The tumor was considered unresectable; a choledocho-duodenostomy was made.

b. DC study, supine position, LPO, after the operation. There is retrograde filling of the biliary tree. The smooth indentation of the duodenal bulb and the gastric antrum has disappeared, proving that this antral pad sign was caused by the dilated gall bladder.

8.7. Miscellaneous

8.7.1. PROLAPSE OF GASTRIC MUCOSA

Prolapse of gastric mucosa through the pylorus is a frequent radiological finding. The clinical significance is a matter of controversy (13, 199).

8.7.2. PROLAPSE OF GASTRIC POLYPS

Prolapse of a gastric polyp may mimic prolapse of the gastric mucosa. The diagnosis can be readily made when a stalk is demonstrated or when the polyp relapses in the stomach in the course of the examination (fig. 185). Symptoms of intermittent obstruction may be present.

8.7.3. DIVERTICULUM

Diverticula are often encountered in the duodenum. The site of predilection is the medial aspect of the descending part of the duodenum. If the folds are seen to progress into the diverticulum, an ulcer niche can be excluded. Diverticula are considered to be clinically unimportant. A juxta-papillary diverticulum containing retained material may obstruct the biliary or pancreatic ducts (60, 198) (fig. 188).

8.7.4. ANNULAR PANCREAS

In annular pancreas a ring of pancreatic tissue encircles the descending part of the duodenum causing a stenotic ring. The main differential diagnosis is stricture caused by post-bulbar peptic ulceration (figs. 189, 190). Because peptic ulceration is not infrequently encountered in cases of annular pancreas (66, 222), this distinction may be impossible. En-

doscopic retrograde pancreatico-cholangiography demonstrating an annular duct, permits a definite diagnosis (5).

8.7.5. DUODENAL SEPTUM

A disorder in the vacuolization of the duodenal lumen during fetal life may manifest in adulthood as a total or partial duodenal septum (fig. 192). The radiological diagnosis is easily made. A septum with an eccentric opening may result in an intraluminal pseudo-diverticulum (215).

8.7.6. CROHN'S DISEASE

Crohn's disease of the duodenum is rare, involving no more than a few per cent of the patients suffering from the disease (154, 231). The appearances are similar to those found in lesions of more distal parts of the small bowel (154), description of which is beyond the scope of this chapter. Recently varioliform erosions in the duodenum were demonstrated as an early manifestation of the disease (64, 117, 153, 159). The diagnosis should be considered whenever multiple stenotic lesions in the duodenum are visualized (187).

8.7.7. EROSIONS

Only erosions of the varioliform type can be reliably diagnosed by the radiologist. Varioliform erosions seem to be less frequent in the duodenum than in the stomach. They occur with or without peptic ulceration. As in the stomach, varioliform erosions may represent the early lesion of Crohn's disease (64, 117, 153, 159).

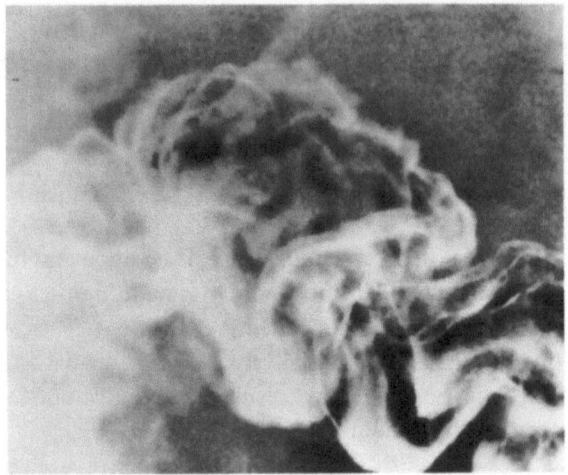

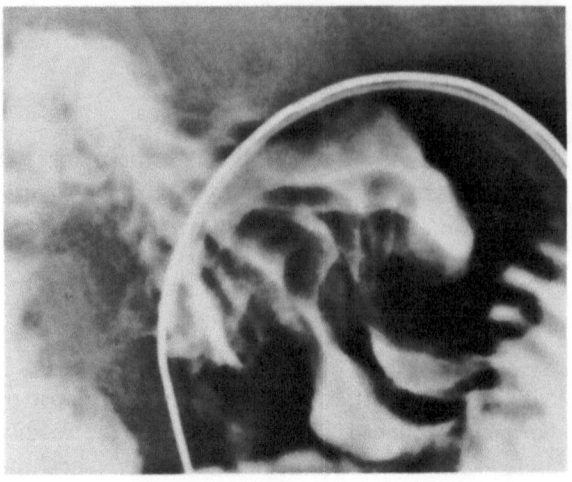

Fig. 184
a. DC study, supine position, LPO.

b. PC compression study, erect position, LPO. Prolapse of gastric mucosa through the pylorus.

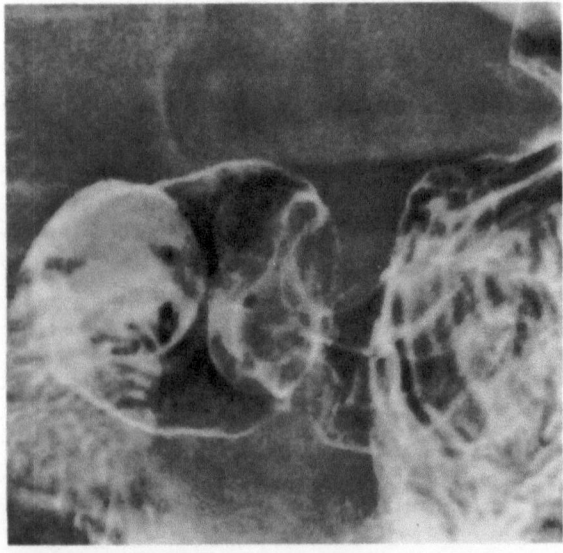

a

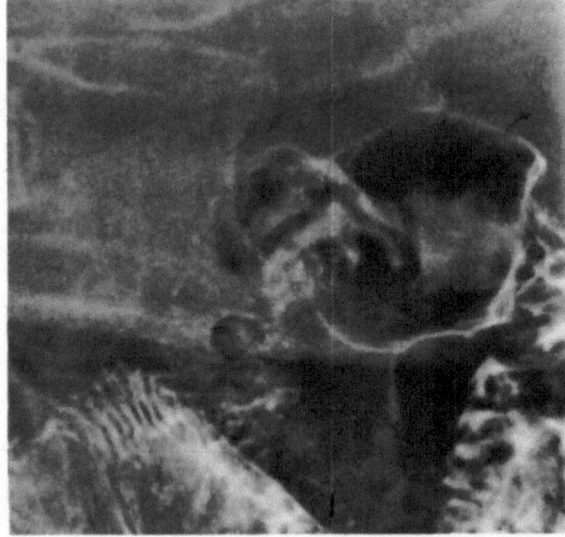

b

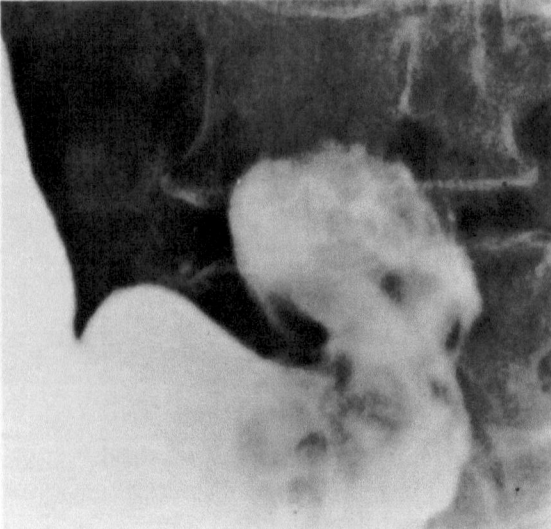

c

Fig. 185
a. DC study, supine position, LPO.
b. DC study, supine position, LPO.
c. PC study, prone position. Prolapse of a gastric polyp in the duodenum. The appearance in fig. a. mimicks a prolapse of gastric mucosa. The diagnosis of a prolapsing gastric polyp could be made because the polyp relapsed in the stomach in the course of the examination as shown in b. and c.

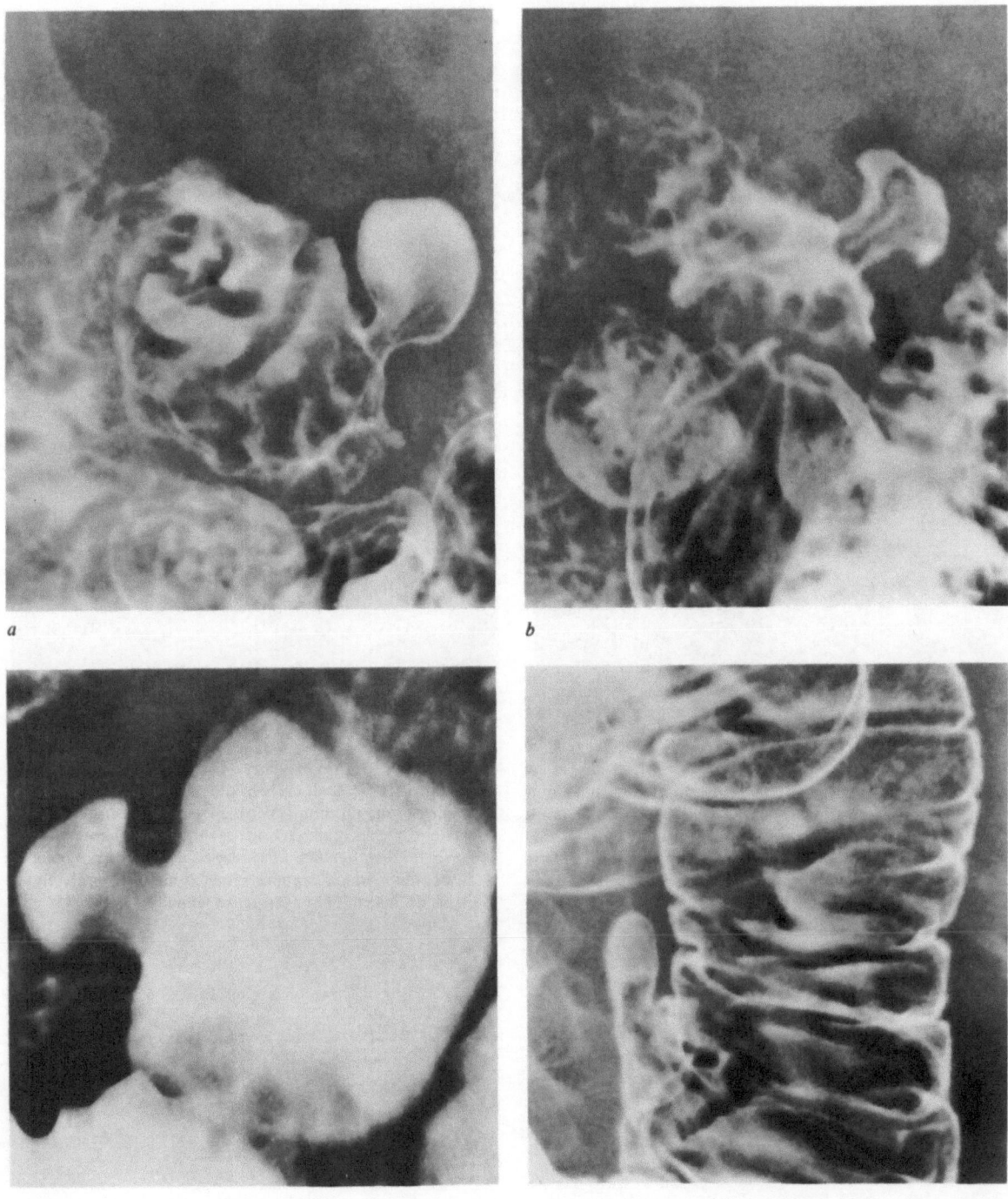

a

b

c

Fig. 186
a & b. DC studies, supine position, LPO.
c. PC study, prone position. Diverticulum of the duodenal bulb;
an ulcer niche could be excluded because the folds are seen to
progress in the outpouching.

Fig. 187
DC hypotonic duodenography, prone position. A juxtapapilllary
diverticulum; a fold is seen to progress into the diverticulum.

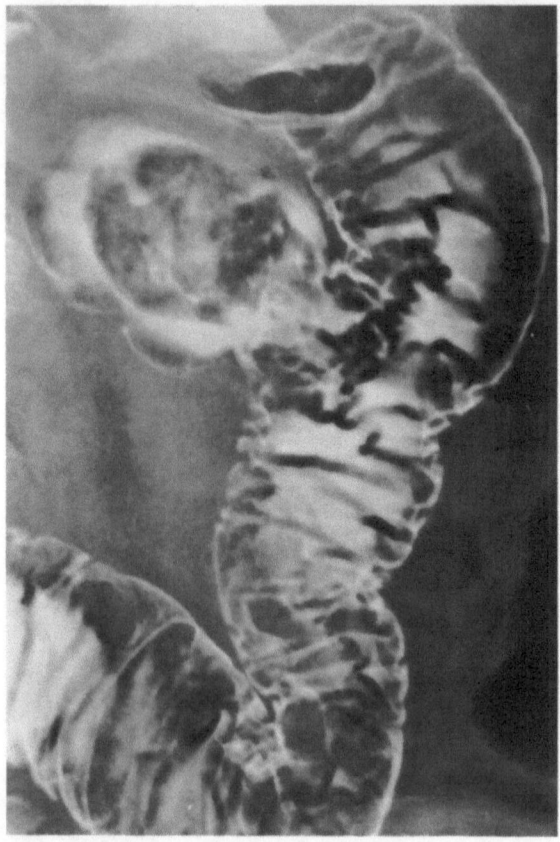 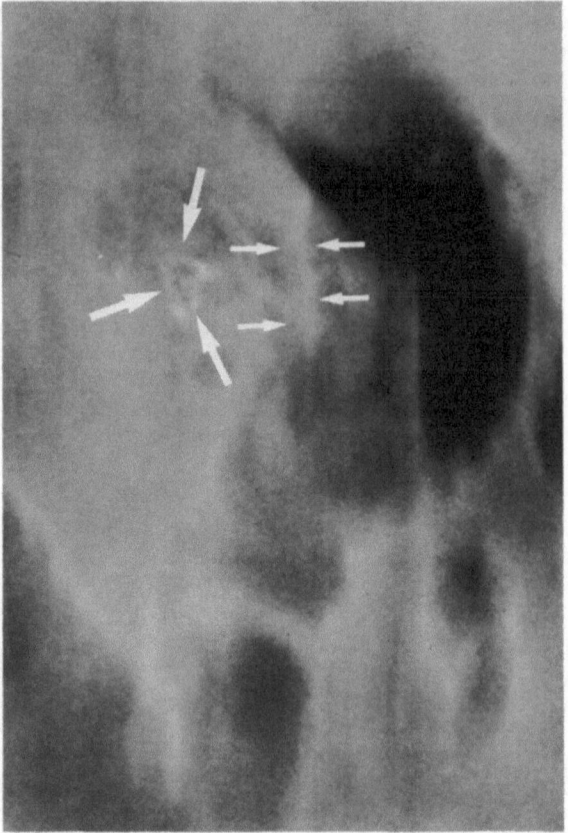

Fig. 188

a. DC hypotonic duodenography, prone position. A huge out-pouching of the medial side of the proximal part of the descending duodenum. A fold is seen to progress in the outpouching which confirms the diagnosis diverticulum. There is a filling defect in the diverticulum, probably caused by retained material. The patient suffered from intermittent obstructive jaundice.

b. Combined IVC and carbon dioxide hypotonic duodenography, prone position. The small arrows point to the distal common bile duct.; the large arrows to retained barium suspension in the diverticulum. The juxta-papillary localization of the diverticulum which contains retained material, probably explains the intermittent obstructive jaundice.

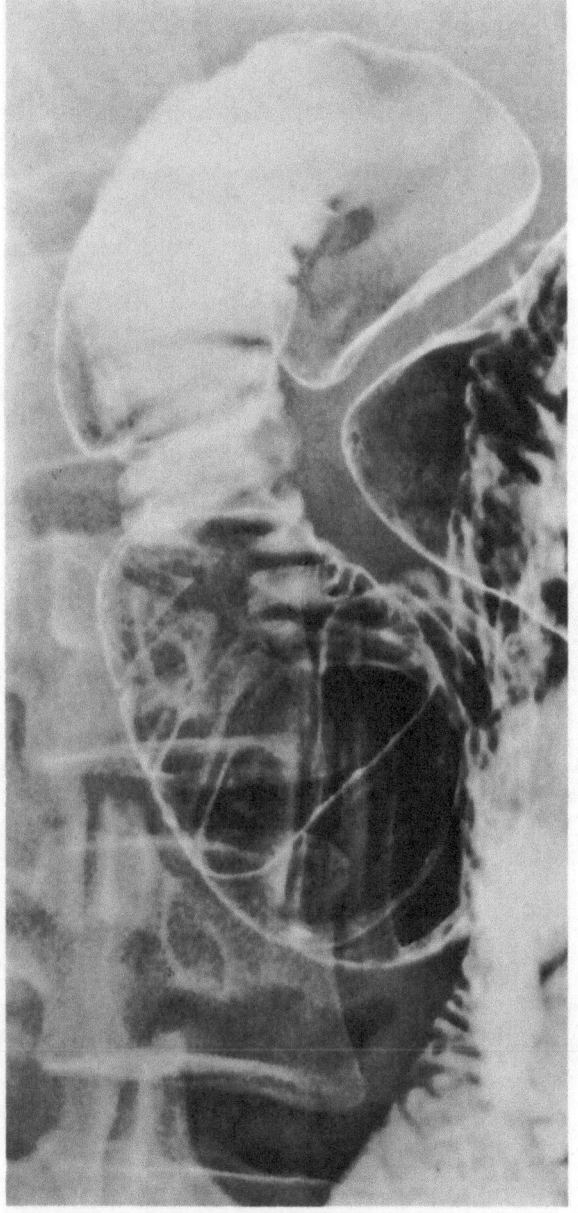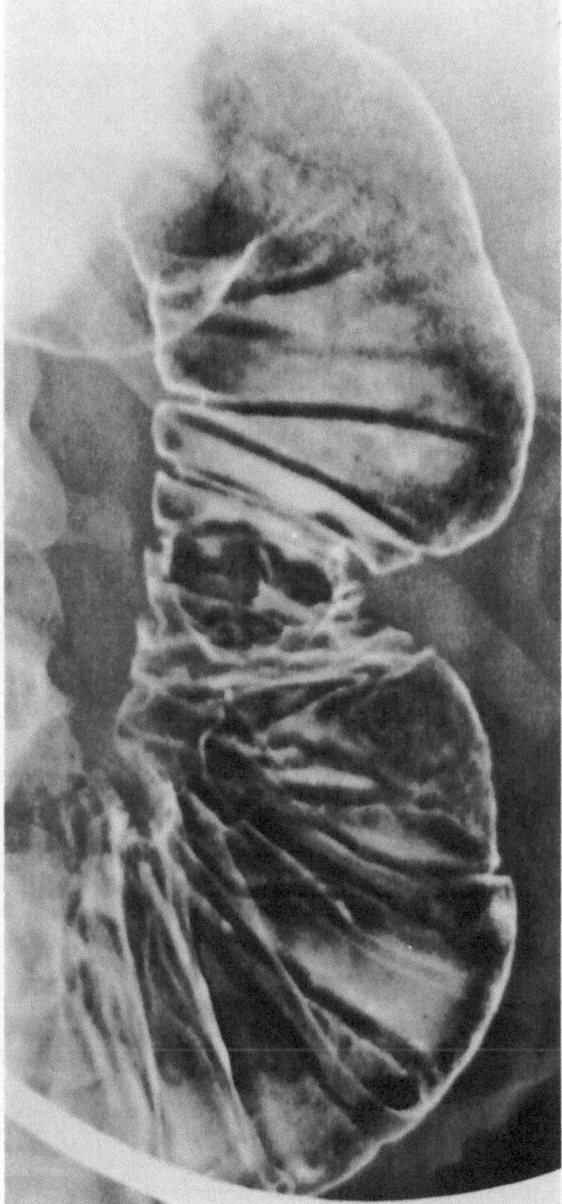

Fig. 189
a. DC hypotonic duodenography, supine position, LPO.
b. DC hypotonic duodenography, prone position. Stenotic ring in
  the descending part of the duodenum. At operation an annular
  pancreas was found.

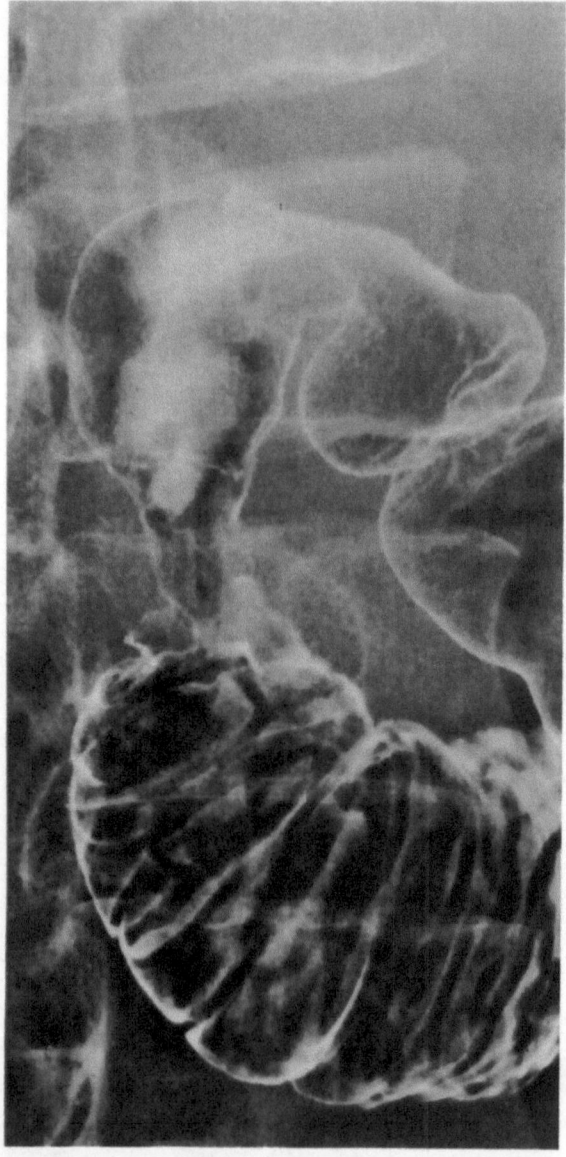 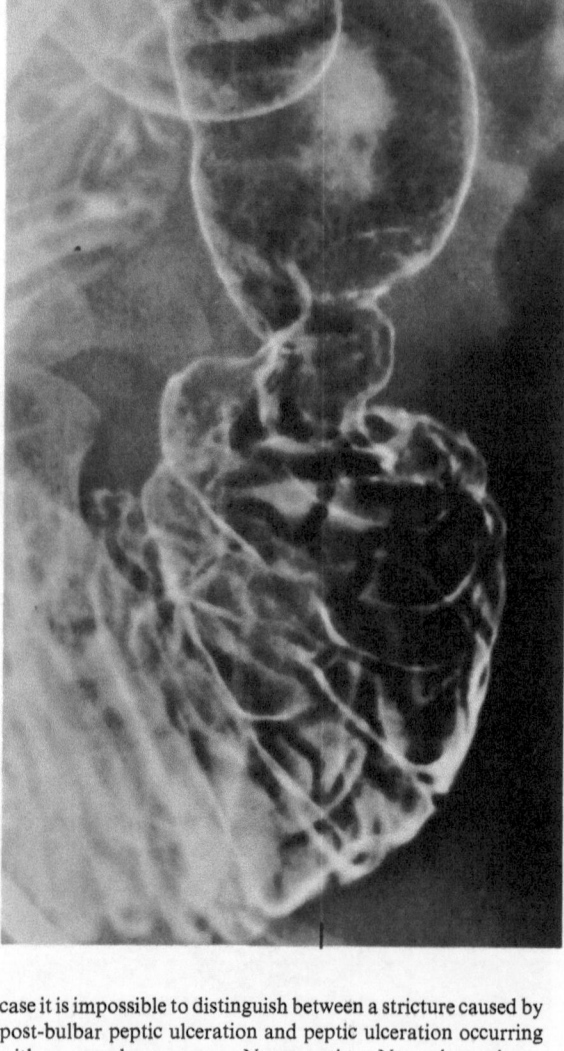

Fig. 190

a. DC hypotonic duodenography, supine position, LPO.

b. DC hypotonic duodenography, prone position. Stenotic ring in the descending part of duodenum. Endoscopy demonstrated a small ulcer niche in the vicinity of the stenosis. In this case it is impossible to distinguish between a stricture caused by post-bulbar peptic ulceration and peptic ulceration occurring with an annular pancreas. No operation. No endoscopic retrograde pancreatico-cholangiography.

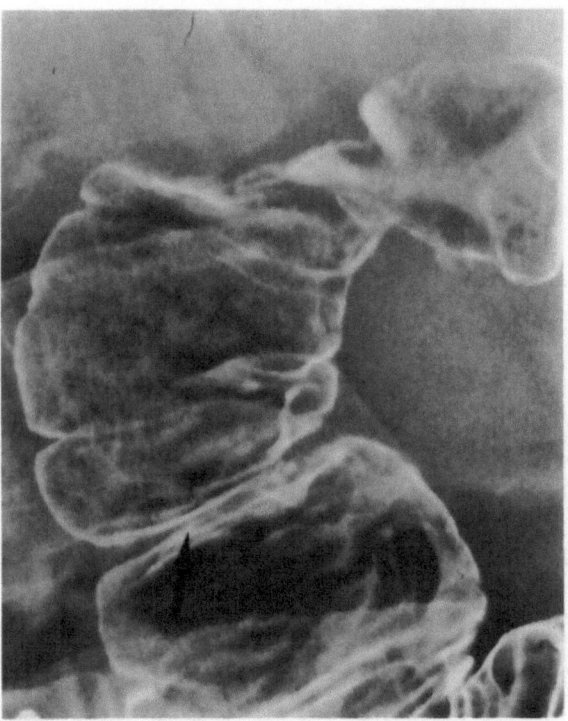 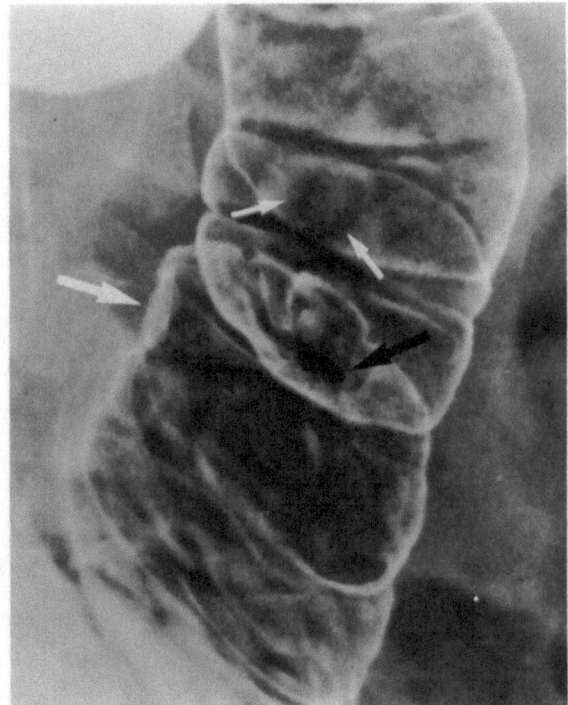

Fig. 191

a. DC hypotonic duodenography, supine position, LPO.

b. DC hypotonic duodenography, prone position. Extreme deformity and scarring in the region of the flexure between the duodenal bulb and the descending duodenum. It was impossible to demonstrate or to exclude an active ulcer in this area. The large black arrow points to the edge of a duodenal septum. The large white arrow points to the major papilla; the small white arrows to the minor papilla. Endoscopy did not show any active ulceration in the post-bulbar region and confirmed the duodenal septum.

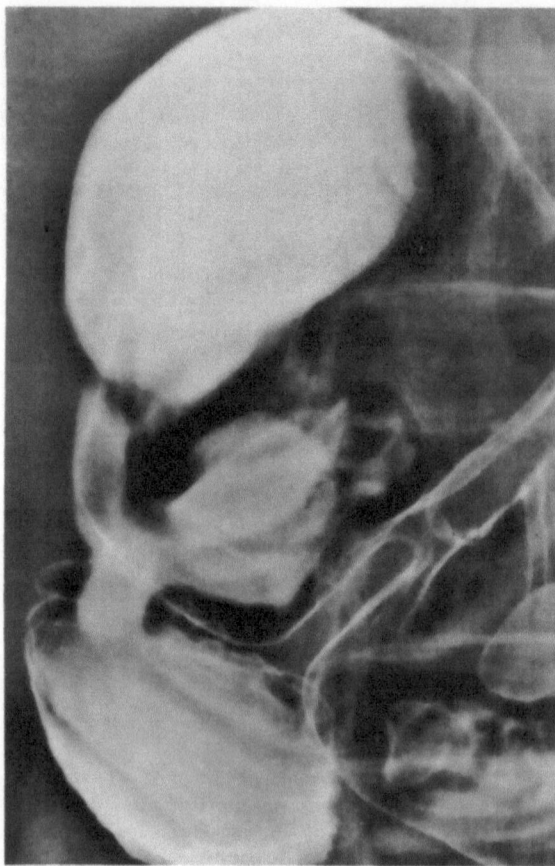

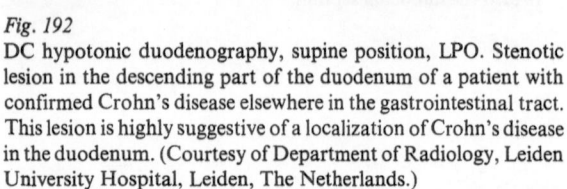

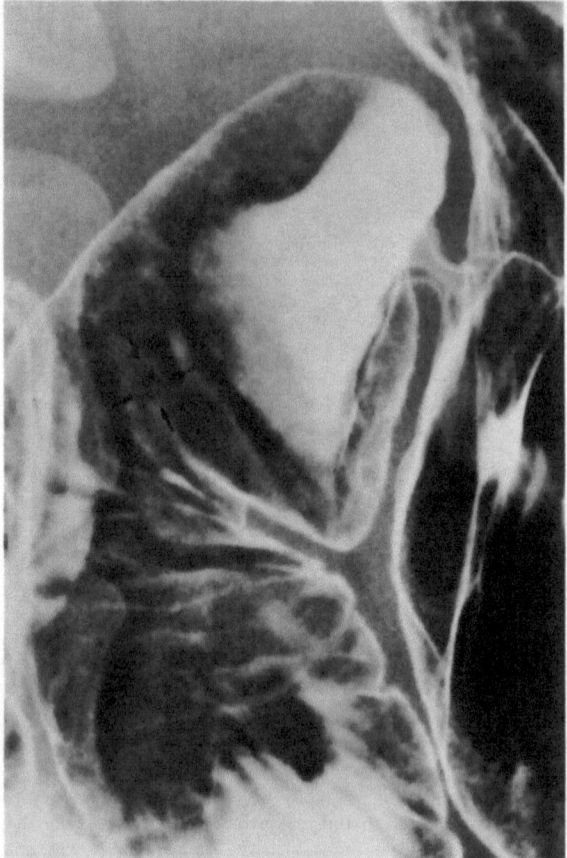

Fig. 192
DC hypotonic duodenography, supine position, LPO. Stenotic lesion in the descending part of the duodenum of a patient with confirmed Crohn's disease elsewhere in the gastrointestinal tract. This lesion is highly suggestive of a localization of Crohn's disease in the duodenum. (Courtesy of Department of Radiology, Leiden University Hospital, Leiden, The Netherlands.)

Fig. 193
DC hypotonic duodenography, supine position, LPO, of a patient with histologically confirmed Crohn's disease of the colon. There is at least one varioliform erosion in the region of the flexure between the duodenal bulb and the descending duodenum (arrows).

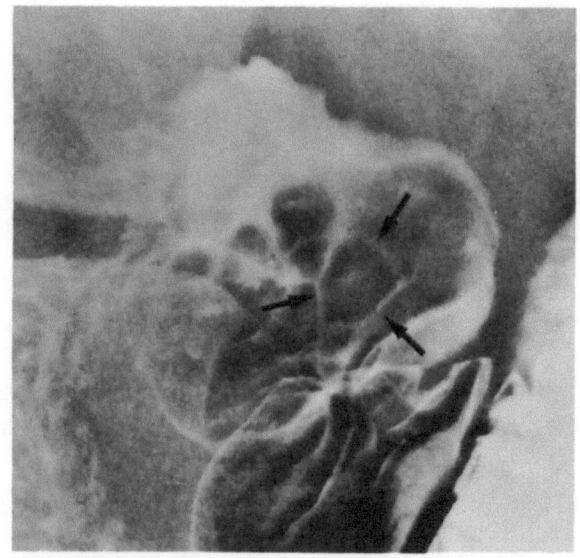

Fig. 194
DC study, supine position, LPO. Typical varioliform erosion on the posterior wall of the duodenal bulb (arrows). Endoscopic confirmation.

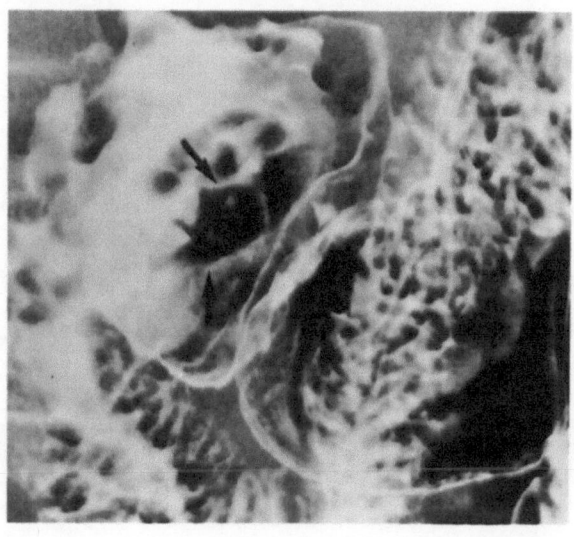

a   *b*

Fig. 195
a & b. DC study, supine position, LPO. 2 erosions in the duodenal bulb, which were verified endoscopically (arrows).

REFERENCES

1. Abel W von: Die Röntgendiagnose der Gastritis erosiva. *Fortschr Röntgenstr* 80: 39-50, 1954.

2. Allman RM, Cavanagh RC, Helwig EB, Lichtenstein JE: RPC (radiologic-pathologic correlation) from the AFIP (Armed Forces Institute of Pathology). Inflammatory fibroid polyp. *Radiology* 127: 69-73, 1978.

3. Amaral NM: Value of the compressive technique associated with pharmacological hypotonia in the diagnosis of erosive gastritis. *Gastrointest Radiol* 3: 161-163, 1978.

4. Amplatz K: A new and simple approach to air-contrast studies of the stomach and duodenum. *Radiology* 70: 392-394, 1958.

5. Anacker H, Weiss HD, Kramann B: *Endoscopic retrograde pancreatico-cholangiography (ERPC)*, Berlin-Heidelberg-New York, Springer-Verlag, 1977, p 57-58.

6. Baastrup ChrI: Roentgenological studies of the inner surface of the stomach and of the movements of the gastric contents. *Acta Radiol* 3: 180-204, 1924.

7. Balikian JP, Nassar NT, Shamma'a MH, Shahid MJ: Primary lymphomas of the small intestine including the duodenum. *Am J Roentgenol* 107: 131-141, 1969.

8. Balthazar EJ, Gade MF: Gastrointestinal edema in cirrhotics, radiologic manifestations and pathogenesis with emphasis on colonic involvement. *Gastrointest Radiol* 1: 215-223, 1976.

9. Bateson EM, Talerman A, Walrond ER: Radiological and pathological observations in a series of seventeen cases of hypertrophic pyloric stenosis of adults. *Br J Radiol* 42: 1-8, 1969.

10. Belber JP: Endoscopic examination of the duodenal bulb: a comparison with X-ray. *Gastroenterology* 61: 55-61, 1971.

11. Berg HM: Antral gastritis. *Radiology* 59: 324-335, 1952.

12. Berk JE: Pyloric muscle hypertrophy in adults. In: *Gastroenterology*, Bockus HL (ed), Philadelphia-London-Toronto, W.B. Saunders Company, 1974, vol I, p 1072-1080.

13. Berk JE: Prolapse of gastric mucosa through the pylorus. In: *Gastroenterology*, Bockus HL (ed), Philadelphia-London-Toronto, W.B. Saunders Company, 1974, vol I, p 1087.

14. Bilbao MK, Frische LH, Rösch J, Benson JA, Dotter CT: Postbulbar duodenal ulcer and ring-structure. *Radiology* 100: 27-35, 1971.

15. Bötticher R, Bünte H, Hermanek P, Rösch W: Magenpolypen, Prognose und Therapie. *Dtsch med Wschr* 5: 167-170, 1975.

16. Bosse G, Neely JA: Roentgenologic findings in primary malignant tumors of the duodenum. *Am J Roentgenol* 107: 111-118, 1969.

17. Bree RL, Flynn RE: Hypotonic duodenography in the evaluation of choledocholithiasis and obstructive jaundice. *Am J Roentgenol* 116: 309-319, 1972.

18. Brombart M, Dony A, Massun P, Dewitte Cl, Serste JP, Toussaint J, Dechreyer M: Les aspects radiologiques et endoscopiques des ulcérations bénignes et malignes de l'estomac. *Acta Gastro-Enterologica Belgica*: 39: 186-202, 1976.

19. Bücker J: Die Antrumgastritis. *Radiologe* 6: 264-270, 1966.

20. Bücker J: Die Erkrankungen des Magens und Zwölffingerdarmes. In: *Handbuch der medizinischen Radiologie*, Diethelm L, Olsson O, Strnad F, Vieten H, Zuppinger A (eds), Berlin-Heidelberg-New York, Springer-Verlag, 1969, vol XI, p 537-550.

21. Büttner D, Pichlmayr R, Seifert E: Das Magenfrühcarcinom. *Chirurg* 46: 65-72, 1975.

22. Burrell M, Toffler R: Flexural pseudolesions of the duodenum. *Radiology* 120: 313-315, 1976.

23. Centraal Bureau voor de Statistiek: *Overledenen naar doodsoorzaak, leeftijd en geslacht in het jaar 1976*. Voorburg, Centraal bureau voor de Statistiek, Hoofdafdeling Gezondheidsstatistieken.

24. Chernish SM, Miller RE, Rosenak BD, Scholz NE: Hypotonic duodenography with the use of glucagon. *Gastroenterology* 63: 392-398, 1972.

25. Chiles JT, Platz CE: The radiographic manifestations of pseudolymphoma of the stomach. *Radiology* 116: 551-556, 1975.

26. Cho KJ: Gastric antral diaphragm. *Gastrointest Radiol* 1: 37-40, 1976.

27. Correll R, Roth F-J, Fuchs HF: Magen. In: *Röntgenologische Differentialdiagnostik*, Teschendorf WW (ed), Stuttgart, Georg Thieme Verlag, 1978, vol II, p 108.

28. Idem, p 117.

29. Idem, p 179.

30. Dekker W: *Fiberendoscopisch-bioptisch onderzoek van maagmaligniteiten*, Amsterdam, Academische Pers, 1976, p 2.

31. Idem, p 2-3.

32. Idem, p 27-29.

33. Dekker W, Op den Orth JO: Early gastric cancer. *Radiologia Clin* 46: 115-129, 1977.

34. Dekker W, Op den Orth JO: *Correlations and discorrelations between endoscopy and radiology of the upper GI tract*, Chicago, The Radiological Society of North America, Inc., 1977, scientific exhibit, space 151.

35. Dekker W, Tytgat GN: Diagnostic accuracy of fiberendoscopy in the detection of upper intestinal malignancy; a follow-up analysis. *Gastroenterology* 73: 710-714, 1977.

36. Demling L, Ottenjann R, Elster K: *Endoskopie und Biopsie der Speiseröhre und des Magens*, Stuttgart-New York, F.K. Schattauer Verlag, 1972, p 77.

37. Idem, p 87-89.

38. Idem, p 107.

39. Dihlmann W: Die ökonomisch-standardisierte Röntgenuntersuchung des Magens. *Dtsch med Wschr* 101: 900-904, 1976.

40. Dodd GD, Sheft D: Diverticulum of the greater curvature of the stomach: a roentgenologic curiosity. *Am J Roentgenol* 107: 102-104, 1969.

41. Dodd GD: Gastric mucosa and submucosa. In: *Syllabus categorical course on radiology of gastrointestinal tract diseases*, Chicago, The Radiological Society of North America Inc., 1974, p 7 (c)-8 (c).

42. Dodds WJ, Goldberg HI, Margulis AR: Leiomyosarcoma of the small intestine. *Am J Roentgenol* 107:-142-149, 1969.

43. Doi H: Radiologic Diagnosis of early gastric cancer. In: *The papers-collection*, presented at the 18th Annual Clinical Conference on Cancer, Houston, University of Texas, System Cancer Center, 1973 p 245-251.

44. Donner MW, Margulies SI: Water Siphonage Test. In: *Gastroesophageal reflux and hiatal hernia*, Skinner DB, Belsey RHR, Hendrix TR, Zuidema GD (eds), Boston, Little, Brown and Company, 1972, p 65.

45. Donner MW, Margulies SI: Radiographic Diagnostic Criteria. In: *Gastroesophageal reflux and hiatal hernia*, Skinner DB, Belsey RHR, Hendrix TR, Zuidema GD (eds), Boston, Little, Brown and Company, 1972, p 71-73.

46. Idem, p 74.

47. Doss JC, Ferrucci JT: Gastric cannonballs: a roentgen sign of hepatic metastases. *Gastroenterology* 67: 519-520, 1974.

48. Eaton SB, Ferrucci JT: *Radiology of the pancreas and duodenum*, Philadelphia-London-Toronto, W.B. Saunders Company, 1973, p 103.

49. Idem, p 110.

50. Idem, p 113.

51. Idem, p 125.

52. Idem, p 126.

53. Idem, p 130.

54. Idem, p 131.

55. Idem, p 132.

56. Idem, p 135.

57. Idem, p 178.

58. Idem, p 292.

59. Idem, p 306-307.

60. Idem, p 335.

61. von Elischer J: Über eine Methode zur Röntgenuntersuchung des Magens. *Fortschr Röntgenstr* 18: 338-340, 1911.

62. D'Eloia AS: Pneumogastroscopy. *Am J of Surgery* 13: 280-283, 1941.

63. Elster K, Kolaczek F, Shimamoto K, Freitag H: Early gastric cancer – experience in Germany. *Endoscopy* 7: 5-10, 1975.

64. Engelholm L, de Toeuf J: Aspects radiologiques des lésions gastroduodénales dans la maladie de Crohn. In: *Collège d'enseignement post-universitaire de radiologie*, Brussels, 1977.

65. Evans DMD, Craven JL, Murphy F, Cleary BK: Comparison of "early gastric cancer" in Britain and Japan. *Gut* 19: 1-9, 1978.

66. Faegenburg D, Bosniak M: Duodenal anomalies in the adult. *Am J Roentgenol* 88: 642-657, 1962.

67. Farman J, Faegenburg D, Dallemand S, Chen C-K: Crohn's disease of the stomach: the "ram's horn" sign. *Am J Roentgenol* 123: 242-251, 1975.

68. Faust H, Hartweg H, Eugenidis N: Zur Differentialdiagnose neoplastischer Prozesse im Duodenum. *Fortschr Röntgenstr* 116: 499-508, 1972.

69. Fays J, Borrelly J, Floquet J, Hennequin F, Rauber G, Tréheux A: Radio-anatomie de la région vatérienne, résultat d'une technique originale. *Comptes Rendus Assoc Anat* 154: 1013-1019, 1972.

70. Felson B: *Chest roentgenology*, Philadelphia, W.B. Saunders Company, 1973, p 24.

71. Ferrucci JT: Hypotonic duodenography. In: *Syllabus categorical course on radiology of gastrointestinal tract diseases*, Chicago, The Radiological Society of North America Inc., 1974, p 11.

72. Fevre DI, Green PHR, Barratt PJ, Nagy GS: Review of five cases of early gastric carcinoma. *Gut* 17: 41-47, 1976.

73. Filippi L, Isliker K: Gastritis varioliformis mit Proteinverlust. *Dtsch med Wschr* 98: 1892-1894, 1973.

74. Fischer AW: Ueber eine neue röntgenologische Untersuchungsmethode des Dickdarms: Kombination von Kontrasteinlauf und Luftaufblähung. *Klin Wschr* 34: 1595-1598, 1923.

75. Frik W, Hesse R: Die röntgenologische Darstellung von Magenerosionen, verbesserte Ergebnisse mit Doppelkontrast-Aufnahmen und Bildverstärker. *Dtsch med Wschr* 28: 1119-1121, 1956.

76. Frik W; Magen. In: *Lehrbuch der Röntgendiagnostik*, Schinz HR, Baensch WE, Frommhold W, Glauner R, Uehlinger E, Wellauer J (eds), Stuttgart, Georg Thieme Verlag, 1965, vol V, p 105-106.

77. Idem, p 119.

78. Idem, p 123.

79. Idem, p 133.

80. Idem, p 265-266.

81. Frik W: Neoplastic diseases of the stomach. In: *Alimentary Tract Roentgenology*, Margulis AR, Burhenne HJ (eds), Saint Louis, The C.V. Mosby Company, 1973, vol I, p 697.

82. Frik W, Fernholz HJ, Spieth W: Die Doppelkontrastuntersuchung des Magens, Begriffsbestimmung, Technik, Indikation. *Z Gastroenterol* 14: 487-497, 1976.

83. Frommhold H, Rohner HG, Koischwitz D, Kühr J: Das Röntgenbild kaustischer Veränderungen des oberen Intestinaltraktes. *Fortschr Röntgenstr* 125: 514-520, 1976.

84. Fuchs HF: Kombinierte radiologische Untersuchungstechnik des Magens mit Direktaufnahmen und verbesserten Indirektaufnahmen. *Leber Magen Darm* 6: 146-153, 1976.

85. Gelfand DW, Hachiya J: The double-contrast examination of the stomach using gas-producing granules and tablets. *Radiology* 93: 1381-1382, 1969.

86. Gelfand DW: The double-contrast upper gastrointestinal examination in the Japanese style. *Am J Gastroenterol* 63: 216-220, 1975.

87. Gelfand DW: Double-contrast examination of the gastrointestinal tract: the Japanese-style double-contrast examination of the stomach. *Gastrointest Radiol* 1: 7-17, 1976.

88. Gerhardt P: Hypotonic duodenography in the diagnosis of pancreatic disease. In: *Endoscopic Retrograde Pancreatico-cholangiography*, Anacker H, Weiss HD, Kramann B (eds), Berlin-Heidelberg-New York, Springer-Verlag, 1977, p 73.

89. Gloor F: Das Oberflächenkarzinom (Frühkarzinom) des Magens. *Schweiz med Wschr* 106: 21-27, 1976.

90. Gohel VK, Dalinka MK, Mandell GA, Azimi F: Pharmacoradiology of the gastrointestinal tract. *Critical Reviews in Clinical Radiology and Nuclear Medicine* 5: 69-110, 1974.

91. Gohel VK, Kressel HY, Laufer I: Double-contrast artifacts. *Gastrointest Radiol* 3: 139-146, 1978.

92. Golden R: Antral gastritis and spasm. *JAMA* 109: 1497-1500, 1937.

93. Goldsmith MR, Paul RE, Poplack WE, Moore JP, Matsue H, Bloom S: Evaluation of routine double contrast views of the anterior wall of the stomach. *Am J Roentgenol* 126: 1159-1163, 1976.

94. Goldstein HM: Double-contrast gastrography. *Digestive Diseases* 21: 797-803, 1976.

95. Gonzalez G, Kennedy T: Crohn's disease of the stomach. *Radiology* 113: 27-29, 1974.

96. Govoni AF: Benign lymphoid hyperplasia of the duodenal bulb. *Gastrointest Radiol* 1: 267-269, 1976.

97. Green PHR, Fevre DI, Barrett PJ, Hunt JH, Gillespie PE, Nagy GS: Chronic erosive (verrucous) gastritis, a study of 108 patients. *Endoscopy* 9: 74-78, 1977.

98. Grundmann E, Grunze H, Witte S: *Early gastric cancer, current status of diagnosis*, Berlin-Heidelberg-New York, Springer-Verlag, 1974.

99. Grundner H-G, Nägele E: Röntgenbefunde bei Tumoren im Duodenum. *Radiologe* 10: 29-35, 1970.

100. Guien C: L'estomac et le duodénum normaux. *Le concours Médical*, C.M. 21-10-1972-94-42: 6815-6828, 1972.

101. Guien C: Mucographie gastro-duodénale en double contraste. Texte présenté aux *Journées Lyonnaises de Radiologie Digestive*, 16-17 mars 1973, p 1467-1472.

102. Gutmann RA: *Le diagnostic du Cancer d'estomac précoce et avancé*, Paris, Editions Doin – Deren & Cie, 1967, p 22-23.

103. Gutmann RA: Forty years of early diagnosis of gastric cancer. In: *Early gastric cancer, current status of diagnosis*, Berlin-Heidelberg-New York, Springer-Verlag, 1974, p 69-75.

104. Habermann M, Windorfer K, Petzel H: Röntgendiagnostische Hinweise auf Morbus Crohn unter besonderer Berücksichtigung von Magenveränderungen (Doppelkontrastmethode). *Fortschr Röntgenstr* 125: 508-510, 1976.

105. Hanelin LG, Margulis AR: Radiologische Diagnostik des Magenkarzinoms. *Leber Magen Darm* 6: 97-107, 1976.

106. Hauzeur F, Moldenhauer W, Arendt R: Röntgenologie und Endoskopie in der Diagnostik des gastroduodenalen Ulkus. *Zschr inn Med* 19: 632-637, 1975.

107. Hedemand N, Mathiasen MS: Double contrast roentgenography of the stomach. *Danish med journ* 136: 1079-1083, 1974.

108. Heitzeberg H, Treichel J: Intensivierte Röntgendiagnostik des Magens mittels Doppelkontrast, Erfahrungsbericht über ein neues Zusatzpräparat zur Kontrastmitteluntersuchung. *Fortschr Röntgenstr* 116: 529-533, 1972.

109. Henning N, Schatzki R: Gastrophotographisches und röntgenologisches Bild der Gastritis ulcerosa. *Fortschr Röntgenstr* 48: 177-182, 1933.

110. Herlinger H, Glanville JN, Kreel L: An evaluation of the double contrast barium meal (DCBM) against endoscopy. *Clin Radiol* 28: 307-314, 1977.

111. Hermanek P: Die Früherkennung des Magenkarzinoms im Spannungsfeld unterschiedlicher Methoden, Klinisch-pathologische Gesichtspunkte. *Med. Welt* 25: 507-511, 1974.

112. Hertzer NR, Hoerr SO: An interpretive review of lymphoma of the stomach. *Surg Gynecol Obstet* 143: 113-124, 1976.

113. Hessler PC, Braunstein E: Adenocarcinoma of the duodenum arising in a villous adenoma. *Gastrointest Radiol* 2: 355-357, 1978.

114. Hilpert F: Das Pneumo-Relief des Magens. *Fortschr Röntgenstr* 38: 80-87 (1929).

115. Hirayama T: Epidemiology of stomach cancer. In: *Early gastric cancer*, Japanese Cancer Association, Murakami T (ed), Baltimore-London-Tokyo, University Park Press, 1972, p 6.

116. Hunt JH, Anderson IF: Double contrast upper gastrointestinal studies. *Clin Radiol* 27: 87-97, 1976.

117. Hyland J, Laufer I, Stevenson GW, Somers S: *Crohn's disease of the stomach and duodenum*, Chicago, The Radiological Society of North America, Inc., 1977, scientific exhibit, space 155.

118. Ichikawa H: *The basic concepts of double-contrast radiography of the stomach*, Tokyo, Fuji Photo Film Co., Ltd., 1973.

119. Ichikawa H: Differential diagnosis between benign and malignant ulcers of the stomach. *Clin Gastroenterol* 2: 329-343, 1973.

120. Jacobson HG, Shapiro JH, Pisano D, Poppel MH: The vaterian and peri-vaterian segments in peptic ulcer. *Am J Roentgenol* 79: 793-798, 1958.

121. Jacquemet P, Liotta D, Mallet-Guy P: *The early radiological diagnosis of diseases of the pancreas and ampulla Vater*, Springfield, Charles C. Thomas, 1965, p 154.

122. Jacquemet P: Potentials and limitations of hypotonic duodenography. In: *Efficiency and limits of radiologic examination of the pancreas*, Anacker H (ed), Stuttgart, Georg Thieme Verlag, 1975.

123. Kalokerinos J: Double contrast barium meal technique. *Aust Radiol* 11: 246-249, 1967.

124. Kawai K, Takada H, Takekoshi T, Misaki F, Mukami K, Masada M, Nishizawa M, Hayakawa H, Shirakabe H: Double contrast radiograph on routine examination of the stomach. *Am J Gastroenterol* 53: 147-153, 1970.

125. Kawai K, Shimamoto K, Misaki F, Murakami K, Masuda M: Erosion of gastric mucosa – pathogenesis, incidence a classification of the erosive gastritis. *Endoscopy* 3: 168-174, 1970.

126. Kawai K: Present results in early detection of stomach cancer by radiologic means. In: *Early gastric cancer, current status of diagnosis*, Grundmann E, Grunze H, Witte S (eds), Berlin-Heidelberg-New York, Springer-Verlag, 1974, p 84.

127. Kawai K, Tanaka H: *Differential Diagnosis of gastric diseases*, Tokyo, Igaku Shoin Ltd. and Berlin-Heidelberg-New York, Springer-Verlag, 1974.

128. Idem, p 51.

129. Idem, p 57.

130. Idem, p 59-60.

131. Idem, p 216.

132. Idem, p 216-220.

133. Keller RJ, Wolf BS, Khilnani MT: Roentgen features of healing and healed benign gastric ulcers. *Radiology* 97: 353-359, 1970.

134. Keto P, Korhola O, Ihamäki T: Faltenwulstungen des Magens bei Akromegaliepatienten. *Fortschr Röntgenstr* 128: 233-234, 1978.

135. Kidokoro T: Frequency of resection, metastasis and five-year survival rate of early gastric carcinoma in a surgical clinic. In: *Early gastric cancer*, Japanese Cancer Association, Murakami T (ed), Baltimore-London-Tokyo, University Park Press, 1972, p 45-49.

136. Kilman WJ, Berk RN: The spectrum of radiographic features of aberrant pancreatic rests involving the stomach. *Radiology* 123: 291-296, 1977.

137. Kirkpatrick JR, Davies GT, Evans KT: The diagnosis of atrophic gastritis. *Ann Clin Res* 5: 39-45, 1973.

138. Kitakabe T, Yokoyama M, Sakka M, Koga S: Estimation of benefits and radiation risks from stomach mass X-ray survey in Japan. *Strahlentherapie* 146: 352-358, 1973.

139. Koehler RE, Hanelin LG, Laing FC, Montgomery CK, Margulis AR: Invasion of the duodenum by carcinoma of the stomach. *Am J Roentgenol* 128: 201-205, 1977.

140. Koga M, Nakata H, Kiyonari H, Inakura M, Tanaka M, Nobe T: Minute mucosal patterns in gastric carcinoma. *Radiology* 120: 199-201, 1976.

141. Koischwitz von D, Brecht G, Gerlach F, Lackner K: Die Manifestation der Enteritis regionalis (M. Crohn) an Magen und Duodenum. *Fortschr Röntgenstr* 125: 501-507, 1976.

142. Kormano M, Mäkelä P, Rossi I: Visualization of the areae gastricae in a double contrast examination – dependence on the contrast medium. *Fortschr Röntgenstr* 128: 52-56, 1978.

143. Kreel L, Herlinger H, Glanville J: Technique of the double contrast barium meal with examples of correlation with endoscopy. *Clin Radiol* 24: 307-314, 1973.

144. Kreel L, Herlinger H, Sandin B, France C: A technique for the in vitro testing of barium preparations. *Radiography* 15: 51-55, 1974.

145. Kreel L: Recent advances in gastroduodenal radiology. *Proc R Soc Med* 68: 111-114, 1975.

146. Kreel L: Pharmaco-radiology in barium examinations with special reference to glucagon. *Br J Radiol* 48: 691-703, 1975.

147. The Lancet: Screening for gastric cancer in the west. *The Lancet* 13: 1023-1024, 1978.

148. Laufer I, Mullens JE, Hamilton J: The diagnostic accuracy of barium studies of the stomach and duodenum – correlation with endoscopy. *Radiology* 115: 569-573, 1975.

149. Laufer I, Hamilton J, Mullens JE: Demonstration of superficial gastric erosions by double contrast radiography. *Gastroenterology* 68: 387-391, 1975.

150. Laufer, I: A simple method for routine double-contrast study of the upper gastrointestinal tract. *Radiology* 117: 513-518, 1975.

151. Laufer I: Assessment of the accuracy of double contrast gastroduodenal radiology. *Gastroenterology* 71: 874-878, 1976.

152. Laufer I, Trueman T: Multiple superficial gastric erosions due to Crohn's disease of the stomach; radiologic and endoscopic diagnosis. *Br J Radiol* 49: 726-728, 1976.

153. Laufer I: *The early lesions of Crohn's disease*, Chicago, The Radiological Society of North America, Inc., 1977, scientific exhibit, space 161.

154. Legge DA, Carlson HC, Judd ES: Roentgenologic features of regional enteritis of the upper gastrointestinal tract. *Am J Roentgenol* 110: 355-360, 1970.

155. Lemmens HA: Crohn's disease of the regio gastroduodenalis. *Arch Chir Neerl* 25: 1-12, 1973.

156. Machado G, Davies JD, Tudway AJC, Salmon PR, Read AE: Superficial carcinoma of the stomach. *Br Med J* 2: 77-79, 1976.

157. Mackintosh CE, Kreel L: Anatomy and radiology of the areae gastricae. *Gut* 18: 855-864, 1977.

158. Maeder H-U, Fuchs HF: Pharmakoradiographie des Gastrointestinaltraktes. *Radiologe* 16: 498-503, 1976.

159. Mainguet P: Endoscopie des lésions gastroduodénales dans la maladie de Crohn. In: *Collège d'enseignement post-universitaire de radiologie*, Brussels, 1977.

160. Marshak RH, Feldman F: Gastric polyps. *Am J of Digestive Diseases* 10: 909-935, 1965.

161. Marshak RH, Lindner AE: *Radiology of the Small Intestine*, Philadelphia-London-Toronto, W.B. Saunders Company, 1976, p 409-451.

162. Merlo RB, Stone M, Baugus P, Martin M: The use of pro-banthine to induce gastrointestinal hypotonia. *Radiology* 127: 61-62, 1978.

163. Menuck LS: Gastric lymphoma, a radiologic diagnosis. *Gastrointest Radiol* 1: 157-161, 1976.

164. Meyers MA, Katzen B, Alonso DR: Transpyloric extension to duodenal bulb in gastric lymphoma. *Radiology* 115: 575-580, 1975.

165. Meyers MA: *Dynamic radiology of the abdomen, normal and pathologic anatomy*, New York-Heidelberg-Berlin, Springer-Verlag, 1976, p 243.

166. Miller G, Kaufmann M: Das Magenfrühkarzinom in Europa. *Dtsch med Wschr* 100: 1946-1949, 1975.

167. Miller G, Kaufmann M: Magenfrühkarzinom; Endoskopie oder Radiologie. *Dtsch med Wschr* 101: 1006-1010, 1976.

168. Miller RE, Chernish SM, Rosenak BD, Rodda BE: Hypotonic duodenography with glucagon. *Radiology* 108: 35-42, 1973.

169. Miller RE, Chernish SM, Skucas J, Rosenak BD, Rodda BE: Hypotonic roentgenography with glucagon. *Am J Roentgenol* 121: 264-274, 1974.

170. Miller RE: Hypotonic radiography with glucagon. In: *Diagnostic Radiology 1977*, Margulis Ar, Gooding CA, St. Louis, The C.V. Mosby Company, 1977, p 61-63.

171. Miller RE, Chernish SM, Brunelle RL, Rosenak BD: Double-blind radiographic study of dose response to intravenous glucagon for hypotonic duodenography. *Radiology* 127: 55-59, 1978.

172. Ming S-C: *Tumors of the esophagus and stomach, atlas of tumor pathology*, Washington, Armed Forces Institute of Pathology, 1973, section II, p 82.

173. Idem, p 120.

174. Idem, p 124.

175. Idem, p 161.

176. Idem, p 174.

177. Idem, p 206.

178. Idem, p 215.

179. Idem, p 231.

180. Idem, p 235.

181. Ming S-C: The adenoma-carcinoma sequence in the stomach and colon: II. malignant potential of gastric polyps. *Gastrointest Radiol* 1: 121-125, 1976.

182. Mortelmans P, Ponette E, Broeckaert L: Erosive gastritis of varioliform type. *J Belge Radiol* 58: 271-274, 1975.

183. Murakami T: *Early gastric cancer*, Japanese Cancer Association, Baltimore-London-Tokyo, University Park Press, 1972.

184. Nelson RS, Lanza FL: Gastroscopic and radiologic patterns in gastric lymphoma. In: *The papers-collection*, presented at the 18th Annual Clinical Conference on Cancer, Houston, University of Texas, System Cancer Center, 1973, p 255-260.

185. Nelson RS: Malignant tumors of the stomach other than carcinoma. In: *Gastroenterology*, Bockus HL (ed), Philadelphia-London-Toronto, W.B. Saunders Company, 1974, vol I, p 998.

186. Nelson SW: The discovery of gastric ulcers and the differential diagnosis between benignancy and malignancy. In: *The radiologic clinics of North America*, symposium on radiology of the alimentary tract, Marshak RH (ed), Philadelphia-London-Toronto, W.B. Saunders Company, 1969, vol VII, p 5-25.

187. Nelson SW: Some interesting and unusual manifestations of Crohn's disease ("regional enteritis") of the stomach, duodenum and small intestine. *Am J Roentgenol* 107: 86-101, 1969.

188. Nelson SW: The effect of pressure on the Carman type lesion. In: *Syllabus categorical course on radiology of gastrointestinal tract diseases*, Chicago, The Radiological Society of North America Inc., 1974, p 28-30.

189. Novak D, Weber J: Gegenwärtiger Stand der Pharmakoradiologie des Magen-Darm-Traktes. *Radiologe* 16: 504-512, 1976.

190. Obata WG: A double-contrast technique for examination of the stomach using barium sulfate with simethicone. *Am J Roentgenol* 115: 275-280, 1972.

191. Oosterkamp WJ: Benefit risk comparisons in diagnostic radiology. *Medicamundi* 21: 2-6, 1976.

192. Op den Orth JO: De dubbelcontrastmethode; een essentieel onderdeel van het röntgenonderzoek van maag en bulbus. *Ned T Geneesk* 115: 535-538, 1971.

193. Op den Orth JO, Ploem S: The stalactite phenomenon in double contrast studies of the stomach. *Radiology* 117: 523-525, 1975.

194. Op den Orth JO, Dekker W: Gastric erosions: radiological and endoscopic aspects. *Radiologia Clin* 45: 88-99, 1976.

195. Op den Orth JO, Ploem S: The standard biphasic-contrast gastric series. *Radiology* 122: 530-532, 1977.

196. Op den Orth JO: Radiologic visualization of the normal duodenal minor papilla. *Fortschr Röntgenstr* 128: 572-576, 1978.

197. Op den Orth JO: Detailed double contrast examination of the post-operative stomach. In: *Double contrast examination of the gastrointestinal tract*, Laufer I (ed), Philadelphia-London-Toronto, W.B. Saunders Company, 1979.

198. Osnes M, Lötveit T: Juxtaminorpapillary diverticulum associated with chronic pancreatitis. *Endoscopy* 8: 106-108, 1976.

199. Palmer WL: General gastroenterologic considerations. In: *Alimentary tract roentgenology*, Margulis AR, Burhenne HJ (eds), Saint Louis, The C.V. Mosby Company, 1973, vol II, p 1665.

200. Paul F, Freyschmidt J: Anwendung von glukagon bei endoskopischen und röntgenologischen Untersuchungen des Gastrointestinaltrakts. *Fortschr Röntgenstr* 125: 31-37, 1976.

201. Pochaczevsky R: "Bubbly barium", a carbonated cocktail for double-contrast examination of the stomach. *Radiology* 107: 461-462, 1973.

202. Poplack W, Paul RE, Goldsmith M, Matsue H, Moore JP, Norton RN: Demonstration of erosive gastritis by the double-contrast technique. *Radiology* 117: 519-521, 1975.

203. Press AJ: Practical significance of gastric rugal folds. *Am J Roentgenol* 125: 172-183, 1975.

204. Prévôt R: Roentgenology of the duodenum. In: *Alimentary tract roentgenology*, Margulis AR, Burhenne HJ (eds), Saint Louis, The C.V. Mosby Company, 1973, vol I, p 719.

205. Pribram BO, Kleiber N: Ein neuer Weg zur röntgenologischen Darstellung des Duodenums (Pneumo-Duodenum). *Fortschr Röntgenstr* 36: 739-744, 1927.

206. Quattromani F, Finby N: Roentgenographic double-contrast examination of stomach and duodenum. *NY State J Med* 72: 1140-1143, 1972.

207. Régent D, Bigard MA, Hodez Cl, Balzer H, Leichtmann G, Roussel J: Intérêt de l'exploration radiologique en double contraste pour l'étude des images pathologiques de la grand courbure gastrique. *J Radiol Electrol* 57: 673-681, 1976.

208. Richter K: Frühdiagnose des Magenkarzinoms aus radiologischer Sicht. *Dt Gesundh-Wesen* 31: 401-404, 1976.

209. Ring EJ, Ferrucci JT, Eaton SB, Clements JL: Villous adenomas of the duodenum. *Radiology* 104: 45-48, 1972.

210. Robbins LL: *Golden's diagnostic radiology*, Baltimore, The Williams & Wilkins Company, 1969, section V, p 5. 194.

211. Idem, p 5. 225.

212. Idem, p 5. 249.

213. Idem, p 5. 272.

214. Rodriguez HP, Aston JK, Richardson CT: Ulcers in the descending duodenum. *Am J Roentgenol* 119: 316-322, 1973.

215. Roelen AD: *Hypotone duodenografie*. Asten, Schriks Drukkerij N.V., 1969, p 179.

216. Rösch W, Elster K, Ottenjann R: Morbus Crohn des Magens unter dem Bild der "kompletten" Erosionen. *Endoscopy* 4: 178-182, 1969.

217. Rösch W: Früherkennung des Magenkarzinoms – Wunsch oder Realität? *Med Welt* 25: 501-503, 1974.

218. Rona A, Sylvestre J: Prepyloric mucosal diaphragm. *J Can Assoc Radiol* 26: 291-294, 1975.

219. Roth JLA: Symptomatology. In: *Gastroenterology*, Bockus HL (ed), Philadelphia-London-Toronto, W.B. Saunders Company, 1974, vol I, p 80.

220. Roussel J, Régent D, Bigard MA: *Radiologie digestive en double contraste*, Paris, Masson, 1976.

221. Rubenstein ZJ, Bank S, Marks IN, Psillos C: Hypotonic duodenography in chronic pancreatitis. *Br J Radiol* 44: 142-149, 1971.

222. Schipperijn AJM: Annular pancreas in the adult. *Gastroenterologia* 101: 95-104, 1964.

223. Schulman A, Simpkins KC: The definition of radiological signs in gastric ulcer and assessment of their validity by inter-observer variation study. *Clin Radiol* 26: 311-316, 1975.

224. Schulman A, Simpkins: The accuracy of radiological diagnosis of benign, primarily and secondarily malignant gastric ulcers and their correlation with three simplified radiological types. *Clin Radiol* 26: 317-325, 1975.

225. Scott-Harden WG: Evaluation of double contrast gastro-duodenal radiology *Br J Radiol* 46: 153, 1973.

226. Seaman WB: The stomach and duodenum. In: *Alimentary tract roentgenology*, Margulis AR, Burhenne HJ (eds), Saint Louis, The C.V. Mosby Company, 1973, vol I, p 604.

227. Idem, p 626.

228. Idem, p 626-627, 641.

229. Seifert E: Die Früherkennung des Magenkarzinoms. *Klinik der Gegenwart* 8: E639-E646, 1973.

230. Sellink JL: *Radiological atlas of common diseases of the small bowel*, Leiden, H.E. Stenfert Kroese B.V., 1976, p 118.

231. Idem, p 175.

232. Idem, p 177.

233. Idem, p 259.

234. Idem, p 259-268.

235. Idem, p 266-267.

236. Seymour EQ, Meredith HC: Antral and esophageal rimple: a normal variation. *Gastrointest Radiol* 3: 147-149, 1978.

237. Shirakabe H: *Atlas of X-ray diagnosis of early gastric cancer*, Philadelphia-Toronto, J.B. Lippincott Company, 1966.

238. Shirakabe H: *Double contrast studies of the stomach*. Stuttgart, Georg Thieme Verlag, 1972.

239. Shirakabe H, Hayakawa H, Itai Y, Takeda N, Hosoi T: A comparison of X-ray, endoscopy and biopsy examinations for the diagnosis of early gastric cancer. *Jap J. Clin Oncol* 12: 93-98, 1972.

240. Shirakabe H, Nishizawa M, Hayakawa H, Maruyama M: Röntgenologisch-endoskopische Diagnostik des Magenfrühkarzinoms. *Leber Magen Darm* 3: 60-63, 1973.

241. Shirakabe H Ichikawa H: Early gastric cancer. In: *The esophagus and stomach, an atlas of tumor radiology*, Stein GN, Finkelstein AK (eds), Chicago, Year Book Medical Publishers, 1973, p 277-283.

242. Skinner DB: Anatomy. In: *Gastroesophageal reflux and hiatal hernia*, Skinner DB, Belsey RHR, Hendrix TR, Zuidema GD (eds), Boston, Little, Brown and Company, 1972, p 16-17.

243. van der Sluys, MA: *Barietcontrastmiddelen*, Almelo, 1970 (circular letter to hospital pharmacists).

244. Smeets R, Op den Orth JO : The gall bladder , a common cause of the antral pad sign. *Am J Roentgenol* in press, 1979.

245. Solanke TF, Kumakura K, Maruyama M, Someya N: Double-contrast method for the evaluation of gastric lesions. *Gut* 10: 436-442, 1969.

246. Spjut HJ, Navarrete A: Pathology of the stomach. In: *Alimentary tract roentgenology*, Margulis AR, Burhenne HJ (eds), Saint Louis, The C.V. Mosby Company, 1973, vol I, p 559.

247. Spjut HJ, Navarrete A: The stomach and duodenum. In: *Alimentary tract roentgenology*, Margulis AR, Burhenne HJ (eds), Saint Louis, The C.V. Mosby Company, 1973, vol I, p 562.

248. Stadelmann O, Miederer SE, Löffler A, Müller R, Käufer C, Elster K: So-called early gastric cancer and its detection. *Endoscopy* 5: 70-76, 1973.

249. Stassa G, Klingensmith WC: Primary tumors of the duodenal bulb. *Am J Roentgenol* 107: 105-110, 1969.

250. Stender H-St, Seifert E, Luska G, Otto P: Vergleichende röntgenologische und endoskopische Diagnostik des Ulcus ventriculi und duodeni. *Fortschr Röntgenstr* 122: 381-385, 1975.

251. Stevenson G: The distribution of gastric ulcers: double contrast barium meal and endoscopy findings. *Clin Radiol* 28: 617-624, 1977.

252. Sun DCH: Etiology and pathology of peptic ulcer. In: *Gastroenterology*, Bockus HL (ed), Philadelphia-London-Toronto, W.B. Saunders Company, 1974, vol I, p 603.

253. Takasugi T, Sasagawa M, Yamada T, Ichikawa H, Kitaoka H, Hirota T: A study on end results of early gastric cancer. *Stomach and Intestine* 12: 933-940, 1977.

254. Tenner R, Kurosawa A: Verfeinerte Magendiagnostik durch das Dünnschichtverfahren bei der Doppelkontrastuntersuchung. *Fortschr Röntgenstr* 125: 490-496, 1976.

255. Tomoda M: Beitrag zur Kenntnis der Geschwürsbildung im Magen und Duodenum. *Archiv klin Chir* 190: 254-290, 1937.

256. Tootla B, Lucas RJ, Bernacki EG, Tabor H: Gastroduodenal Crohn disease. *Arch Surg* 111: 855-857, 1976.

257. Treichel J: L'examen radiologique de l'estomac à l'aide d'une nouvelle technique de double contraste. *J Radiol Electrol* 53: 857-859, 1972.

258. Treichel J, Oeser H: Die Doppelkontrastmethode: optimale Technik der röntgenologischen Magenuntersuchung. *Dtsch med Wschr* 100: 2226-2229, 1975.

259. Treichel J, Gerstenberg E, Palme G, Klemm T: Diagnosis of partial gastric diverticula. *Radiology* 119: 13-18, 1976.

260. Tschaikowski KL: Zur Doppelkontrastuntersuchung des Magens: Vorschlag einer Routinemethode. *Röntgen-Bl* 29:399-404, 1976.

261. Tubiana JM, Rouger Ph, Chalut J: Etude critique comparant la valeur relative de l'endoscopie et de la radiologie dans les ulcères gastro-duodénaux. *Ann Radiol* 20: 173-177, 1977.

262. Turner CJ, Lipits LR, Pastore RA: Antral gastritis. *Radiology* 113: 305-312, 1974.

263. Valdes-Dapena A: In: *Gastroenterology*, Bockus HL (ed), Philadelphia-London-Toronto, W.B. Saunders Company, 1974, vol I, p 1014-1015.

264. Vallebona A: Nuovo metodo di esame radiologico del tubo digerente. *Radiol Med* 13: 241-248, 1926.

265. Veen HF, Oscarson JEA, Malt RA: Alien cancers of the duodenum. *Surg Gynecol Obstet* 143: 39-42, 1976.

266. Walk L: The roentgen signs of gastritis, clinical analysis. *Am J Roentgenol* 74: 567-579, 1955.

267. Walk L: Erosive gastritis. *Gastroenterologia* 84: 87-98, 1955.

268. Walk L: Polyps caused by gastric erosions. *Radiologe* 15: 354-355, 1975.

269. Walk L: Long-term prognosis of idiopathic gastric erosions. *Radiologe* 15: 356-359, 1975.

270. Wehunt WD, Olmsted WW, Neiman HL, Phillips JF: RPC (Radiologic-pathologic correlation) from the AFIP (Armed Forces Institute of Pathology): Eosinophilic gastritis. *Radiology* 120: 85-89, 1976.

271. Wiener SN, Vertes V, Shapiro H: The upper gastrointestinal tract in patients undergoing chronic dialysis. *Radiology* 92: 110-114, 1969.

272. Wilson WJ, Templeton AW, Turner AH, Lodwick GS: The computer analysis and diagnosis of gastric ulcers. *Radiology* 85: 1064-1073, 1965.

273. Wolf BS: Observations on roentgen features of benign and malignant gastric ulcers. *Sem Roentgenol* 6: 140-150, 1971.

274. Wood DA: *Tumors of the intestines, atlas of tumor pathology*, Washington, Armed Forces Institute of Pathology, 1965, section VI, p F22-37.

275. Yamada T, Ichikawa H: X-ray diagnosis of elevated lesions of the stomach. *Radiology* 110: 79-83, 1974.

180

INDEX

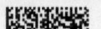